# Chordoma of the Spine

Daniel M. Sciubba • Joseph H. Schwab
Editors

# Chordoma of the Spine

## A Comprehensive Review

Springer

*Editors*
Daniel M. Sciubba
Department of Neurosurgery
Johns Hopkins University School of Medicine
Baltimore, MD
USA

Joseph H. Schwab
Department of Orthopaedic Surgery
Massachusetts General Hospital
Harvard Medical School
Boston, MA
USA

ISBN 978-3-030-76200-1 ISBN 978-3-030-76201-8 (eBook)
https://doi.org/10.1007/978-3-030-76201-8



This Springer imprint is published by the registered company Springer Nature Switzerland AG
The registered company address is: Gewerbestrasse 11, 6330 Cham, Switzerland

# Foreword

Everyone affected by chordoma is able to overcome the disease and maintain his or her quality of life: that's the vision of the Chordoma Foundation, and the future that this book seeks to help bring closer. Current population-wide statistics for patients with chordomas of the spine and sacrum suggest a wide gap between that future and the present. Hence, better treatments are urgently needed, particularly for patients with large or biologically aggressive tumors.

On the other hand, for many chordoma patients, an excellent outcome is already possible with state-of-the-art care. But, while achievable in principle, in practice, it is not simple, requiring sophisticated techniques and tight coordination among a well-informed, multi-disciplinary team of multiple surgical specialists, radiation oncologists, medical oncologists, and more.

Historically, knowledge about how to deliver such state-of-the-art care has not been widespread, resulting in inconsistent treatment, and, all too often, suboptimal outcomes for chordoma patients. This book is an important step towards broadening that knowledge, and, in turn, improving the care provided to chordoma patients. At the Chordoma Foundation, we see that, combined with better treatments for tumors that cannot be controlled with existing approaches and ample support for patients throughout their journey with the disease, as the keys to making chordoma a disease that can be lived with, if not cured. I am, therefore, delighted to see this book come to fruition and am confident that its impact will be felt, whether knowingly or not, by countless fellow patients.

Josh Sommer
Chordoma Foundation
Durham, NC, USA

# Preface

Chordoma of the spinal column is an extremely rare clinical pathology, considered to be one of a handful of orphan disease that is amenable to surgical intervention. Given its rarity, the opportunity to acquire the experience necessary to treat chordomas safely is one that has been confined to only a few comprehensive cancer centers. However, improved awareness of the disease because of multi-institutional organizations such as *AOSpine* and patient advocacy groups such as the *Chordoma Foundation* have led to greater awareness of this clinical pathology. With this increased awareness has come a concordantly increased desire to discover the molecular underpinnings of chordoma and the optimal management paradigms for this disease.

In this text, we attempt to provide a comprehensive review of the epidemiology, pathogenesis, diagnosis, and management of chordomas of the mobile spine and sacrum. The book is divided into 4 parts comprising 16 chapters. The first part focuses on the pathophysiology and molecular drivers of chordoma. The second focuses on the epidemiology and clinical history, as well as the histological, oncologic, and radiographic work-up of chordoma. The third part focuses primarily on the technical aspects of surgery for chordoma. It is broken down by anatomic region, with the final two chapters focusing on the soft tissue and bony reconstruction following chordoma resection. The last part focuses on the exciting field of adjuvant therapies for chordoma. This includes both radiation therapies and novel chemotherapeutic options for recurrent, metastatic, and dedifferentiated chordoma.

Though we attempt to cover the gamut of chordoma treatment, we realize that ongoing advances in the science of chordoma will inevitably make this book obsolete. Nevertheless, we believe that in recruiting world experts from leading chordoma centers, including the Johns Hopkins Hospital, the Massachusetts General Hospital, the Mayo Clinic, Memorial Sloan Kettering, and others, we have been able to construct a central reference for spinal oncologists and general spine surgeons who may encounter chordoma patients in their practice. We greatly appreciate our colleagues who donated the time to make this book possible and to the patients whose experience with this rare disease have taught us along the way.

Baltimore, MD, USA — Daniel M. Sciubba
Boston, MA, USA — Joseph H. Schwab

# Acknowledgments

Heartfelt thanks to Karrie, Hayley, Camryn, and Duncan for all of their love; appreciation to Andy and Zach for their generosity and tireless grit in getting this book completed; admiration to Joe for his wisdom and friendship; and eternal gratitude to our patients who share their journeys and trust us with their lives.

Daniel M. Sciubba, MD

Thank you to Cristina, Peter, Annamaria, and Joe! As with all great efforts there are great teams. Caring for patients with chordomas requires a committed, capable team and I am lucky to be part of such a team at MGH. Thank you Zach and Andy, whose work sincerely made this book possible. Thank you Dan for your positive energy and keen insight.

Joseph H. Schwab, MD, MS

# Contents

# Contributors

**Oliver G. S. Ayling, MD, MSc** Combined Neurosurgical and Orthopedic Spine Program, Vancouver General Hospital, University of British Columbia, Vancouver, BC, Canada

**Chetan Bettegowda, MD, PhD** Department of Neurosurgery, Johns Hopkins University School of Medicine, Baltimore, MD, USA

**David C. Clever, MD, PhD** Department of Orthopedics, Washington University in St Louis, St Louis, MO, USA

**Matthew W. Colman, MD** Department of Orthopedic Surgery, Midwest Orthopaedics at Rush University Medical Center, Chicago, IL, USA

**Cory G. Couch, MD** Department of Orthopaedic Surgery, Mayo Clinic, Rochester, MN, USA

**Nicolas Dea, MD, MSc** Combined Neurosurgical and Orthopedic Spine Program, Vancouver General Hospital, University of British Columbia, Vancouver, BC, Canada

**Thomas F. DeLaney, MD** Department of Radiation Oncology, Massachusetts General Hospital, Harvard Medical School, Boston, MA, USA

**Jeff Ehresman, BS** Department of Neurosurgery, Johns Hopkins University School of Medicine, Baltimore, MD, USA

**Matthew L. Goodwin, MD, PhD** Department of Orthopedics, Washington University in St Louis, St Louis, MO, USA

**John M. Gross, MD** Department of Orthopaedic Pathology, Johns Hopkins Hospital, Baltimore, MD, USA

**Matthew T. Houdek, MD** Department of Orthopaedic Surgery, Mayo Clinic, Rochester, MN, USA

**Reiko Imai, MD** QST Hospital, Quantum Medical Science Directorate, National Institute for Quantum and Radiological Sciences and Technology, Chiba, Japan

**Chunzi Jenny Jin, MD, MSc** Division of Radiation Oncology, The Ottawa Hospital Cancer Centre, Ottawa, ON, Canada

**Majid Khan, MD** Division of Nonvascular Interventional Neuroradiology, Thomas Jefferson University Hospital, Philadelphia, PA, USA

**David J. Konieczkowski, MD, PhD** Department of Radiation Oncology, Arthur G. James Cancer Center and Richard J. Solove Research Institute, The Ohio State University Comprehensive Cancer Center, Columbus, OH, USA

**Ann Liu, MD** Department of Neurosurgery, Johns Hopkins University School of Medicine, Baltimore, MD, USA

**Connor Liu, BS** Department of Neurosurgery, Washington University School of Medicine, St. Louis, MO, USA

**Sheng-Fu Larry Lo, MD** Department of Neurosurgery, Johns Hopkins University School of Medicine, Baltimore, MD, USA

**Edward F. McCarthy, MD** Department of Orthopaedic Pathology, Johns Hopkins Hospital, Baltimore, MD, USA

**Christian Meyer, MD, PhD, MS** Department of Medical Oncology, The Johns Hopkins Sidney Kimmel Comprehensive Cancer Center, Baltimore, MD, USA

**Sutipat Pairojboriboon, MD** Department of Neurosurgery, Johns Hopkins University School of Medicine, Baltimore, MD, USA

Department of Orthopaedic Surgery, Phramongkutklao Hospital and College of Medicine, Bangkok, Thailand

**Zach Pennington, BS** Department of Neurosurgery, Johns Hopkins University School of Medicine, Baltimore, MD, USA

**Peter S. Rose, MD** Department of Orthopaedic Surgery, Mayo Clinic, Rochester, MN, USA

**Daniel Ryan, MD** Russel H. Morgan Department of Radiology and Radiological Science, Johns Hopkins Hospital, Baltimore, MD, USA

**Amanda Sacino, MD, PhD** Department of Neurosurgery, Johns Hopkins University School of Medicine, Baltimore, MD, USA

**Justin M. Sacks, MD, MBA, FACS** Division of Plastic and Reconstructive Surgery, Washington University in St. Louis School of Medicine, St. Louis, MO, USA

**Andrew Schilling, AB** Department of Neurosurgery, Johns Hopkins University School of Medicine, Baltimore, MD, USA

**Joseph H. Schwab, MD, MS** Department of Orthopaedic Surgery, Massachusetts General Hospital, Harvard Medical School, Boston, MA, USA

**Daniel M. Sciubba, MD** Department of Neurosurgery, Johns Hopkins University School of Medicine, Baltimore, MD, USA

**Nicholas A. Shepard, MD** Department of Orthopedic Surgery, Midwest Orthopaedics at Rush University Medical Center, Chicago, IL, USA

**John H. Shin, MD** Department of Neurologic Surgery, Massachusetts General Hospital, Harvard Medical School, Boston, MA, USA

**Rachel Skladman, MD** Division of Plastic and Reconstructive Surgery, Washington University in St. Louis School of Medicine, St. Louis, MO, USA

**Daniel G. Tobert, MD** Department of Orthopaedic Surgery, Massachusetts General Hospital, Harvard Medical School, Boston, MA, USA

**Yoshiya Josh Yamada, MD, FRCPC** Department of Radiation Oncology, Memorial Sloan Kettering Cancer Center, New York, NY, USA

**Daniel J. Zabransky, MD, PhD** Department of Medical Oncology, The Johns Hopkins Sidney Kimmel Comprehensive Cancer Center, Baltimore, MD, USA

# Abbreviations

| | |
|---|---|
| ADC | Apparent diffusion coefficient |
| ALL | Anterior longitudinal ligament |
| ASA | Anterior spinal artery |
| ASIS | Anterior superior iliac spine |
| BMI | Body mass index |
| BNCT | Benign notochordal cell tumor |
| BSSMO | Bilateral-sagittal split mandibular osteotomy |
| C | Cervical |
| CBVA | Chin-brown vertical angle |
| CDK4/6 | Cyclin-dependent kinases 4 and 6 |
| CDKN2A | Cyclin-dependent kinase inhibitor 2A |
| CGE | Cobalt gray equivalent |
| CGH | Comparative genomic hybridization |
| CI | Confidence interval |
| CIRT | Carbon ion radiotherapy |
| CK | Cytokeratin |
| cm | Centimeter |
| CSC | Cancer stem cell |
| CT | Computed tomography |
| CTCAE | Common terminology criteria for adverse events |
| CTV | Clinical target volume |
| DFS | Disease-free survival |
| DNA | Deoxyribonucleic acid |
| DS | Double scatter |
| DSS | Disease-specific survival |
| EA | Enneking appropriate |
| EBR | En bloc resection |
| EGFR | Epidermal growth factor receptor |
| EI | Enneking inappropriate |
| EMA | Epithelial membrane antigen |
| EZH2 | Enhancer of zeste 2 |
| FDA | Food and Drug Administration |
| FISH | Fluorescence in situ hybridization |

| | |
|---|---|
| FVFG | Free vascularized fibular graft |
| Fx | Fraction |
| GM | Gluteus maximus |
| GTV | Gross tumor volume |
| GVNR | Giant vertebral notochordal rest |
| Gy | Gray |
| GyRBE | Gray-equivalent relative biologic effectiveness |
| HADM | human acellular dermal matrix |
| HER2 | Human epidermal growth factor receptor 2 |
| HR | Hazard ratio |
| HR | Homologous recombination |
| hTERT | Human telomerase reverse transcriptase |
| ICA | Internal carotid artery |
| ICU | Intensive care unit |
| IGRT | Image-guided radiation therapy |
| IHC | Immunohistochemistry |
| IMRT | Intensity modulated radiation therapy |
| IOBL | Intraoperative blood loss |
| JAK | Janus kinase |
| KIT | Tyrosine-protein kinase KIT |
| LAG-3 | Lymphocyte-activation gene 3 |
| LC | Local control |
| LD | Latissimus dorsi |
| LECA | Lateral extracavitary approach |
| LMG | Labial-mandibular-glossotomy |
| LR | Local recurrence |
| LRFS | Local relapse-free survival |
| MAP | Mean arterial pressure |
| MGH | Massachusetts General Hospital |
| miRNA | microRNA |
| MRI | Magnetic resonance imaging |
| mRNA | messenger RNA |
| MSKCC | Memorial Sloan Kettering Cancer Center |
| mTOR | mammalian target of rapamycin |
| MUC1 | Polymorphic epithelial mucin/Mucin 1 |
| NCDB | National Cancer Database |
| NCI | National Cancer Institute |
| OC | Occipitocervical |
| OER | Oxygen enhancement ratio |
| ORR | Overall response rate |
| OS | Overall survival |
| P32 | Phosphorus-32 |
| PARP | Poly(ADP)-ribose polymerase |
| PBS | Pencil-beam scanning |

| | |
|---|---|
| PD1 | Programmed cell death protein 1 |
| PDGFB | Platelet-derived growth factor β |
| PDGFR | Platelet-derived growth factor receptor |
| PDGFRA | Platelet-derived growth factor receptor α |
| PDGFRB | Platelet-derived growth factor receptor β |
| PD-L1 | Program cell death ligand 1 |
| PFS | Progression free survival |
| PI3K | Phosphoinositide-3-kinase (PI3K) |
| PLL | Posterior longitudinal ligament |
| PR | Partial response |
| PRC2 | Polycomb repressive complex 2 |
| PSIS | Posterior superior iliac spine |
| PTEN | Phosphatase and tensin homolog deleted on chromosome 10 |
| PTV | Planned tumor volume |
| Rb | Retinoblastoma |
| RBE | Relative biological effectiveness |
| RFS | Recurrence-free survival |
| RT | Radiation therapy |
| RTK(s) | Receptor tyrosine kinase(s) |
| S-100 | Low molecular weight protein soluble in 100% ammonium sulfate at neutral pH |
| S2AI | S2-alar-iliac |
| SBRT | Stereotactic body radiation therapy |
| SD | Stable disease |
| SEER | Surveillance, epidemiology, and end results |
| SHH | Sonic hedgehog |
| SI | Sacroiliac |
| SMARCB1 | SWI/SNF related, matrix associated, actin dependent regulator of chromatin, subfamily b, member 1 |
| SNP | Single nucleotide polymorphism |
| SRS | Stereotactic radiosurgery |
| STAT | Signal transducer activator of transcription |
| SVA | Sagittal vertical axis |
| SWI/SNF | Switch/sucrose non-fermentable |
| T | Thoracic |
| TBXT | T-box transcription factor T |
| TCR | T cell receptor |
| TCR | Transmandibular-circumglossal-retropharyngeal |
| TES | Total en bloc spondylectomy |
| TKI(s) | Tyrosine kinase inhibitor(s) |
| TMC | titanium mesh cage |
| US | United States |
| VBR | Vertebral body replacement |
| VEGFR | Vascular endothelial growth factor receptor |

| | |
|---|---|
| VMAT | Volumetric arc therapy |
| VP-16 | Etoposide |
| VRAM | Vertical rectus abdominis muscle |
| WBB | Weinstein-Boriani-Biagini |
| XRT | X-ray therapy |
| YAP | Yes-associated protein |

# Part I

# Pathophysiology and Molecular Mechanisms of Chordoma

# 1 Notochordal Morphogenesis and the Origin of Chordoma

Matthew L. Goodwin and David C. Clever

## Abbreviations

| | |
|---|---|
| BNCT | Benign notochordal tumor |
| GVNR | Giant vertebral notochordal rest |
| SEER | Surveillance, epidemiology, and end results (program) |
| SHH | Sonic hedgehog |

## Introduction and Epidemiology

Chordomas are slow-growing, locally aggressive tumors thought to be derived from remnants of the notochord [1]. Based upon this, much of the knowledge regarding the clinical behavior of chordoma, in terms of lesion localization and tumorigenesis, is informed by animal studies of notochordal development. Here, we review the basic science of notochordal morphogenesis, which will serve as a basis for understanding chordoma, its potential origins, and clinical behavior.

## Notochordogenesis

In vertebrate embryos, the notochord is an evolutionarily preserved midline structure that is thought to play a critical role in left-right development as well as regulation of local tissue development during embryogenesis [2, 3]. The embryonic notochord is a rod-shaped structure that lies just ventral to the neural tube. Abnormal

M. L. Goodwin (✉) · D. C. Clever
Department of Orthopedics, Washington University in St Louis, St Louis, MO, USA



D. M. Sciubba, J. H. Schwab (eds.), *Chordoma of the Spine*,
https://doi.org/10.1007/978-3-030-76201-8_1

development of the notochord structure may lead to malformation of the neural tube, spine, and gut [4, 5].

Descriptions of the process of notochord formation vary slightly from reference to reference, undoubtedly due to the variety of experimental models used to study notochord development. In an effort to consolidate varying views on the notochordal process as it pertains to humans, de Bakker et al. employed a 3D reconstruction of multiple histological sections from 2 to 6 weeks in human embryos [6, 7]. The resultant description of human notochord formation is one of the more comprehensive descriptions of notochordal development (Fig. 1.1).

Beginning at days 17–19, what is described as the "notochordal process" begins. The notochordal process initially is characterized by an accumulation of cells on the ventral surface of the endoderm in an epithelial pattern. Just cranial, these same cells form a broader and thicker network deemed the prechordal plate [8]. Except for at its most caudal end, these midline cells gradually become the notochordal

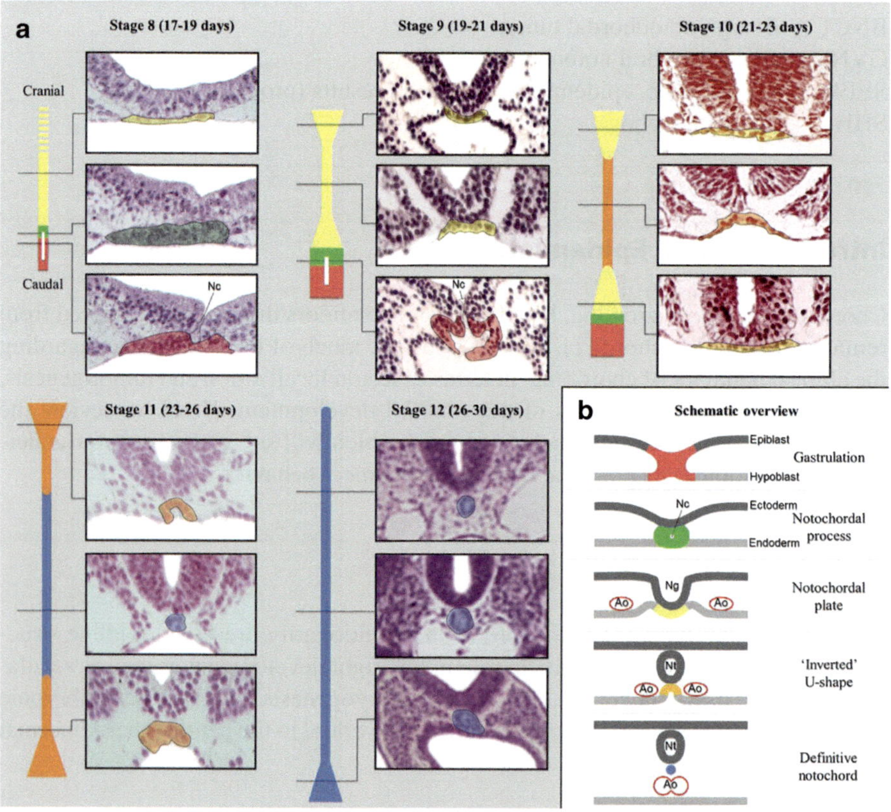


**Fig. 1.1** Development of the notochord. (**a**) Taken from numerous human tissue samples, this cartoon and corresponding histology displays perhaps the most accurate and complete view of notochordal development, from days 17 to 30. (**b**) The five stages of notochord development. (Used with permission from de Bakker et al. [7])

plate during days 19–23. By definition, the early notochord is a one-cell thick layer structure along the neural tube that is intercalated with the roof of the developing gut. During days 23–26, a notochordal plate is present along the entirety of the cranial-caudal axis, and notochordal ridges begin the formation of what will be the definitive notochord, completed in days 26–30. This definitive notochord becomes incorporated into the mesoderm, migrating away from the gut and maintaining its neural tube association. The mature notochord is then thought of as a factory of signaling molecules and chemical moieties that play a multitude of essential roles in directing further embryonic development and tissue maturation and differentiation.

Among several important functions, the mature notochord plays an important role in directing vertebral column formation and segmentation. The bony elements of the spinal column are derived from the sclerotome components of each segmental somite [9]. Each sclerotome migrates to surround the notochord. An intimate relationship largely driven by *Homeobox (Hox)* and *Sonic Hedgehog (SHH)* signaling pathways exists between the embryonic notochord and each sclerotome to maintain appropriate vertebral column development and segmentation along the cranial-caudal axis from skull base to sacrum [10]. In this process, segments of the notochord become embedded within the developing vertebral column, specifically in the regions that ultimately become the intervertebral disk [11].

## Fate of Notochord Cells

The intervertebral disk (Fig. 1.2) consists of a nucleus pulposus, or the softer inner part, and the annulus fibrosus, or the tougher outer layer. Utilizing methods that "fate map" cells, the nucleus pulposus appears likely to develop from the embryonic notochord [12, 13]. How these cells transition from notochord to nucleus pulposus has not been fully determined, although some combination of physical restraints from the developing vertebrae and attractive/repulsive signaling has been proposed [14]. While the distinct molecular and environmental cues are likely multifaceted and incompletely elucidated, recent gene expression studies have implicated the sonic hedgehog and transforming growth factor-beta pathways as important regulators in notochordal maturation into the mature nucleus pulposus [15].

While all cellular components of the nucleus pulposus cells appear to be of notochordal origin, not all notochordal cells end up transitioning to nucleus pulposus cells. In fact, some notochordal cells can be found within the bony aspects of adult vertebrae [14]. In a study of human cadavers, nearly all adult vertebrae were found to contain evidence of remnant notochordal cells [16, 17]. The vast majority of these notochordal remnant cells remain dormant. Yet it is these "notochordal islands" within the axial skeleton that are thought to be the cells of origin for both benign notochordal cell tumors and malignant chordoma tumors [18]. Given the ubiquitous nature of notochordal remnants within the axial skeleton, it is unclear why the vast minority progress to form both benign and malignant lesions. In the next section, we will explore the various tumor types thought to be derived from notochordal remnants as well as the proposed molecular mechanisms driving their development.

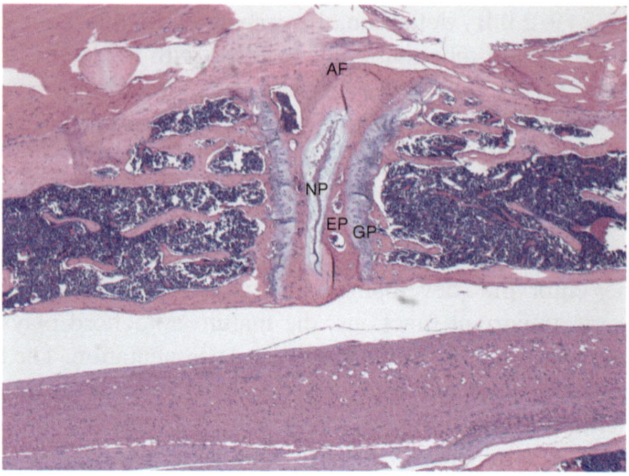


**Fig. 1.2** Typical H&E stain of an endplate-disk-endplate. Note the nucleus pulposus (NP) at the center of the intervertebral disk. In this case, the tissue was taken from 7-month-old C57BL/6J mice. NP nucleus pulposus, EP endplate, AF annulus fibrosis, GP growth plate. (Image courtesy of Dr. Mieradili Mulati, Goodwin Lab (Washington University, St. Louis))

## Benign Notochordal Tumors (BNCTs)

Benign notochordal tumors (BNCTs) are collections of unencapsulated sheets of vacuolated cells contained within axial bones (most commonly in vertebral bodies) that are thought to arise from notochordal remnants [19–21]. BNCTs have also been referred to as notochordal rests (and giant vertebral notochordal rests (GVNRs)), giant notochordal hamartomas, and benign notochordal cell lesions, giving credence to their presumed notochordal origin. These benign tumor-like lesions uniformly lack local bony destruction, soft tissue extension, or malignant/proliferative properties [1, 22]. While both chordoma and BNCTs are thought to arise from notochordal remnants, they have some important differences. Chordomas manifest as slow-growing yet destructive lesions that often grow beyond the bone, may be lytic in nature with variable enhancement on MRI, and often have an intrinsic capacity for extra-osseous metastasis. Like chordomas, BNCTs are found in the bones of the axial skeleton and skull base. Often incidentally noted on MRI, BNCTs are typically (but not always) small, well-demarcated, and lack soft tissue extension. On imaging, they may be sclerotic on CT and often lack significant post-contrast enhancement on MRI [23, 24].

One of the more controversial aspects of BNCTs is the hypothesis that they represent a precursor to chordoma development with biological potential for oncogenic transformation into malignant chordoma. As such, these lesions might represent an intermediate stage between a dormant notochordal remnant and a full blown malignant chordoma. This view stems from data showing that the anatomic distribution of BNCTs in the spine mirrors that of chordoma, and in excised sacral chordomas, 7.3% have nearby co-existent BNCTs [19, 25]. While attractive in principle given their similarities in location, histologic appearance, and cellular origin, the pre-clinical and clinical data supporting BNCTs as a precursor to chordoma development are limited. There has been no documented BNCT-to-chordoma transition to date [20, 21]. Given this uncertainty and the rarity of BNCTs, they are currently treated in a variety of acceptable ways that range from serial imaging to complete *en bloc* excision [26]. In this setting, treatment choice is often driven by patient symptomatology.

## The Ontogeny of Chordoma

While the presence of notochordal elements within the mature human axial skeleton seems to be a ubiquitous phenomenon, the transformation to malignant chordoma is an exceedingly rare process. Chordomas are rare tumors, accounting for 1.4% of all primary malignant bone tumors, and just 0.2% of spinal tumors, working out to <1 case/1,000,000 of the US population [27]. Data from the Surveillance, Epidemiology, and End Results program (SEER) database from 1973 to 2005 revealed that around 1/3 were found in the skull base, 1/3 in the spine, 1/3 in the sacrum, and the remaining ≈5% outside the neuroaxis [28, 29]. The average age of diagnosis is approximately 60 years, although cases of pediatric chordoma have been described and typically portend a very poor prognosis [30]. Moreover, chordomas of the skull base tend to present in younger patients relative to those tumors involving the sacrum or other areas of the axial skeleton [27]. Overall, survival in the SEER database at 5 years was 64% for all chordoma patients, with tumor size at diagnosis, the presence of distant metastases, local recurrence, and older age (excluding pediatric chordomas) all being poor prognostic factors [31]. Despite high rates of local recurrence, surgical resection is a mainstay of most chordoma treatment paradigms [32], as resection with appropriate margins typically leads to improved survival and decreased local recurrence [33].

The molecular processes involved in promoting chordoma ontogeny, proliferation, and biologic activity are heterogeneous. However, recurrent aberrations in a few conserved molecular pathways have been identified in familial and sporadic chordoma. The overall somatic mutational frequency in chordomas is modest. The pattern of somatic mutations observed in chordomas is common across several cancer histologies and shows age-associated accumulation, suggesting that these mutations are likely passenger phenomena as opposed to the driving mechanism in chordoma development [34].

Recently, the expression of the transcription factor brachyury has been established as a distinguishing feature of chordoma [35]. Brachyury is a transcription factor member of the T-box family. It is involved in coordinating a multitude of cellular processes, including cell migration and motility and preventing cellular senescence. Uniformly expressed in the developing notochord, pathologic analysis of brachyury has demonstrated its expression in nearly all chordoma samples, and its absence in other musculoskeletal tumor types [36]. This observation further establishes the link between the developing notochord and chordoma. It should be noted that BNCTs also appear to express brachyury, although the pattern seems to be more focally positive areas surrounded by less positive areas, as compared to the diffuse positive brachyury staining seen in chordomas [1, 20, 37]. While one of the early reports of "notochordal rests" reports them as being brachyury negative [38], several studies that followed demonstrated that BNCTs do indeed express brachyury, albeit in what appears to be a slightly different histological pattern, as noted previously (focal vs diffuse) [1, 20, 37, 38].

The molecular mechanism supporting brachyury expression in chordoma is duplication of the chromosomal region containing the brachyury gene, rather than a de novo mutation within the brachyury gene coding region [34, 35]. This brachyury gene duplication phenomenon is present in many cases of both familial and sporadic chordomas. Brachyury is predominantly expressed in malignant tissues and not in mature normal tissues, making it an ideal target for anti-neoplastic therapies. While there has not been a drug developed to specifically target brachyury, recent clinical trials utilizing a vaccine targeted against brachyury have deemed this strategy safe, and in several cases, potentially effective [39]. Further investigation of therapies targeting brachyury, pharmacologically, and/or immunologically remain an active and interesting area of ongoing research.

Histologically, chordomas have a classic and consistent histomorphological appearance (Fig. 1.3), with "physaliphorous" cells throughout (from the Greek for physalis (bubble) and phorous (bearing)) [26]. These unique cells have abundant eosinophilic cytoplasm and intracytoplasmic vacuoles [40], possibly related to dysfunctional lysosomes [34, 41, 42]. While lysosomes are important in notochordal development [43], it is unclear if the vacuolar cytoplasmic appearance of malignant chordoma cells is a passive remnant of their notochordal origin or an important component of their transformation, proliferation, and survival. Interestingly, recent

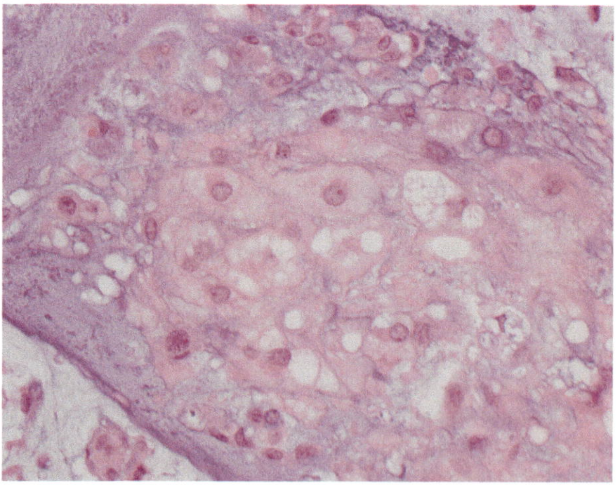

**Fig. 1.3** Typical appearance of H&E stain of chordoma, featuring the classic physaliphorous cells. (Image courtesy of Dr. John Chrisinger (Washington University, St. Louis))

studies have identified recurrent inactivating mutations in the *Lyst* gene, which encodes the lysosomal trafficking regulator protein [34]. Whether targeting the lysosomal machinery represents a novel therapeutic strategy for the pharmacologic treatment of chordoma remains to be determined, but represents a promising area of future investigation.

In response to various mechanical and environmental stresses, cellular components of the nucleus pulposus are driven toward biologic senescence. Activation of cellular senescence programs within cells of the nucleus pulposus has been implicated in the molecular pathogenesis of degenerative disk disease [44]. Given the common notochordal origin between the nucleus pulposus and notochordal remnant chordoma precursor cells, it is suspected that chordoma precursor cells possess appropriate machinery for cellular senescence to take place. One might propose, then, that the pathogenesis of chordoma development depends on the subversion of programmed cellular senescence. The *CDKN2a* gene has also been demonstrated to be recurrently mutated at a significantly high frequency in human chordomas [34, 45]. *CDKN2a* is a well-known tumor suppressor gene that encodes two proteins through alternative splicing: $p16^{INK4a}$ and $p14^{ARF}$. Interestingly, p16 is absent in >50% of chordomas [46]. The loss of a potent mediator of cellular senescence at such a high frequency in human chordomas further supports the notion that the core pathogenesis of chordoma development is the failure of cellular senescence. Whether activation of cellular senescence pathways provides a future therapeutic strategy for chordoma treatment remains to be shown, but should be an active area of future research.

Finally, it should be noted that extra-axial soft tissue chordomas, although rare, do exist, and have led to questions on the origin of chordoma [47]. These very rare tumors are histologically indistinguishable from axial chordomas, and express brachyury much like their more common axial counterparts [47]. However, unlike axial chordomas, there are no BNCTs found in extra-axial locations, suggesting the BNCT-to-chordoma pathway may be sufficient but not necessary for chordoma genesis [47]. On the other hand, expression of brachyury mRNA has been previously found outside of the axial skeleton in noncancerous adult tissues (in the absence of the protein) [48, 49]. Thus, it is possible that nonaxial cells may develop a mutation that leads to aberrant expression of the brachyury gene, and eventual chordoma formation.

## Summary

Chordomas, locally aggressive slow-growing tumors, are thought to typically be derived from notochord remnants. The notochord, a critical midline structure featured prominently in the early weeks of embryogenesis, plays a critical role in left-right development as well as regulation of local structural development. In adult humans, the nucleus pulposus in the intervertebral disk appears to derive from this notochord, although remnant notochordal cells are found throughout adult vertebrae as well. The development of chordomas likely arises from these remnants, although many of the underlying mechanisms remain elusive. Among factors involved in this transition to a chordoma, expression of the brachyury gene appears central, as non-chordoma tumors and normal adult tissues lack the significant overexpression of this gene characteristic of chordoma. While wide resection remains the "gold standard" when possible (with or without radiation), advances in our understanding of chordoma and its origins are leading to more targeted, and potentially more efficacious, therapies.

## References

1. Yamaguchi T, Imada H, Iida S, Szuhai K. Notochordal tumors: an update on molecular pathology with therapeutic implications. Surg Pathol Clin. 2017;10:637–56.
2. Schneider H, Brueckner M. Of mice and men: dissecting the genetic pathway that controls left-right asymmetry in mice and humans. Am J Med Genet. 2000;97:258–70.
3. Lee JD, Anderson KV. Morphogenesis of the node and notochord: the cellular basis for the establishment and maintenance of left-right asymmetry in the mouse. Dev Dyn. 2008;237:3464–76.
4. Babić MS. Development of the notochord in normal and malformed human embryos and fetuses. Int J Dev Biol. 1991;35:345–52.
5. Cleaver O, Krieg PA. Notochord patterning of the endoderm. Dev Biol. 2001;234:1–12.
6. de Bree K, de Bakker BS, Oostra R-J. The development of the human notochord. PLoS One. 2018;13:e0205752.
7. de Bakker BS, de Jong KH, Hagoort J, et al. An interactive three-dimensional digital atlas and quantitative database of human development. Science. 2016;354:aag0053.
8. Müller F, O'Rahilly R. The prechordal plate, the rostral end of the notochord and nearby median features in staged human embryos. Cells Tissues Organs. 2003;173:1–20.
9. Kaplan KM, Spivak JM, Bendo JA. Embryology of the spine and associated congenital abnormalities. Spine J. 2005;5:564–76.
10. Chen Y, Liu Z, Chen J, et al. The genetic landscape and clinical implications of vertebral anomalies in VACTERL association. J Med Genet. 2016;53:431–7.
11. Ward L, Pang ASW, Evans SE, Stern CD. The role of the notochord in amniote vertebral column segmentation. Dev Biol. 2018;439:3–18.
12. Choi K-S, Cohn MJ, Harfe BD. Identification of nucleus pulposus precursor cells and notochordal remnants in the mouse: implications for disk degeneration and chordoma formation. Dev Dyn. 2008;237:3953–8.
13. McCann MR, Tamplin OJ, Rossant J, Seguin CA. Tracing notochord-derived cells using a Noto-cre mouse: implications for intervertebral disc development. Dis Model Mech. 2012;5:73–82.
14. Lawson L, Harfe BD. Notochord to nucleus pulposus transition. Curr Osteoporos Rep. 2015;13:336–41.
15. Peck SH, McKee KK, Tobias JW, Malhotra NR, Harfe BD, Smith LJ. Whole transcriptome analysis of notochord-derived cells during embryonic formation of the nucleus pulposus. Sci Rep. 2017;7:10504.
16. McCann M, Séguin C. Notochord cells in intervertebral disc development and degeneration. J Dev Biol. 2016;4:3.
17. Yamaguchi T, Suzuki S, Ishiiwa H, Shimizu K, Ueda Y. Benign notochordal cell tumors: a comparative histological study of benign notochordal cell tumors, classic chordomas, and notochordal vestiges of fetal intervertebral discs. Am J Surg Pathol. 2004;28:756–61.
18. Risbud MV, Shapiro IM. Notochordal cells in the adult intervertebral disc: new perspective on an old question. Crit Rev Eukaryot Gene Expr. 2011;21:29–41.

19. Yamaguchi T, Suzuki S, Ishiiwa H, Ueda Y. Intraosseous benign notochordal cell tumours: overlooked precursors of classic chordomas? Histopathology. 2004;44:597–602.
20. Du J, Xu L, Cui Y, Liu Z, Su Y, Li G. Benign notochordal cell tumour: clinicopathology and molecular profiling of 13 cases. J Clin Pathol. 2019;72:66–74.
21. Carter JM, Wenger DE, Rose PS, Inwards CY. Atypical notochordal cell tumors: a series of notochordal-derived tumors that defy current classification schemes. Am J Surg Pathol. 2017;41:39–48.
22. Terzi S, Mobarec S, Bandiera S, Gasbarrini A, Barbanti-Bròdano G, Alberghini M, Boriani S. Diagnosis and treatment of benign notochordal cell tumors of the spine. Spine. 2012;37:E1356–60.
23. Oner AY, Akpek S, Tali T, Ucar M. Giant vertebral notochordal rest: magnetic resonance and diffusion weighted imaging findings. Korean J Radiol. 2009;10:303.
24. Sayyid SK, Wong PK, Read W, Monson DK, Umpierrez M, Gonzalez F, Kakarala A, Singer AD. The clincoradiologic spectrum of notochordal derived masses. Clin Imaging. 2019;56:124–34.
25. Deshpande V, Petur Nielsen G, Rosenthal DI, Rosenberg AE. Intraosseous Benign Notochord Cell Tumors (BNCT): further evidence supporting a relationship to chordoma. Am J Surg Pathol. 2007;31:1573–7.
26. Karpathiou G, Dumollard JM, Dridi M, Dal Col P, Barral F-G, Boutonnat J, Peoc'h M. Chordomas: a review with emphasis on their pathophysiology, pathology, molecular biology, and genetics. Pathol Res Pract. 2020;216:153089.
27. George B, Bresson D, Herman P, Froelich S. Chordomas: a review. Neurosurg Clin N Am. 2015;26:437–52.
28. McMaster M, Goldstein A, Bromley C, Ishibe N, Parry D. Chordoma: incidence and survival patterns in the United States, 1973–1995. Cancer Causes Control. 2001;12:1–11.
29. Righi A, Sbaraglia M, Gambarotti M, Cocchi S, Drago G, Casadei R, Picci P, Vanel D, Dei Tos AP. Extra-axial chordoma: a clinicopathologic analysis of six cases. Virchows Arch. 2018;472:1015–20.
30. Beccaria K, Tauziède-Espariat A, Monnien F, et al. Pediatric chordomas: results of a multicentric study of 40 children and proposal for a histopathological prognostic grading system and new therapeutic strategies. J Neuropathol Exp Neurol. 2018;77:207–15.
31. Lee IJ, Lee RJ, Fahim DK. Prognostic factors and survival outcome in patients with chordoma in the United States: a population-based analysis. World Neurosurg. 2017;104:346–55.
32. Jawad MU, Scully SP. Surgery significantly improves survival in patients with chordoma. Spine. 2010;35:117–23.
33. Gokaslan ZL, Zadnik PL, Sciubba DM, et al. Mobile spine chordoma: results of 166 patients from the AOSpine Knowledge Forum Tumor database. J Neurosurg Spine. 2016;24:644–51.
34. Tarpey PS, Behjati S, Young MD, et al. The driver landscape of sporadic chordoma. Nat Commun. 2017;8:890.
35. Yang XR, Ng D, Alcorta DA, Liebsch NJ, Sheridan E, Li S, Goldstein AM, Parry DM, Kelley MJ. T (brachyury) gene duplication confers major susceptibility to familial chordoma. Nat Genet. 2009;41:1176–8.
36. Vujovic S, Henderson S, Presneau N, Odell E, Jacques T, Tirabosco R, Boshoff C, Flanagan A. Brachyury, a crucial regulator of notochordal development, is a novel biomarker for chordomas. J Pathol. 2006;209:157–65.
37. Usher I, Flanagan AM, Choi D. Systematic review of clinical, radiologic, and histologic features of benign notochordal cell tumors: implications for patient management. World Neurosurg. 2019;130:13–23.
38. Shen J, Shi Q, Lu J, Wang D-L, Zou T-M, Yang H-L, Zhu G-Q. Histological study of chordoma origin from fetal notochordal cell rests. Spine. 2013;38:2165–70.
39. Collins JM, Donahue RN, Tsai Y-T, et al. Phase I trial of a modified vaccinia Ankara priming vaccine followed by a Fowlpox virus boosting vaccine modified to express brachyury and costimulatory molecules in advanced solid tumors. Oncologist. 2020;25:560.

40. Wasserman JK, Gravel D, Purgina B. Chordoma of the head and neck: a review. Head Neck Pathol. 2018;12:261–8.
41. Resutek L, Hsieh AH. The vacuolated morphology of chordoma cells is dependent on cytokeratin intermediate filaments. J Cell Physiol. 2019;234:3458–68.
42. Kolb-Lenz D, Fuchs R, Lohberger B, et al. Characterization of the endolysosomal system in human chordoma cell lines: is there a role of lysosomes in chemoresistance of this rare bone tumor? Histochem Cell Biol. 2018;150:83–92.
43. Ellis K, Bagwell J, Bagnat M. Notochord vacuoles are lysosome-related organelles that function in axis and spine morphogenesis. J Cell Biol. 2013;200:667–79.
44. Che H, Li J, Li Y, et al. p16 deficiency attenuates intervertebral disc degeneration by adjusting oxidative stress and nucleus pulposus cell cycle. elife. 2020;9:e52570.
45. Choy E, MacConaill LE, Cote GM, Le LP, Shen JK, Nielsen GP, Iafrate AJ, Garraway LA, Hornicek FJ, Duan Z. Genotyping cancer-associated genes in chordoma identifies mutations in oncogenes and areas of chromosomal loss involving CDKN2A, PTEN, and SMARCB1. PLoS One. 2014;9:e101283.
46. Cottone L, Eden N, Usher I, et al. Frequent alterations in p16/CDKN2A identified by immunohistochemistry and FISH in chordoma. J Pathol Clin Res. 2020;6:113–23.
47. Lauer SR, Edgar MA, Gardner JM, Sebastian A, Weiss SW. Soft tissue chordomas: a clinicopathologic analysis of 11 cases. Am J Surg Pathol. 2013;37:719–26.
48. Tirabosco R, Mangham DC, Rosenberg AE, et al. Brachyury expression in extra-axial skeletal and soft tissue chordomas: a marker that distinguishes chordoma from mixed tumor/myoepithelioma/parachordoma in soft tissue. Am J Surg Pathol. 2008;32:572–80.
49. Palena C, Polev DE, Tsang KY, Fernando RI, Litzinger M, Krukovskaya LL, Baranova AV, Kozlov AP, Schlom J. The human T-box mesodermal transcription factor brachyury is a candidate target for T-cell–mediated cancer immunotherapy. Clin Cancer Res. 2007;13:2471–8.

# Molecular Morphogenesis and Genetic Mechanisms of Spinal Chordoma

# 2

Connor Liu, Ann Liu, and Chetan Bettegowda

## Abbreviations

| | |
|---|---|
| CGH | comparative genomic hybridization |
| CSC | cancer stem cell |
| FISH | fluorescent in-situ hybridization |
| HR | homologous recombination |
| hTERT | human telomerase reverse transcriptase |
| miRNA | microRNA |
| mRNA | messenger RNA |
| OS | overall survival |
| PARP | poly(ADP)-ribose polymerase |
| PFS | progression-free survival |
| Rb | retinoblastoma |
| SNP | single nucleotide polymorphism |
| YAP | Yes-associated protein |

C. Liu
Department of Neurosurgery, Washington University School of Medicine, St. Louis, MO, USA

A. Liu · C. Bettegowda (✉)
Department of Neurosurgery, Johns Hopkins University School of Medicine, Baltimore, MD, USA
e-mail: cbetteg1@jhmi.edu



D. M. Sciubba, J. H. Schwab (eds.), *Chordoma of the Spine*,
https://doi.org/10.1007/978-3-030-76201-8_2

## Introduction

Chordoma is a rare malignant primary tumor of the axial skeleton. Accounting for 1–4% of primary malignant bone tumors and the most common primary tumor of the spine [1, 2], chordomas most commonly arise in sacrococcygeal areas, skull base, and mobile spine [3, 4]. Unlike other malignant tumors, chordomas demonstrate a characteristic slow growth pattern with a propensity for local invasion of critical bony and neural structures [4]. Although unusual, metastases can occur years after initial diagnosis. Given the frequently large tumor burden at time of diagnosis and proximity of these tumors to vital structures, appropriate surgical excision represents a considerable challenge. Furthermore, these lesions are resistant to conventional chemotherapy and radiotherapy [5]. As a result of the challenges facing clinical chordoma management, local disease recurrence is common, ranging from 30% to 85%, with median 5- and 10-year survival rates at 67.6% and 39.9%, respectively [4].

Recently, scientific progress in understanding the genetic and molecular events underpinning chordoma tumorigenesis has provided insight into avenues for more effective targeted therapies. Indeed, the use of contemporary techniques such as comparative genomic hybridization (CGH), fluorescent in-situ hybridization (FISH), methylation assays, single nucleotide polymorphism (SNP) microarrays, and, more recently, whole-genome sequencing has advanced current understanding of the chordoma genomic and epigenetic landscape. Understanding these processes is important as they govern the biological behavior of the neoplasm and may harbor potential relevant targets for therapy. In this review, we highlight current concepts in the molecular morphogenesis and genetic landscape of spinal chordomas.

## Genetic Hallmarks of Chordoma

### Cytogenetics

Chordomas are cytogenetically heterogenous tumors that display complex karyotypes. While most chordomas display near diploid or moderately hypodiploid karyotypes, they feature complex genomic rearrangements including deletions and gains of chromosomal segments, gene copy number changes, and chromothripsis. Despite the diversity of chromosome abnormalities documented in the literature, molecular techniques such as G-banding, CGH, and FISH have been used to detect recurrent chromosomal aberrations including gains and losses at various regions throughout the genome (Table 2.1) [6]. Deletions affecting all chromosomes, except chromosome 5, have been identified in chordoma [7]. In 2011, Le and colleagues used genome-wide oligonucleotide microarrays to analyze copy number changes in 21 sporadic chordoma samples (2 clival, 7 spinal, 11 sacral) [6]. Consistent with previous results published by Hallor and colleagues (2 spinal, 24 sacral), they identified frequent losses in chromosomes 3, 4, 9p, 9q, 10, 13, 14, 18, and 22, and common gains in chromosomes 7 and 19 [6, 7].

**Table 2.1** Common genomic alterations identified in chordoma

| Locus | Genomic alteration | Associated genes | Gene functions | Clinical significance | References |
|---|---|---|---|---|---|
| 1p36 | Deletion | RUNX3 | Tumor suppressor, chondrocyte maturation | 1p36 LOH correlates with worse prognosis in skull base chordoma [8]. 1p36 loss associated with familial chordoma [9, 10]. | [7, 11] |
| | Deletion | TNFRSF8, TNFRSF9, TNFRSF14 | Apoptotic signaling | | [8] |
| 1q42.3 | Truncating mutations | LYST | Lysosomal trafficking regulation | | [33] |
| 3p21 | Deletion | PBRM1 | Chromatin remodeling | | [24, 33] |
| 3p21 | Deletion | SETD2 | | | |
| 3p21 | Deletion | BAP1 | | | |
| 3q26 | Deletion | PIK3CA | Tumor suppressor | | |
| 5p15 | Promoter mutations | TERT | Telomerase activity | Promoter mutations associated with better survival [31]. | [28, 31] |
| 6q25 | Deletion | ARID1B | Chromatin remodeling | | [24] |
| 6q27 | Gain | Brachyury | Notochordal development | rs2305089 SNP associated with increased risk of chordoma development and improved survival [48, 53]. | [33, 36, 39] |
| 7q31 | Gain | MET | Receptor tyrosine kinase | | [81, 82] |
| 9p21 | Deletion/ LOH | CDKN2A | G1-S cell cycle checkpoint | 9p LOH associated with shorter OS [80]. | [33, 80, 83] |
| | Deletion | CDKN2B | | | |
| 9p21 | Deletion | MTAP | Purine salvage metabolism | MTAP deficient cells are sensitive to purine synthesis inhibitors [84]. | [18] |
| 10q23 | Deletion | PTEN | Tumor suppressor | Lower PTEN expression correlates with shorter PFS and OS [20]. PTEN loss associated with degree of bone invasion [85]. | [6, 15, 20] |
| 11q22 | Deletion | ATM | Cell cycle checkpoint kinase | | [7] |

(continued)

**Table 2.1** (continued)

| Locus | Genomic alteration | Associated genes | Gene functions | Clinical significance | References |
|---|---|---|---|---|---|
| 22q12 | Deletion | CHEK2 | Homologous recombination DNA repair | | [7, 35] |
| 22q11 | Deletion | SMARCB1 | Chromatin remodeling, cell cycle regulation | SMARCB1 loss associated with decreased OS in patients with poorly differentiated chordoma [86–88]. | [15, 88] |

*LOH* Loss of heterozygosity, *SNP* Single nucleotide polymorphism, *OS* Overall survival, *PFS* Progression-free survival

Among the samples studied by Le et al., the 1p36 chromosomal segment was either partially or completely lost in the majority of samples [6]. The 1p36 region contains a myriad of cancer-associated genes and is one of the most frequently altered regions in other cancer types such as oligodendrogliomas, yolk sac tumors, melanoma, and squamous cell carcinomas [8]. Genetic mapping studies have identified 1p36 as a key site of loss in cases of familial and sporadic chordoma [9, 10]. 1p36 loss is also common in sporadic chordomas and has been shown to be associated with a worse prognosis in skull base chordomas [8]. Furthermore, the mapping of genes involved in chondrocyte maturation and osteogenesis to the 1p36 loci provides a potential link to chordoma tumorigenesis. Specifically, 1p36 contains *RUNX3*, a transcription factor essential for hematopoiesis, osteogenesis, and neurogenesis, and an important regulator of chondrocyte maturation [11].

Deletions involving chromosome segment 9p21 represent the second most common chromosomal abnormality in chordoma, occurring in 50–80% of tumors [6, 7]. Chromosome 9p21 houses the *CDKN2A* and *CDKN2B* genes encoding for p14/16 and p15 proteins, respectively. p14 and p16 are both involved in cell cycle control through their function as modulators of the retinoblastoma (Rb) and p53 pathways for cell renewal and aging. p14 promotes the p53 pathway whereas p16 inhibits cell cycle progression at the G1/S phase by blocking Rb phosphorylation. At that same locus, *CDKN2B* encodes for p15, a tumor suppressor which regulates the complexes CDK4 and CDK6-cyclin D, two serine-threonine kinases that modulate progression through the G1 cell cycle phase. Thus, aberrant regulation of these pathways is central to the progression of many cancer types and is frequently mediated through homozygous deletions or promoter hypermethylation [12]. The *CDKN2A* gene locus is deleted and p16 protein expression is lost in a number of chordoma cell lines [13]. Although a small percentage of chordomas contain homozygous *CDKN2A* deletions [7, 14], single nucleotide variants and promoter hypermethylation of this locus are rare [6, 15]. In one study, *CDKN2A* homozygous deletion detected by FISH was associated with p16 protein loss, but only contributed to 33% of cases that were p16-negative [14]. The remainder of p16-negative cases were attributed to mechanisms involving disomy (27%), monosomy (12%), heterozygous loss (20%), and copy number gain (7%) of *CDKN2A*. The authors suggest that their findings could be explained by prominent epigenetic or post-transcriptional mechanisms regulating p16 expression. p16 loss has been shown to sensitize cancer cell lines to CDK4/6 inhibitors, making the expression of p16 a potential biomarker for patient stratification and prognosis [13, 16]. In addition to *CDKN2A* and *CDKN2B*, another adjacent gene, *MTAP*, is lost in a significant percentage of chordomas [17]. *MTAP*, an essential enzyme in the purine salvage pathway, and its subsequent loss in chordoma represent a potential therapeutic target as *MTAP*-deficient cells are vulnerable to purine synthesis inhibitors [17, 18].

Other common deletions in chordoma include loss of 10q23 [6, 19]. *PTEN*, a tumor suppressor gene located on chromosome region 10q23, is commonly inactivated in a wide range of neoplasms including chordomas. In chordoma, *PTEN* deletions occur in 60–80% of cases [6, 15, 20, 21]. *PTEN* has two well-described biochemical functions including lipid and protein phosphatase activity. Through negative regulation of the growth factor *PI3K* pathway, lipid phosphatase downregulates *AKT* activity and promotes proapoptotic caspase signaling. *PTEN's* protein phosphatase function is to regulate cell migration via inhibition of focal adhesions and *MAPK* signaling. Therefore, the loss of *PTEN* in chordoma likely promotes cell proliferation and migration via activation of *PI3K*, *AKT*, and *mTOR* pathways. In a study of sacral chordoma, decreased levels of *PTEN* expression correlated with *mTOR* overexpression and was associated with more severe tumor invasion into surrounding tissues [21]. Furthermore, this study revealed that *PTEN* negative expression and *mTOR* positive expression were associated with significantly lower continuous disease-free survival. In another study, chordoma patients with lower *PTEN* expression had a significantly shorter progression-free survival (PFS) and overall survival (OS) than those with higher *PTEN* expression [20].

## Chromothripsis

In 2011, a large study of cancer cell lines and primary tumors of various origins described a new genomic event termed chromothripsis, involving tens to hundreds of chromosomal rearrangements occurring as a result of a single cellular catastrophe [22]. Thus, chromothripsis can induce repeated switches in copy numbers along the length of a chromosome and is thought to be a potential initiating event in tumor development. While contributing to the pathogenesis in 2–3% of all cancers, chromothripsis occurs in up to 25% of bone cancers including chordomas [23]. In one of the chordoma samples studied, they detected 147 somatic genomic rearrangements linking together regions of chromosomes 3q, 4q, 7q, 8p, and 9p [23]. In a separate study, Wang and colleagues detected a similar chromothripsis event rate (18%, 4 out of 22 samples) in chordoma, with 1–2 chromosomes affected per sample [24].

Recently, investigations into the role of human telomerase reverse transcriptase (hTERT) in chordoma progression provide potential explanations for the origin of chromosomal instability. hTERT is the rate-limiting component in the formation of the telomerase complex and replenishes telomeric DNA at chromosomal ends by synthesizing telomeric sequences via an RNA template. *hTERT* expression is absent in normal somatic cells but is often exploited by cancer to promote uncontrolled cell proliferation. Ernst and colleagues showed significant differences in telomere lengths and stabilization mechanisms when comparing before and after chromothripsis-like genomic events [25]. A number of studies have now demonstrated *hTERT* expression in chordoma and have shown that *hTERT* expressing chordomas have reduced in vitro doubling times [26, 27]. Zou and colleagues identified *hTERT* expression in 54 spinal chordomas but absent expression in 20 nucleus pulposus samples [28]. *hTERT* expression was significantly associated with poor local recurrence-free survival but had no correlation with overall survival. Similarly, Hu et al. showed that higher telomerase expression was a predictor of sacral chordoma recurrence [29]. In skull base chordomas, *hTERT* expression is associated with shorter tumor doubling time, increased proliferation, and disease recurrence [27, 30]. However, while telomerase activity is present in a proportion of chordoma cases and has prognostic value, the basic mechanisms underlying *hTERT* and further downstream effects remain unclear. While *hTERT* promoter mutations and subsequent increases in *hTERT* expression are typically associated with worse prognosis in many cancers, recently Bettegowda et al. found that the presence of *hTERT* promoter mutations C228T and C250T were associated with statistically significant overall survival benefit in spinal chordoma patients [31]. Thus, the link between these specific *hTERT* promoter mutations (present in 8.7% of spinal chordomas) and survival benefit likely represent the result of complex interactions between *hTERT* and other genetic driver events. Future studies investigating *hTERT* in chordoma will provide important insight into the utility of this biomarker in predicting patient prognosis or as a potential therapeutic target.

## Whole-Genome Approaches

In recent years, new high-throughput sequencing technologies have enabled unbiased investigations of chordoma at a genetic level. These studies offer new insight into the genomic and transcriptomic landscape of chordoma with potentially actionable alterations. Fischer and colleagues used deep sequencing analysis to evaluate somatic mutations in 9 chordoma samples (3 skull base, 4 spinal, 2 sacral) [32]. Consistent with prior studies [15, 24], they did not observe any highly recurrent somatic mutations with the exception of non-protein altering variants in the known cancer genes *KDR*, *KIT*, and *TP53*. Similarly, whole-genome sequencing approaches demonstrate that chordomas harbor low mutational burdens. Tarpey and colleagues identified potentially causative somatic mutations in only 40% of tumors [33]. These results likely indicate that epigenetic and structural genomic rearrangements contribute to the bulk of key driver events in chordomagenesis. Liang et al. observed genomic alterations amenable to off-label FDA-approved treatments in three patients with sacral chordoma [34]. These targetable mutations included *FGFR1* overexpression, and *CDK4* and *ERBB3* copy-number duplication events, all of which have FDA-approved therapies (ponatinib, palbociclib, and gefitinib, respectively) [34]. Groschel and colleagues used whole-genome sequencing to characterize the genomes of advanced and heavily pretreated chordomas ($n$ = 11) [35]. In their study, they found genomic patterns consistent with defective homologous recombination (HR) DNA repair and identified pathogenic germline variants in HR-related genes including *BRCA2*, *NBN*, and *CHEK2*. Similar mutational patterns can be observed in the genomes of breast, ovarian, and prostate cancer, where HR deficiency increases sensitivity to poly(ADP)-ribose polymerase (PARP) inhibitors. Significantly, they report a patient with refractory chordoma that experienced a prolonged clinical response after treatment with the PARP inhibitor, olaparib [35]. These studies underscore the importance of comprehensive genomic analysis in the development of rational personalized therapies for chordoma.

## Brachyury

Given the presumed notochordal origin of chordomas, intense interest has been focused on studying genes and pathways implicated in the maintenance of this embryological structure. These experiments have generated interesting results, with one of the earlier studies by Vujovic and colleagues in 2006 showing that high expression of the transcription factor, brachyury, was present in notochord tissues and chordomas, while absent in over 300 other neoplasms and normal tissues studied [36]. The *brachyury* gene, located on 6q27, encodes an evolutionary conserved T-box transcription factor that regulates essential notochord functions including posterior mesoderm formation. Specifically, *brachyury* regulates several downstream stem cell-related genes and has even been shown to promote epithelial-mesenchymal transition in other human carcinomas [37]. Miettinen et al. showed that out of 5229 tumors of diverse origin including 76 chordomas, nuclear *brachyury* expression was a sensitive and specific marker for chordoma [38]. *Brachyury* expression has also been demonstrated in germ cell tumors, small cell carcinomas, teratomas, as well as lung cancers, indicating a more central role in tumorigenesis [39–44].

Further evidence implicating *brachyury* overexpression in chordoma pathogenesis has come from studies of familial chordoma. Specifically, germline *brachyury* duplication has been identified as a major susceptibility factor for familial chordoma [45, 46]. In 2009, Yang et al. analyzed several families with chordoma predispositions using high-resolution array-based comparative genomic hybridization and combined genetic linkage analyses [45]. Out of 7 familial chordoma groups, 4 demonstrated germline duplications of 6q27 containing the *brachyury* gene [45]. Using FISH and qPCR, another study showed that among 181 sporadic chordoma samples, nearly half demonstrated a gain of chromosome band 6q27 [39]. In those cases, the majority of the somatic copy number gains were the result of polysomy of the entire chromosome 6, whereas only 4.5% and 7% were due to *brachyury* locus minor allelic gain and amplification, respectively. Interestingly, of the remaining half that contained a normal *brachyury* gene copy number, all expressed *brachyury* mRNA and protein at levels equivalent to those with *brachyury* copy number gains. The authors also showed that in the U-CH1 chordoma cell line which harbors polysomy of chromosome 6q27, knockdown of the *brachyury* gene resulted in a significant decrease in cell proliferation and marked changes in morphological features toward a senescent phenotype [39]. In a study of skull base chordomas ($n$ = 27), Otani et al. found that patients with tumors expressing high levels of *brachyury* had significantly shorter progression-free survival compared to those with lower *brachyury* expression [47]. While earlier studies looking at brachyury duplication in chordoma concluded that it was a genetic event more specific to familial cases, recent evidence suggests that somatic *brachyury* duplication is also a common occurrence in sporadic chordoma [39, 46, 48, 49]. Tarpey et al. identified somatic duplications of brachyury in 27% of sporadic chordoma cases [33]. Furthermore, 16% had recurrent mutations in *PI3K* signaling and 10% had inactivating mutations in the novel *LYST* gene [33].

As *brachyury* overexpression appears to play a critical role in chordoma tumorigenesis and does not solely rely on chromosomal alterations, perturbations in upstream regulatory events may influence *brachyury* overexpression. Upstream control of *brachyury* is principally regulated by *FGF* signaling and it has been shown in Xenopus that *FGF* signaling and brachyury expression are tightly coupled in a feedback loop [50]. However, in a study by Shalaby and colleagues, no mutations in the *FGF* receptor or its downstream targets including *KRAS*, *RAF*, and *ERK* 1/2 were found despite 94% of the chordomas samples studied expressing at least one member of the *FGF* receptor family [51].

Other groups have identified heritable genetic variants of the *brachyury* gene associated with increased risk of chordoma development. In 2012, Pillay and colleagues identified the germline rs2305089 allele of the *brachyury* gene resulting in a Gly177Asp alteration that was strongly associated with chordoma risk (allelic odds ratio = 6.1) [48]. The rs2305089 variant is a common nonsynonymous SNP located in exon 4 of the *brachyury* gene, which encodes for the DNA binding domain of the brachyury transcription factor, thus making it a potential causal variant for developing chordoma [52]. They further showed that the rs2305089 allele was associated with higher levels of *brachyury* mRNA expression as well as of its downstream targets. In a separate follow-up study by Kelley et al., the rs2305089 allele was also present in cases of familial chordoma and was associated with a similar susceptibility risk as in sporadic cases [46]. Additionally, in cases of sporadic chordomas, they found that the rs3816300 allele, when analyzed jointly with rs2305089, had a significant disease association, suggesting that multivariant analysis may provide more accurate risk assessments. Among familial chordoma cases (61 skull base, 19 spinal, 23 sacral), the rs1056048 allele was identified as a susceptibility variant and was highly associated with brachyury duplications in those patients. The authors note that rs1056048, a nonsynonymous SNP, is located at a splice site with potential downstream consequences on sumoylation and nuclear localization and is also bound by the region containing a *SUZ12*-binding site required for polycomb repressive complex 2-mediated gene silencing [46]. While the exact role of each variant in chordomagenesis remains unclear, the high incidence of these common variants and the rarity of chordomas suggests complex multifactorial genetic networks at play.

However, leveraging these *brachyury* gene variants has already shown some promise as prognostic indicators. In a study of over 300 spinal chordoma patients stratified by their rs2305089 genotype, overall survival was significantly greater in patients with the rs2305089 variant compared to wildtype [53]. The authors postulate that although rs2305089 is associated with increased brachyury expression, it may also increase the chordoma sensitivity to treatment or other antitumor mechanisms. Similarly, chordomas without the variant may rely on alternative, more aggressive mechanisms of upregulating brachyury pathways. Interestingly, a recent study of skull-based chordoma patients in China showed that rs2305089 was not associated with chordoma risk suggesting that the increased susceptibility may not be conserved across different ethnicities [54].

Subsequently, the generation of a patient-derived chordoma cell line, JHC7 [55], has enabled functional investigations into the role brachyury plays in tumorigenesis. In particular, both shRNA and liposomal-nanoparticle methods have been used to silence *brachyury* expression in JHC7, resulting in chordoma cell differentiation and complete growth arrest [55, 56]. Indeed, these promising preclinical correlates have led to a number of clinical trials testing brachyury targeted therapies in chordoma patients. In a phase I trial of 7 advanced chordoma patients, treatment with a yeast-brachyury vaccine was safe and resulted in brachyury-specific T-cell responses [49]. The corresponding phase II trial assessing the overall response rate to brachyury vaccination is currently underway (NCT02383498).

## Epigenetics: DNA Methylation and Chromatin Remodeling

While aberrant genetic mechanisms play a key role in chordoma tumorigenesis, increasing evidence implicates epigenetic deregulation with chordoma development and progression. Epigenetics, the study of heritable changes in gene expression without any alterations to underlying DNA sequences, has increasingly been implicated in the pathological processes of many cancer types [57]. Epigenetic mechanisms can be broadly categorized into DNA methylation, histone modifications, and post-transcriptional regulation by non-coding RNA. Specifically, DNA methylation has provided a wealth of information in establishing useful biomarkers for cancer diagnosis, prognosis, and disease monitoring. DNA methylation is a well-described mechanism of cancer progression through both hyper and hypomethylation of specific loci, including tumor suppressor genes. For example, methylation of promoter CpG islands results in transcriptional inactivation and has been implicated in malignancies including chordoma. Tarpey et al. identified a subset of somatic mutations altering the SWI/SNF chromatin remodeling complex, suggesting that epigenetic changes may play a more prominent role in chordoma tumorigenesis than previously thought [33]. Wang and colleagues applied a similar approach using targeted next-generation sequencing of 24 chordoma tumors (3 spinal, 18 sacral, 3 pelvic) [24]. They found that nearly half of the observed mutation events occurred in chromatin regulatory genes including *SETD2*, *PBRM1*, and *ARID1B*. Subsequent copy number analysis revealed the histone-modifying enzyme gene *SETD2* to be the single most affected gene in chordoma. This represents a potentially actionable alteration as cancer cell lines deficient for *SETD2* are sensitive to inhibition of *WEE1*, a G2 checkpoint kinase [58].

Rinner et al. compared DNA methylation patterns of blood from healthy individuals and chordoma patients and found 20 significantly differentially methylated genes, including *RASSF1*, *KL*, and *HIC1*, three tumor suppressor genes with well-described mechanisms in cancer pathogenesis [59]. *RASSF1* encodes for a RAS-like protein, which is a cell cycle regulator and is frequently transcriptionally inactivated by promoter methylation in breast and colorectal cancers. KL, acting as a tumor suppressor in a variety of malignancies, functions as a modulator of IGF-1 and FGF pathways – both of which have been found to be activated in chordomas. Similarly, HIC1, a downstream transcriptional target of p53, is a target of hypermethylation in solid tumors.

Alholle and colleagues also reported on their findings implicating methylation perturbations in chordoma [60]. Comparing chordomas to nucleus pulposus tissue, they found evidence of cancer-specific hypermethylation in chordomas including four of the hypermethylated genes previously identified by Rinner et al. (*RASSF1*, *IRF4*, *DLEC1*, and *HSD17B4*) [60]. Furthermore, they identified eight gene loci that were differentially methylated between chordomas that recurred and those that did not. In addition to providing insight into epigenetic events associated with chordoma development, these findings suggest that in the future it may be possible to develop diagnostic markers for early detection and intervention of chordoma management. For example, MGMT methylation status is a well-established indicator of responsiveness to temozolomide therapy in glioma. Marucci et al. found that MGMT methylation is present in 26% of recurrent clival chordomas but is not a feature of non-recurrent tumors [61]. These results suggest that select patients with recurrent chordomas may benefit from temozolomide adjuvant therapy and warrants further investigation.

## MicroRNA

Mounting evidence implicates aberrant expression of microRNA (miRNA) in the pathogenesis of many human cancers [62]. MiRNA represents a type of non-protein-coding RNA that modulates gene expression by binding messenger RNA (mRNA) and leading to transcript degradation. Duan et al. demonstrated that *Met* and *HDAC-4*, two downstream targets of miRNA-1, are overexpressed in chordoma, and that transfection of chordoma cells with miRNA-1 results in suppression of these oncogenic transcripts [63]. Furthermore, they found that miRNA-1 expression was significantly reduced in a majority of chordoma samples and that miRNA expression correlated with clinical prognosis [64]. One of the principal mechanisms of miRNA-1 appears to be the regulation of *Slug* gene expression, which chordoma cells rely on to promote cell migration and invasion of surrounding tissues [65].

Thus, the miRNA-1 pathway is involved in multiple critical pathways in chordomagenesis that may serve as potential therapeutic targets. Indeed, the growing number of miRNAs differentially expressed in chordoma warrants further investigation. Zou et al. identified 29 differentially expressed miRNA in spinal chordoma patients ($n = 42$) and showed that reduced expression of miRNA-1237-3p was associated with worse tumor invasion and shorter recurrence-free survival [66]. A separate study confirmed similar findings with miRNA-140-3p in spinal chordoma [67]. Furthermore, miRNA-1290 and miRNA-155 expression were predictive of patient outcomes in sacral chordomas [68, 69].

## Chordoma Cancer Stem Cells

There is growing evidence that chordomas may harbor a cancer stem cell (CSC) population that drives disease progression and recurrence. In addition to their origins from embryological tissues, chordomas also exhibit marked radio- and chemotherapy resistance and a predilection to seed new tumors upon surgical violation of the capsule, both of which are characteristic features of CSCs [70]. More evidence now suggests that cancer stem cells may be present in chordoma. Aydemir and colleagues were the first to describe CSC-related observations in chordoma [71]. They identified expression of specific stem cell surface markers (CD133 and CD15) in chordoma and the U-CH1 chordoma cell line, and demonstrated these cells could differentiate into another osteogenic lineage and were able to live in nonadherent soft agar medium requiring self-renewal capability. Furthermore, Hsu et al. generated sarcospheres from a chordoma cell line expressing classic chordoma markers including brachyury, keratin, and S-100 [72]. The chordoma sarcospheres expressed high levels of the ALDH1 stem cell marker compared to other chordoma cells, were able to self-perpetuate, and could differentiate into neuroepithelial and mesodermal cell types [72].

While the exact mechanisms through which chordoma stem cells propagate are not precisely understood, they likely involve numerous downstream brachyury targets. Shah et al. showed the patient-derived JCH7 chordoma cell line exhibits a variety of stem-cell features including expression of vimentin, CD90, CD105, Oct4, and nestin, transdifferentiation capacity, and the ability to undergo serial tumor formation in mice [73]. Notably, shRNA silencing of *brachyury* expression resulted in a significant reduction in all of the stem-cell capacities [73]. The study authors then show that *brachyury* regulation of a stem-cell phenotype is mediated through one of its downstream targets, the transcriptional co-activator Yes-associated protein (YAP) [73]. They found that brachyury tightly regulates YAP expression and signaling by binding to the proximal region of the YAP promoter. Similarly, shRNA knockdown of YAP resulted in a significant reduction of self-renewal capacity and expression of stem-cell markers. YAP, a transcriptional activator of genes involved in cell survival as well as organ development [74], is also overexpressed in a variety of cancer types and thus presents an intriguing therapeutic target [75].

## Conclusion

Despite modern challenges in the treatment of chordoma, recent advancements in the understanding of key molecular and genetic events in the pathogenesis of this disease have paved the way for clinical trials testing promising targeted therapies [76]. For instance, the discovery of brachyury as an essential regulator of notochordal development and as a specific biomarker in chordoma has yielded human trials investigating the efficacy of a brachyury vaccine in chordoma patients [77]. Furthermore, as the genomic technologies that have yielded these insights become more widely available, the interplay of genetic and epigenetic events driving disease progression will lead to a more complete understanding of chordoma pathophysiology. To date, numerous studies have demonstrated the utility of high-resolution genomic studies in identifying genetic biomarkers for clinical prognostication in chordoma patients [31, 64, 78–80]. Given the heterogenous genomic architecture observed in chordoma, future studies aiming to build off of this work will likely look towards multidimensional biomarker analysis in order to tailor disease treatment and management for individual patients.

## References

1. Sun X, Hornicek F, Schwab JH. Chordoma: an update on the pathophysiology and molecular mechanisms. Curr Rev Musculoskelet Med. 2015;8(4):344–52. https://doi.org/10.1007/s12178-015-9311-x.
2. Boriani S, Bandiera S, Biagini R, et al. Chordoma of the mobile spine: fifty years of experience. Spine. 2006;31(4):493–503. https://doi.org/10.1097/01.brs.0000200038.30869.27.
3. Eriksson B, Gunterberg B, Kindblom LG. Chordoma: a clinicopathologic and prognostic study of a swedish national series. Acta Orthop. 1981;52(1):49–58. https://doi.org/10.3109/17453678108991758.
4. Mcmaster ML, Goldstein AM, Bromley CM, Ishibe N, et al. Chordoma: incidence and survival patterns in the United States, 1973 ± 1995. Cancer Causes Control. 2001;12(1):1–11.
5. Casali PG, Stacchiotti S, Sangalli C, Olmi P, Gronchi A. Chordoma. Curr Opin Oncol. 2007;19(4):367–70. https://doi.org/10.1097/CCO.0b013e3281214448.
6. Le LP, Nielsen GP, Rosenberg AE, et al. Recurrent chromosomal copy number alterations in sporadic chordomas. PLoS One. 2011;6(5):e18846. https://doi.org/10.1371/journal.pone.0018846.
7. Hallor KH, Staaf J, Jönsson G, et al. Frequent deletion of the CDKN2A locus in chordoma: analysis of chromosomal imbalances using array comparative genomic hybridisation. Br J Cancer. 2008;98(2):434–42. https://doi.org/10.1038/sj.bjc.6604130.
8. Longoni M, Orzan F, Stroppi M, Boari N, Mortini P, Riva P. Evaluation of 1p36 markers and clinical outcome in a skull base chordoma study. Neuro-Oncology. 2008;10(1):52–60. https://doi.org/10.1215/15228517-2007-048.
9. Miozzo M, Dalprà L, Riva P, et al. A tumor suppressor locus in familial and sporadic chordoma maps to 1p36. Int J Cancer. 2000;87(1):68–72. https://doi.org/10.1002/1097-0215(20000701)87:1<68::AID-IJC10>3.0.CO;2-V.
10. Riva P, Crosti F, Orzan F, et al. Mapping of candidate region for chordoma development to 1p36.13 by LOH analysis. Int J Cancer. 2003;107(3):493–7. https://doi.org/10.1002/ijc.11421.
11. Blyth K, Cameron ER, Neil JC. The RUNX genes: gain or loss of function in cancer. Nat Rev Cancer. 2005;5(5):376–87. https://doi.org/10.1038/nrc1607.

12. Zhao R, Choi BY, Lee MH, Bode AM, Dong Z. Implications of genetic and epigenetic alterations of CDKN2A (p16INK4a) in cancer. EBioMedicine. 2016;8:30–9. https://doi.org/10.1016/j.ebiom.2016.04.017.
13. von Witzleben A, Goerttler LT, Marienfeld R, et al. Preclinical characterization of novel Chordoma cell systems and their targeting by pharmocological inhibitors of the CDK4/6 cell-cycle pathway. Cancer Res. 2015;75(18):3823–31. https://doi.org/10.1158/0008-5472.CAN-14-3270.
14. Cottone L, Eden N, Usher I, et al. Frequent alterations in p16/CDKN2A identified by immunohistochemistry and FISH in chordoma. J Pathol Clin Res. 2020;6(2):113–23. https://doi.org/10.1002/cjp2.156.
15. Choy E, MacConaill LE, Cote GM, et al. Genotyping cancer-associated genes in chordoma identifies mutations in oncogenes and areas of chromosomal loss involving CDKN2A, PTEN, and SMARCB1. PLoS One. 2014;9(7):e101283. https://doi.org/10.1371/journal.pone.0101283.
16. Dickson MA. Molecular pathways: CDK4 inhibitors for cancer therapy. Clin Cancer Res. 2014;20(13):3379–83. https://doi.org/10.1158/1078-0432.CCR-13-1551.
17. Duan Z, Feng Y, Shen J, Hornicek F. Genomic and epigenetic instability in chordoma: current insights. Adv Genomics Genet. 2014;4:67. https://doi.org/10.2147/agg.s50523.
18. Sommer J, Itani DM, Homlar KC, et al. Methylthioadenosine phosphorylase and activated insulin-like growth actor-1 receptor/insulin receptor: potential therapeutic targets in chordoma. J Pathol. 2010;220(5):608–17. https://doi.org/10.1002/path.2679.
19. Lee D-H, Zhang Y, Kassam AB, et al. Combined PDGFR and HDAC inhibition overcomes PTEN disruption in chordoma. PLoS One. 2015;10(8):e0134426. https://doi.org/10.1371/journal.pone.0134426.
20. Yang C, Sun J, Yong L, et al. Deficiency of PTEN and CDKN2A tumor-suppressor genes in conventional and chondroid chordomas: molecular characteristics and clinical relevance. Onco Targets Ther. 2020;13:4649–63. https://doi.org/10.2147/OTT.S252990.
21. Chen K, Mo J, Zhou M, et al. Expression of PTEN and mTOR in sacral chordoma and association with poor prognosis. Med Oncol. 2014;31(4):1–5. https://doi.org/10.1007/s12032-014-0886-7.
22. Meyerson M, Pellman D. Cancer genomes evolve by pulverizing single chromosomes. Cell. 2011;144(1):9–10. https://doi.org/10.1016/j.cell.2010.12.025.
23. Stephens PJ, Greenman CD, Fu B, et al. Massive genomic rearrangement acquired in a single catastrophic event during cancer development. Cell. 2011;144(1):27–40. https://doi.org/10.1016/j.cell.2010.11.055.
24. Wang L, Zehir A, Nafa K, et al. Genomic aberrations frequently alter chromatin regulatory genes in chordoma. Genes Chromosomes Cancer. 2016;55(7):591–600. https://doi.org/10.1002/gcc.22362.
25. Ernst A, Jones DTW, Maass KK, et al. Telomere dysfunction and chromothripsis. Int J Cancer. 2016;138(12):2905–14. https://doi.org/10.1002/ijc.30033.
26. Butler MG, Dahir GA, Hedges LK, Juliao SF, Sciadini MF, Schwartz HS. Cytogenetic, telomere, and telomerase studies in five surgically managed lumbosacral chordomas. Cancer Genet Cytogenet. 1995;85(1):51–7. https://doi.org/10.1016/0165-4608(95)00127-1.
27. Pallini R, Maira G, Pierconti F, et al. Chordoma of the skull base: predictors of tumor recurrence. J Neurosurg. 2003;98(4):812–22. https://doi.org/10.3171/jns.2003.98.4.0812.
28. Zou MX, Lv GH, Li J, She XL, Jiang Y. Upregulated human telomerase reverse transcriptase (hTERT) expression is associated with spinal chordoma growth, invasion and poor prognosis. Am J Transl Res. 2016;8(2):516–29. Accessed 1 Nov 2020. www.ajtr.org
29. Hu H, Yang HL, Lu J, et al. Association of telomerase expression with recurrence of sacral chordoma. Ann Oncol. 2012;23(10):2772. https://doi.org/10.1093/annonc/mds462.
30. Ricci-Vitiani L, Pierconti F, Falchetti ML, et al. Establishing tumor cell lines from aggressive telomerase-positive chordomas of the skull base: technical note. J Neurosurg. 2006;105(3):482–4. https://doi.org/10.3171/jns.2006.105.3.482.

31. Bettegowda C, Yip S, Jiang B, et al. Prognostic significance of human telomerase reverse transcriptase promoter region mutations C228T and C250T for overall survival in spinal chordomas. Neuro-Oncology. 2019;21(8):1005–15. https://doi.org/10.1093/neuonc/noz066.
32. Fischer C, Scheipl S, Zopf A, et al. Mutation analysis of nine chordoma specimens by targeted next-generation cancer panel sequencing. J Cancer. 2015;6(10):984–9. https://doi.org/10.7150/jca.11371.
33. Tarpey PS, Behjati S, Young MD, et al. The driver landscape of sporadic chordoma. Nat Commun. 2017;8(1):890. https://doi.org/10.1038/s41467-017-01026-0.
34. Liang WS, Dardis C, Helland A, et al. Identification of therapeutic targets in chordoma through comprehensive genomic and transcriptomic analyses. Cold Spring Harb Mol Case Stud. 2018;4(6):a003418. https://doi.org/10.1101/mcs.a003418.
35. Gröschel S, Hübschmann D, Raimondi F, et al. Defective homologous recombination DNA repair as therapeutic target in advanced chordoma. Nat Commun. 2019;10(1):1635. https://doi.org/10.1038/s41467-019-09633-9.
36. Vujovic S, Henderson S, Presneau N, et al. Brachyury, a crucial regulator of notochordal development, is a novel biomarker for chordomas. J Pathol. 2006;209(2):157–65. https://doi.org/10.1002/path.1969.
37. Behr R, Heneweer C, Viebahn C, Denker H-W, Thie M. Epithelial-mesenchymal transition in colonies of rhesus monkey embryonic stem cells: a model for processes involved in gastrulation. Stem Cells. 2005;23(6):805–16. https://doi.org/10.1634/stemcells.2004-0234.
38. Miettinen M, Wang Z, Lasota J, Heery C, Schlom J, Palena C. Nuclear brachyury expression is consistent in chordoma, common in germ cell tumors and small cell carcinomas, and rare in other carcinomas and sarcomas: an immunohistochemical study of 5229 cases. Am J Surg Pathol. 2015;39(10):1305–12. https://doi.org/10.1097/PAS.0000000000000462.
39. Presneau N, Shalaby A, Ye H, et al. Role of the transcription factor T (brachyury) in the pathogenesis of sporadic chordoma: a genetic and functional-based study. J Pathol. 2011;223(3):327–35. https://doi.org/10.1002/path.2816.
40. Kilic N, Feldhaus S, Kilic E, et al. Brachyury expression predicts poor prognosis at early stages of colorectal cancer. Eur J Cancer. 2011;47(7):1080–5. https://doi.org/10.1016/j.ejca.2010.11.015.
41. Jezkova J, Williams JS, Jones-Hutchins F, et al. Brachyury regulates proliferation of cancer cells via a p27Kip1-dependent pathway. Oncotarget. 2014;5(11):3813–22. https://doi.org/10.18632/oncotarget.1999.
42. Pinto F, Gomes NP, Vizcaíno JR, Andrade RP, Cárcano FM, Reis RM. Brachyury as a potential modulator of androgen receptor activity and a key player in therapy resistance in prostate cancer. Oncotarget. 2016;7(20):28891–902. https://doi.org/10.18632/oncotarget.8499.
43. Li K, Ying M, Feng D, et al. Brachyury promotes tamoxifen resistance in breast cancer by targeting SIRT1. Biomed Pharmacother. 2016;84:28–33. https://doi.org/10.1016/j.biopha.2016.09.011.
44. Hamilton DH, Roselli M, Ferroni P, et al. Brachyury, a vaccine target, is overexpressed in triple-negative breast cancer. Endocr Relat Cancer. 2016;23(10):783–96. https://doi.org/10.1530/ERC-16-0037.
45. Yang XR, Ng D, Alcorta DA, et al. T (brachyury) gene duplication confers major susceptibility to familial chordoma. Nat Genet. 2009;41(11):1176–8. https://doi.org/10.1038/ng.454.
46. Kelley MJ, Shi J, Ballew B, et al. Characterization of T gene sequence variants and germline duplications in familial and sporadic chordoma. Hum Genet. 2014;133(10):1289–97. https://doi.org/10.1007/s00439-014-1463-z.
47. Otani R, Mukasa A, Shin M, et al. Brachyury gene copy number gain and activation of the PI3K/Akt pathway: association with upregulation of oncogenic Brachyury expression in skull base chordoma. J Neurosurg. 2018;128(5):1428–37. https://doi.org/10.3171/2016.12.JNS161444.

48. Pillay N, Plagnol V, Tarpey PS, et al. A common single-nucleotide variant in T is strongly associated with chordoma. Nat Genet. 2012;44(11):1185–7. https://doi.org/10.1038/ng.2419.
49. Heery CR, Singh BH, Rauckhorst M, et al. Phase I trial of a yeast-based therapeutic cancer vaccine (GI-6301) targeting the transcription factor brachyury. Cancer Immunol Res. 2015;3(11):1248–56. https://doi.org/10.1158/2326-6066.CIR-15-0119.
50. Hu Y, Mintz A, Shah SR, Quinones-Hinojosa A, Hsu W. The FGFR/MEK/ERK/brachyury pathway is critical for chordoma cell growth and survival. Carcinogenesis. 2014;35(7):1491–9. https://doi.org/10.1093/carcin/bgu014.
51. Shalaby AA, Presneau N, Idowu BD, et al. Analysis of the fibroblastic growth factor receptor-RAS/RAF/MEK/ERK-ETS2/ brachyury signalling pathway in chordomas. Mod Pathol. 2009;22(8):996–1005. https://doi.org/10.1038/modpathol.2009.63.
52. Papapetrou C, Edwards YH, Sowden JC. The T transcription factor functions as a dimer and exhibits a common human polymorphism Gly-177-Asp in the conserved DNA-binding domain. FEBS Lett. 1997;409(2):201–6.
53. Bettegowda C, Yip S, Lo SFL, et al. Spinal column chordoma: prognostic significance of clinical variables and T (brachyury) gene SNP rs2305089 for local recurrence and overall survival. Neuro-Oncology. 2017;19(3):405–13. https://doi.org/10.1093/neuonc/now156.
54. Wu Z, Wang K, Wang L, et al. The brachyury Gly177Asp SNP is not associated with a risk of skull base chordoma in the Chinese population. Int J Mol Sci. 2013;14(11):21258–65. https://doi.org/10.3390/ijms141121258.
55. Hsu W, Mohyeldin A, Shah SR, et al. Generation of chordoma cell line JHC7 and the identification of Brachyury as a novel molecular target: laboratory investigation. J Neurosurg. 2011;115(4):760–9. https://doi.org/10.3171/2011.5.JNS11185.
56. Hu Y, Singh R, Deng Z, Mintz A, Hsu W. Liposome-protamine-DNA nanoparticle-mediated delivery of short hairpin RNA targeting brachyury inhibits chordoma cell growth. J Biomed Nanotechnol. 2016;12(10):1952–61. https://doi.org/10.1166/jbn.2016.2236.
57. Sharma S, Kelly TK, Jones PA. Epigenetics in cancer. Carcinogenesis. 2009;31(1):27–36. https://doi.org/10.1093/carcin/bgp220.
58. Pfister SX, Markkanen E, Jiang Y, et al. Inhibiting WEE1 selectively kills histone H3K36me3-deficient cancers by dNTP starvation. Cancer Cell. 2015;28(5):557–68. https://doi.org/10.1016/j.ccell.2015.09.015.
59. Rinner B, Weinhaeusel A, Lohberger B, et al. Chordoma characterization of significant changes of the DNA methylation pattern. PLoS One. 2013;8(3):e56609. https://doi.org/10.1371/journal.pone.0056609.
60. Alholle A, Brini AT, Bauer J, et al. Genome-wide DNA methylation profiling of recurrent and non-recurrent chordomas. Epigenetics. 2015;10(3):213–20. https://doi.org/10.1080/15592294.2015.1006497.
61. Marucci G, Morandi L, Mazzatenta D, Frank G, Pasquini E, Foschini MP. MGMT promoter methylation status in clival chordoma. J Neuro-Oncol. 2014;118(2):271–6. https://doi.org/10.1007/s11060-014-1445-y.
62. Yu X, Li Z. Epigenetic deregulations in chordoma. Cell Prolif. 2015;48(5):497–502. https://doi.org/10.1111/cpr.12204.
63. Duan Z, Choy E, Petur Nielsen G, et al. Differential expression of microRNA (miRNA) in chordoma reveals a role for miRNA-1 in met expression. J Orthop Res. 2010;28(6):746–52. https://doi.org/10.1002/jor.21055.
64. Duan Z, Shen J, Yang X, et al. Prognostic significance of miRNA-1 (miR-1) expression in patients with chordoma. J Orthop Res. 2014;32(5):695–701. https://doi.org/10.1002/jor.22589.
65. Osaka E, Yang X, Shen JK, et al. MicroRNA-1 (miR-1) inhibits chordoma cell migration and invasion by targeting slug. J Orthop Res. 2014;32(8):1075–82. https://doi.org/10.1002/jor.22632.

66. Zou M, Huang W, Wang X, et al. Reduced expression of miRNA-1237-3p associated with poor survival of spinal chordoma patients. Eur Spine J. 2015;24(8):1738–46. https://doi.org/10.1007/s00586-015-3927-9.
67. Zou MX, Huang W, Wang X, et al. Identification of miR-140-3p as a marker associated with poor prognosis in spinal chordoma. Int J Clin Exp Pathol. 2014;7(8):4877–85. Accessed November 3, 2020. www.ijcep.com/
68. Wang Y, Chen K, Chen H, et al. Low expression of miRNA-1290 associated with local invasion and recurrence in sacral chordoma. Int J Clin Exp Pathol. 2017;10(11):10934–40. Accessed November 3, 2020. http://www.ncbi.nlm.nih.gov/pubmed/31966437
69. Osaka E, Kelly AD, Spentzos D, et al. MicroRNA-155 expression is independently predictive of outcome in chordoma. Oncotarget. 2015;6(11):9125–39. https://doi.org/10.18632/oncotarget.3273.
70. Hsu W, Mohyeldin A, Shah SR, Gokaslan ZL, Quinones-Hinojosa A. Role of cancer stem cells in spine tumors: review of current literature. Neurosurgery. 2012;71(1):117–25. https://doi.org/10.1227/NEU.0b013e3182532e71.
71. Aydemir E, Bayrak OF, Sahin F, et al. Characterization of cancer stem-like cells in chordoma. Laboratory investigation. J Neurosurg. 2012;116(4):810–20. https://doi.org/10.3171/2011.12.JNS11430.
72. Hsu W, Mohyeldin A, Shah SR, et al. Generation of chordoma cell line, JHC7, and the identification of brachyury as a novel molecular target. In: 27th Annual Meeting of the AANS/CNS Section on Disorders of the Spine and Peripheral Nerves; 2011.
73. Shah SR, David JM, Tippens ND, et al. Brachyury-YAP regulatory axis drives stemness and growth in cancer. Cell Rep. 2017;21(2):495–507. https://doi.org/10.1016/j.celrep.2017.09.057.
74. Dong J, Feldmann G, Huang J, et al. Elucidation of a universal size-control mechanism in drosophila and mammals. Cell. 2007;130(6):1120–33. https://doi.org/10.1016/j.cell.2007.07.019.
75. Zanconato F, Cordenonsi M, Piccolo S. YAP/TAZ at the roots of Cancer. Cancer Cell. 2016;29(6):783–803. https://doi.org/10.1016/j.ccell.2016.05.005.
76. Gill CM, Fowkes M, Shrivastava RK. Emerging therapeutic targets in chordomas: a review of the literature in the genomic era. Neurosurgery. 2020;86(2):E118–23. https://doi.org/10.1093/neuros/nyz342.
77. A phase 1 open label trial of intravenous administration of MVA-BN-brachyury vaccine in patients with advanced cancer – Full text view – ClinicalTrials.gov. Accessed 24 Nov 2020. https://clinicaltrials.gov/ct2/show/NCT04134312
78. Zenonos GA, Fernandez-Miranda JC, Mukherjee D, et al. Prospective validation of a molecular prognostication panel for clival chordoma. J Neurosurg. 2019;130(5):1528–37. https://doi.org/10.3171/2018.3.JNS172321.
79. Tauziède-Espariat A, Bresson D, Polivka M, et al. Prognostic and therapeutic markers in chordomas: a study of 287 tumors. J Neuropathol Exp Neurol. 2016;75(2):111–20. https://doi.org/10.1093/jnen/nlv010.
80. Horbinski C, Oakley GJ, Cieply K, et al. The prognostic value of Ki-67, p53, epidermal growth factor receptor, 1p36, 9p21, 10q23, and 17p13 in skull base chordomas. Arch Pathol Lab Med. 2010;134(8):1170–6. https://doi.org/10.1043/2009-0380-OA.1.
81. Brandal P, Bjerkehagen B, Danielsen H, Heim S. Chromosome 7 abnormalities are common in chordomas. Cancer Genet Cytogenet. 2005;160(1):15–21. https://doi.org/10.1016/j.cancergencyto.2004.11.016.
82. Walter BA, Begnami M, Valera VA, Santi M, Rushing EJ, Quezado M. Gain of chromosome 7 by chromogenic in situ hybridization (CISH) in chordomas is correlated to c-MET expression. J Neuro-Oncol. 2011;101(2):199–206. https://doi.org/10.1007/s11060-010-0250-5.
83. Scheil S, Brüderlein S, Liehr T, et al. Genome-wide analysis of sixteen chordomas by comparative genomic hybridization and cytogenetics of the first human chordoma cell line, U-CHI. Genes Chromosomes Cancer. 2001;32(3):203–11. https://doi.org/10.1002/gcc.1184.
84. Tang B, Testa JR, Kruger WD. Increasing the therapeutic index of 5-fluorouracil and 6-thioguanine by targeting loss of MTAP in tumor cells. Cancer Biol Ther. 2012;13(11):1082–90. https://doi.org/10.4161/cbt.21115.

85. Wu Z, Wang L, Guo Z, et al. Experimental study on differences in clivus chordoma bone invasion: an iTRAQ-based quantitative proteomic analysis. PLoS One. 2015;10(3):e0119523. https://doi.org/10.1371/journal.pone.0119523.
86. Nachwalter RN, Rothrock RJ, Katsoulakis E, et al. Treatment of dedifferentiated chordoma: a retrospective study from a large volume cancer center. J Neuro-Oncol. 2019;144(2):369–76. https://doi.org/10.1007/s11060-019-03239-3.
87. Shih AR, Cote GM, Chebib I, et al. Clinicopathologic characteristics of poorly differentiated chordoma. Mod Pathol. 2018;31(8):1237–45. https://doi.org/10.1038/s41379-018-0002-1.
88. Mobley BC, McKenney JK, Bangs CD, et al. Loss of SMARCB1/INI1 expression in poorly differentiated chordomas. Acta Neuropathol. 2010;120(6):745–53. https://doi.org/10.1007/s00401-010-0767-x.

# Part II

# Epidemiology, Clinical History, and Work-Up for Chordoma

# Historical Overview, Demographics, and Clinical Presentation of Spinal Chordoma

# 3

Zach Pennington, Andrew Schilling, Joseph H. Schwab, and Daniel M. Sciubba

## Abbreviations

| | |
|---|---|
| BNCT | Benign notochordal cell tumor |
| CGE | Cobalt gray equivalent |
| Gy | Gray |
| MGH | Massachusetts General Hospital |
| NCI | National Cancer Institute |
| SEER | Surveillance, Epidemiology, and End Results |
| US | United States |

## Introduction

As discussed in Chap. 1, chordomas are malignant tumors derived from the notochord, a mesoderm-derived structure essential for normal embryonic patterning [1]. Originally described by Rudolph Virchow in the 1840s [2], chordomas are slow-growing lesions that commonly present with oncologic pain, mechanical pain (pain associated with movement), or neurologic dysfunction secondary to mass effect (e.g., urinary incontinence) [3]. Symptoms may be accompanied by a palpable mass. However, this is generally only seen in sacrococcygeal lesions [3] as the

Z. Pennington · A. Schilling · D. M. Sciubba (✉)
Department of Neurosurgery, Johns Hopkins University School of Medicine, Baltimore, MD, USA
e-mail: dsciubba1@northwell.edu

J. H. Schwab
Department of Orthopaedic Surgery, Massachusetts General Hospital, Harvard Medical School, Boston, MA, USA



D. M. Sciubba, J. H. Schwab (eds.), *Chordoma of the Spine*,
https://doi.org/10.1007/978-3-030-76201-8_3

notochordal remnants giving rise to chordomas of the mobile spine and skull base occupy deep positions within the axial skeleton. Consequently, the majority of patients with mobile spine lesions present with nonspecific back pain of insidious onset [4, 5]. Failure of conservative management then leads to radiographic workup, revealing a large mass of the ventral sacrum or vertebral bodies, oftentimes expanding outside the anatomic compartment defined by the vertebral body [5]. Involvement of multiple contiguous levels is also common [4].

Despite the fact that chordomas commonly present with localized pain, they are an overall uncommon cause of spine pain. In this chapter, we discuss the history of chordoma, its epidemiology, and its clinical presentation.

## History of Chordoma

### Pathologic and Embryonic Characterization

The first histologic description of chordoma was made by German pathologist Rudolf Virchow in 1846 based upon an incidentally discovered, small, myxoid exophytic lesion of the dorsum sella [2]. Virchow described the lesion as soft, transparent, and multi-lobulated with an underlying myxoid structure that appeared "slimy" [1]. Subsequently in 1856, a second German physician, Hubert Luschka [6], described a similar translucent mass invading the sella turcica. This led Virchow to further investigate these "chordomata" [2], that he described as "ecchondrosis physalifora spheno-occipitalis" – cartilaginous physaliphorous (bubbly) lesions arising from the spheno-occipital junction. Virchow posited that these lesions were cartilaginous in nature and resulted from hydropic degeneration of the spheno-occipital junction with concomitant softening of the cartilage matrix [7]. He posited that this hydropic degeneration led to the formation of vacuoles, which characterize the physaliphorous cell of chordoma [8].

The next year [9], Johnannes Müller – Virchow's doctoral advisor – argued that these chordomata were of notochordal origin, citing the persistence of notochordal tissue within the cartilaginous portions of the sacrum and skull base. This perspective was rejected by Virchow and contemporaries, sparking interest in determining the development of chordoma. Work published in 1880 by Leboucq suggesting all notochordal tissue involutes antenatally [10, 11] was cited as support for the cartilaginous origin of chordoma. However, work by others, including Kölliker [12] and Löwe [13] suggested that the nucleus pulposus of the intervertebral disc was derived from the embryonic notochord. Therefore, ongoing disagreement about the origin of chordoma persisted through the latter half of the nineteenth century [7].

In 1894, Hermann Steiner published a case of a spheno-occipital tumor demonstrating that chordomas were likely of notochordal origin [14]. This was followed shortly thereafter by laboratory support from Steiner's senior collaborator, Moritz Ribbert [15]. Using a rabbit model, Ribbert demonstrated that chordoma-like lesions could be reproduced by puncturing the intervertebral ligament and releasing a portion of the nucleus pulposus. The released tissue was noted to expand and form a tumor histologically identical to the Ecchondrosis physalifora of Virchow, which Ribbert later called "chordoma" [16]. More than a half-century later, the findings of this experiment were replicated by Congdon working at the University of Michigan [17].

Ribbert additionally pointed out that the gelatinous texture of chordoma was wholly inconsistent with that expected of cartilaginous tumors. In aggregate, this evidence argued strongly for a notochordal origin and silenced debate about the embryological origin of chordoma [18, 19]. Shortly thereafter, Fischer and Steiner, working within Ribbert's group, described the occurrence of a malignant notochordal tumor [20], indicating that chordoma belonged to a family of notochord-derived tumors. In 1926, Stewart and Morin [21] made the formal proposal that benign notochord-derived lesions be called *ecchordosis physaliphora*, to differentiate them from chordoma. In modern descriptions, notochord-derived lesions are grouped as malignant chordomas and benign notochordal rests, now termed benign notochordal cell tumors (BNCTs) [22].

## Clinical Descriptions

The first clinical description was made by Dr. Edwin Klebs of Berlin in 1864, who relayed a case of a probable chordoma of the spheno-occipital junction [23]. Shortly thereafter Trélat published on the first cervical chordoma, which was diagnosed as an "ecchondrome muqueux" [24]. The second case was subsequently published by Klebs in his text, "Die Allgemeine Pathologie" [25, 26]. In this case, the patient had presented with increased medullary pressure [8]; it was only later that the mass was determined to be malignant. The first sacrococcygeal lesion was diagnosed by Lothar Henning, who described its occurrence in a 7-month-old in 1900 [27]. Roughly 4 years later, Ribbert reported on findings from an autopsy series of 500 patients [16]. He reported notochord-derived lesions of the clivus in 2% of these patients, suggesting that said lesions might be present in a nontrivial proportion of the population.

The first large clinical review was published in 1923 by Burrow and Stewart [28], who reported the case of a 30-year-old man with an intrasellar chordoma along with a summary of 16 previously reported cases. Among these was the case of Grahl [29], who in 1903 reported the first death from chordoma. The patient, a 51-year-old woman, had presented with cranial polyneuropathy (deficits of cranial nerves 3, 4, 7, 9, and 10), headaches, and visual impairment consistent with elevated intracranial pressure. The patient's death was ultimately deemed secondary to medullary compression. Similar findings were reported shortly thereafter by Seiffer (1905) [30], Fischer and Steiner (1907) [20], Frenkel and Bassal (1910) [31], Eitel (1911) [32], and Wegelin (1911) [33]. In all cases, patients succumbed to pontine or medullary compression by their lesion.

Operative cases were notably sparse within the series, as the majority of described cases localized to the skull base. Most contemporary surgeons felt surgical resection of skull base masses was too dangerous. However, one operative case was noted in the review of Burrow and Stewart – that of Linck, who in 1909 described the operative management of a clival chordoma [34]. The patient – a middle-aged man – originally presented with a pharyngeal swelling and right middle ear disease. He was treated with two open biopsies which revealed pathology consistent with chordoma. He later developed the progression of his tumor leading to multiple cranial neuropathies. Contemporaneously, three sacrococcygeal cases were reported [35–37]. Feldmann described the excision of a presacral chordoma in a 46-year-old female; the tumor was resected without issue and the patient was deemed "well" at 3 months postoperatively. Long-term follow-up was not reported. Mazzia [36] reported the case of a 54-year-old man who presented with a large (17 × 8 cm) coccygeal tumor associated with insidious-onset perirectal pain and discomfort. The lesion was excised but recurred at 19 months; local recurrence also occurred after the second operation, at which point the patient's lesion was felt to be inoperable. The next year Curtis and Le Fort [37] reported on the management of a 58-year-old man with a 10 × 8 cm presacral tumor. The lesion was treated with resection of the tumor and coccyx, but locally recurred with the patient passing at 30 months following initial resection. Of note, Moynihan treated a coccygeal chordoma at the same time as these reports; however, the mass was initially misdiagnosed as carcinoma with colloidal degeneration. It was only upon re-investigation of the pathology 9 years subsequent to resection that the mass was recognized as chordoma [38]. Unlike the prior reports, Moynihan's patient appears to have experienced good long-term local control following surgical resection.

The next surgically treated case was reported by Alézais and Peyron [39], who relayed the course of a 68-year-old woman presenting with a swelling of superior occipital lesion and cervicalgia. The occipital tumor was several inches in diameter and was noted to be eroding through the bone. Following resection, she had complete remission of her symptoms; no recurrence was noted. The subsequent year Albert [40] reported on the operative management of a 26-year-old man who presented with perirectal aching following a fall that was worsened by defecation. He was found to have a 10 × 6 × 5 cm sacrococcygeal chordoma compressing the rectum. The patient underwent multiple subtotal resections and ultimately succumbed 14 months after the presentation.

In 1919, Daland described the management of a 30-year-old woman who presented with hoarseness, headaches, and a retro auricular mass "the size of a hen's egg" [41]. The mass was treated with curettage, which resulted in the resolution of the patient's headaches. The patient also received adjuvant radiotherapy. In spite of this multimodal management, the mass recurred by 7-month follow-up, consistent with the known natural history of chordoma. The same year, Pototschnig [42] reported the first instance of metastatic chordoma. The patient was initially treated with surgical resection of his sacrococcygeal mass, but passed 2 days after his operation. On autopsy, the lesion was found to have spread to the regional lymph nodes and liver. Stewart subsequently described the spread of a sacrococcygeal chordoma to the right scapula 8 years after gross total excision [38]. At this point, it became apparent that chordoma had metastatic potential and was not simply limited to locally invasive disease.

As the pathology of chordoma became better defined, several authors began publishing reviews of the literature, including Coenen (1925) [43], Corsy and Sumont (1927) [44], and Mabrey (1935) [25]. The review of Mabrey has been widely cited and included the first 150 published cases with descriptions of tumor localization, patient epidemiology, clinical presentation, and pattern of metastatic spread. Among the reported cases, Mabrey noted a roughly 2:1 male predominance and a predilection for disease onset in the fifth or sixth decade of life. Additionally, lesions most commonly localized to either the spheno-occipital (33%) or sacrococcygeal regions (58%); mobile spine lesions were uncommon.

Extra-axial chordomas have also been described. The first such instance was the case of Alezais and Peyron, above, who described a chordoma of the left superior occipital region in 1914 [39]. Subsequent extra-axial cases have included those of Koritzki (alveolar process of mandible and maxilla) [45], Rubaschow (superior maxilla) [46], Hirsch (tonsillar region) [47], and Higinbotham et al. (scapula) [48]. Intradural [49] and purely epidural lesions of the spine [50–53] and intradural lesions [54–56] of the cranial vault have also been reported. Current radiographic and histopathologic diagnosis are discussed in Chaps. 4 and 5, respectively.

## Management

### Surgery for Skull Base Chordoma

As the majority of initial descriptions of chordoma were of lesions arising from the clivus and skull base, the majority of early case reports described histologic and pathologic findings on autopsy. Surgery was by-in-large felt to be a too high risk given the close proximity to the brainstem. However, with improvements in surgical techniques, case reports began to be published in the second and third decades of the twentieth century. The first by Linck [34] reported on the usage of open biopsies for a patient with clival chordoma. However, it was not until Daland in 1919 that an attempt at curative excision of a skull base chordoma was reported. As mentioned previously, this young woman experienced rapid local recurrence and death at 7 months in spite of complete excision of the mass and adjuvant radiotherapy. The same year Fabricius-Möller [57] and Argaud [58] described the treatment of retropharyngeal and clival chordomas, respectively. In the case of Fabricius-Möller, the patient experienced local recurrence after only a few months. As the 1920s progressed, additional reports of the surgical management of skull base chordomas were described. These include those of Hirsch, who in 1923 reported the use of palate splitting to treat a nasopharyngeal chordoma; the lesion recurred locally after 1 year of follow-up [7, 19]. Additionally, Argaud and Clermont [59] described resection of a small nasopharyngeal tumor via a transsinusofacial route without complications. Unfortunately, the lesion recurred after only a few months. The same year Loebell [60] reported the use of a transantral approach through the maxillary sinus to treat a nasopharyngeal chordoma involving the left nostril and obstructing the left Eustachian tube. The patient additionally received radium adjuvant brachytherapy; however, the lesion recurred after 1.5 years, leading to death.

These cases, among others, were reviewed by Mabrey, who documented an extremely high perioperative mortality, noted at 31% for large lesions. Congdon echoed similar findings in his series of 18 surgically treated patients [61]. Of the four patients treated for clival lesions, three died intraoperatively or within 1 day of attempted resection. A subsequent review of the spheno-occipital chordoma literature by Zoltán and Fényes in 1960 [62] also painted a morbid picture of surgery for skull base chordomas. They described surgical resection as "most discouraging" due to "the impossibility of complete surgical removal" and stated that conventional radiotherapy was "quite hopeless" [62]. They consequently recommended consideration of brachytherapy with yttrium-90 to help obtain local control. Surgical techniques improved steadily through the second half of the twentieth century though [63–65] and surgical resection became considered a standard part of treatment for most lesions. Al-Mefty and Borba [66] reported their experience with 23 patients treated in the early 1990s. All patients were treated with skull base approaches, of which 17 received adjuvant proton-photon radiotherapy; radiographic cure was seen in 71% of patients at a mean of 25 months. Subsequent follow-up using an expanded series found a 5-year recurrence-free survival rate of 50.7% and 5-year overall survival of 86% [67]. Gay et al. [68] reported similarly good results in their series of 60 patients with skull base chordomas or chondrosarcomas treated with surgical resection and adjuvant high-dose radiotherapy between 1983 and 1994. Five-year recurrence-free survival was 65% for patients with chordoma. Of note, it was also during the late 1980s and early 1990s that the first descriptions of transsphenoidal approaches for clival chordomas were described [69–72]. These evolved into the endoscopic transsphenoidal approaches [73–75] that are considered by some to be the approach of choice for clival chordomas [76, 77].

## Surgery for Mobile Spine Chordoma

The first likely report of a chordoma of the mobile spine was reported by Trélat and Ranvier in 1868, who described a chordoma-like mass involving the cervical spine [78]. The mass was noted to be extremely large and extended from the angle of the mandible to the posterior pharyngeal wall. Resection was attempted, but the mass proved extremely adherent and surgery was aborted. The patient passed from pulmonary complication on post-operative day 2.

Then in 1924, the first confirmed case of mobile spine chordoma was made by Raul and Diss [79]. This was shortly followed by the reports of Cameron in 1926 [80], Syme and Cappell in 1926 [78], and Cappell in 1928 [81]. The case of Syme and Cappell [78], represents the first case of mobile spine chordoma treated by surgical management with histologic confirmation. They described a 59-year-old man presenting with neck stiffness, dysarthria, and dysphagia who was treated with curettage for a chordoma involving the anterior cervical spine. The patient experienced recurrence 6 months after resection and underwent repeat resection of the mass, which now extended from the occiput to C5 vertebral body. The patient, unfortunately, succumbed to septic pneumonia postoperatively and died on the third postoperative day. This high surgical morbidity was noted by Mabrey in his 1935 review [25]. Of the 14 patients in the literature who had undergone surgical treatment of mobile spine chordomas, three (21%) had died in the perioperative period [25].

Surgery for mobile spine chordomas remained a contentious issue into the late-twentieth century as procedural morbidity remained high and was felt to be unjustified if cure could not be achieved. Through the 1960s and 1970s, surgery was almost exclusively performed for the relief of neurological symptoms rather than oncologic cure [82–86]. Then in 1981, Stener made the first report of *en* bloc vertebrectomy for mobile spine chordoma [87]. In this case, he resected an L3 chordoma causing cauda equina syndrome. The patient not only regained ambulatory function postoperatively, but she remained disease-free at last follow-up, 7 years post-resection. Such long-term control was particularly notable, as a contemporary series of 51 patients with chordoma showed extremely poor disease-free survival [88]. Of the treated patients, metastatic spread was observed in 25% of those treated for mobile spine lesions and 45% of those treated for sacrococcygeal lesions. The poor control seen in tumors treated with intralesional resection may have led Stener to subsequently argue for more aggressive resection of primary vertebral column lesions [87].

Several years passed before the additional description of these *en bloc* spondylectomies was issued [89]. By the early 1990s though, advances in modern imaging and surgical techniques allowed many groups to begin reporting favorable outcomes following *en bloc* resection of mobile spine lesions [89–92]. Of note are the contributions of Boriani and colleagues at the Rizzoli Orthopaedic Institute in Bologna, Italy [93]. Their experience with *en bloc* resection led to the formulation of the Weinstein-Boriani-Biagini staging system (see Chap. 6) that has become a standard part of surgical evaluation for patients with mobile spine lesions. Modern series, including the large multicenter AOSpine series [4], have indicated that while morbid, *en bloc* resection of mobile spine lesions is feasible. Additionally, where negative margins are achieved, *en bloc* surgical resection improves post-operative survival and local control; it is consequently considered to be the standard of care for these lesions. Current surgical approaches to lesions of the mobile spine are discussed in Chap. 7 (occipitocervical junction), Chap. 8 (cervical spine), Chap. 9 (thoracic spine), and Chap. 10 (lumbar spine).

## Surgery for Sacrococcygeal Chordoma

Descriptions of total excision of sacrococcygeal chordoma started with the reports of Massia [36] and Curtis and Le Fort [37]. In both cases, gross total excision was thought to have been obtained, yet serial follow-up demonstrated local recurrence. The propensity for local recurrence among surgically treated tumors was subsequently noted by multiple authors [94]. Given the apparent proclivity for local recurrence, Stewart argued as early as 1922 that such lesions should be treated via total excision to achieve long-term control or even cure [38]. However, early surgical management was associated with high morbidity and mortality. In his 1935 review of the chordoma literature, Mabrey reported that perioperative mortality across all anatomic sites was 27% [25]. Additionally, local recurrence was seen in 66% of the 59 patients who survived the perioperative period, with an average time to recurrence of 17.5 months [25]. Based upon this, Mabrey author argued for the surgical resection of sacrococcygeal chordomas, focusing on wide excision and without disruption of the tumor, if possible.

Such a treatment paradigm was later espoused in literature reviews by Mixter and Mixter in 1940 [94] and Shackelford and Rhode in 1955 [95]. Both author groups noted that lesions treated with gross total excision had longer times to local recurrence than other lesions and were far likelier to achieve cure. Additionally, Shackelford and Rhodes [95] noted that in cases where there was local recurrence, the intraosseous portion of the tumor had appeared to have been shelled out. In other words, local recurrence occurred more often in cases where excision had involved violation of the tumor capsule. Consequently, they argued that the best outcomes for sacrococcygeal chordoma were achieved through an *en bloc* resection that did not violate the integrity of the tumor capsule.

Subsequent studies demonstrated the superiority of this *en bloc* excision with negative margins in terms of local recurrence and post-operative survival [4, 5, 48, 96–99]. This led other groups to argue for *en bloc* resection with negative margins as the definitive treatment surgically amenable lesions beginning in the 1950s [95, 100]. Such studies serve as the evidentiary base for the treatment paradigm originally described by Enneking in 1980, which recommends *en bloc* resection with negative margins for chordoma [101, 102]. The Enneking system, also known as the Musculoskeletal Sarcoma Tumor Society (MSTS) System, remains the gold standard today for guiding the management of primary bone tumors of the mobile spine and sacrum [1]. More recently, Sim and colleagues provided further support for *en bloc* R0 resection with their experience treating 52 patients for sacrococcygeal chordoma at the Mayo Clinic [103]. When comparing patients treated with a wide margin resection (defined as a healthy cuff of tissue >1–2 cm) to those treated with marginal or intralesional margins, overall survival and local control were significantly better among those treated with wide margin resection. Interestingly though, a more recent 31-year experience published by the Rizzoli Institute [104] noted that long-term recurrence rates may be high even for patients treated with R0 resection. In their series of 99 patients, local control was seen in less than 25% of patients at 15-year follow-up. The reason for this is unclear, however, it may be due to the presence of "micro-skip" metastases – small tumor microfoci situated outside the tumor pseudocapsule. This was suggested by Akiyama et al. [105] who observed micro-skip lesions in over 40% of patients on histological examination. Consistent with this, the group at the Massachusetts General Hospital (MGH) [106] found that the use of adjuvant or neoadjuvant radiation, not surgical margin was the strongest predictor of local control among sacrococcygeal chordomas undergoing index surgery. It is unclear if the superior local recurrence was because the micro-skip lesions were covered by the adjuvant radiation though, and this remains an ongoing area of investigation. Current surgical techniques for sacrococcygeal chordomas are discussed in Chap. 11. Soft tissue and bony defect reconstruction techniques are described in Chaps. 12 and 13, respectively.

## Radiotherapy for Chordoma

Radiation as adjuvant or primary therapy for chordoma has been described repeatedly since the earliest clinical patient series. The first such description was made by Daland [41] in his treatment of a skull base chordoma. The patient was initially treated with surgical resection, which was followed by "two massive x-ray treatments."

By the mid-1950s, most groups began to describe chordoma as highly radioresistant [62, 95, 107, 108] and indicated that radiotherapy was only of "palliative value" [107]. However, in the subsequent decade, it was suggested that extremely high doses of radiation could, in fact, reduce local recurrence. In 1964, Kamrin et al. reported a series of 30 patients treated for chordoma with a combination of biopsy or surgical resection and adjuvant radiation (3600–17,500 rad) [109]. They concluded that only sacrococcygeal chordoma could be reasonably be treated with surgical resection, and that mobile spine and intracranial chordoma should be biopsied and treated with "large tumor doses of therapeutic radiotherapy." They defined large doses as 5000 rad or greater and reported that their practice was to dose with 3000–5000 rad followed by 2000–3000 rad doses at each instance of recurrence. Shortly thereafter, Higinbotham and colleagues reported a 35-year experience of treating chordoma at Memorial Sloan Kettering [48]. Similar to Kamrin et al., the authors argued that high-dose radiation could be used to improve local chordoma control. The authors argued for an even more aggressive dosing schema, arguing that doses of 7000 rad or above were required for substantial benefit, although they acknowledged that such doses were associated with "acute radiation reactions."

Other series in the 1970s [86, 100, 110] and 1980s [111–113] argued for increasingly large radiation doses (60–70 Gy total dose over 6–7 weeks). Based upon the result in their series of 15 patients, Pearlman and Friedman [100] argued for tumor doses of 8000 rad or more; they found that doses ≤4000 rad were ineffective at killing tumor cells. Similar to Kamrin et al., the authors acknowledged the significant toxicities associated with such high levels of radiation and therefore stipulated that such lesions should likely be reserved for sacrococcygeal tumors. Unlike the Kamrin et al. though, Pearlman and Friedman argued against repeat radiation dosing, indicating that it would be unlikely to control the residual chordoma but would almost assuredly cause significant, irreparable radiation damage. The next decade, Amendola et al. [111] reported on the effectiveness of adjuvant hypofractionated radiation with 50–66 Gy in 180–220 cGy fractions for surgically managed chordoma. Though their experience was small, the authors reported that all nine of their cranial chordoma patients were able to tolerate radiotherapy without issue.

Beginning in the 1980s, several authors began to describe the benefits of proton therapy for chordoma [113]. The first report appears to have been by Suit and colleagues at the MGH, who described the use of high-dose proton radiotherapy in 10 patients with chordoma or chondrosarcoma of the skull base or cervical spine [113]. Patients in their series were treated with a combination of high-energy photons and 160-MV proton beams in 1.8–2.0CGE fractions to a total dose of 65.3–76.2CGE between the two modalities. Nine of the ten patients experienced acute radiation reactions though, most commonly mucositis or skin changes (e.g., desquamation, erythema). None of the patients experienced recurrence over a follow-up period that ranged from 2 months to 6 years. Other early experiences included the expanded MGH series published by Fagundes et al. [114] and the experiences of Al-Mefty and Borba [66], Castro et al. [115], and Hug et al. [116]. Doses all ranged from 60 to 77CGE and a recent review of the chordoma literature supports superior outcomes in patients receiving high-dose (>65 Gy) radiotherapy with charged particles or stereotactic photon radiosurgery [117]. More modern experiences have since been described [118–120] and preliminary experiences using carbon ion and other charged particle radiotherapy modalities have been published [121–125]. Experiences with adjuvant stereotactic radiosurgery for chordoma have also been described, dating to the early 1990s [126–131]. The most recent consensus statements recommend the use of adjuvant high-dose charged particle therapy or stereotactic radiosurgery for local tumor control [132, 133]. Current usage of radiotherapy is discussed in Chap. 14 (photon therapy) and Chap. 15 (protons and charged particle therapy).

## Chemotherapy

Owing to its relatively slow-growing nature, chordoma has generally not been considered to be a malignancy that is amenable to systemic chemotherapy [1]. Use of systemic therapy was first described by McSweeney and Sholl [134], who in 1959 published their use of mechlorethamine – a nitrogen mustard – in the treatment of a 78-year-old woman with metastatic sacrococcygeal chordoma. The mechlorethamine treatments led to improvement of the patient's sacrococcygeal pain; however, she progressed on therapy with new metastases to the forearm noted within 8 months of initiating therapy.

The next published description followed 5 years later with the series of Kamrin et al. in 1964 [109]. The authors described using intracarotid perfusion of methotrexate as a treatment adjuvant in two patients. One patient died within 8 days of treatment and the other experienced local recurrence within 1 year, making it unclear if there was any benefit. This was followed by the reports of Rissanen and Holsti in 1967 [135], and Pearlman et al. in 1972 [136] who reported the use of cyclophosphamide and actinomycin D, respectively, for recurrent disease. Both agents were found to be ineffective.

At the same time, these reports were published, Razis et al. [137] described the use of vincristine sulfate (2 mg week) in a patient with recurrent chordoma of the cervical spine. The patient experienced roughly 4 months of systematic improvement, but ultimately succumbed to their disease. Harwick and Miller [138] employed vincristine (1.4 mg/m$^2$ weekly) with similar results. The patient enjoyed symptomatic improvement after the first several doses; however, there was no clear survival benefit. Spratt et al. [139] published their case of a 49-year-old woman with recurrent sacrococcygeal chordoma who failed multiple regimens, including cyclophosphamide-doxorubicin-methotrexate triple therapy, cyclophosphamide-actinomycin D-dacarbazine triple therapy, cyclophosphamide-dacarbazine-vincristine triple therapy, and lomustine-doxorubicin-vincristine-bleomycin quadruple therapy.

The patient had a moderate radiographic benefit on the last line regimen, but was unable to tolerate associated toxicities and succumbed to *Pseudomonas* sepsis 2 years after initiating chemotherapy. Platinum-based agents were similarly found to be ineffective at producing long-term benefits [140].

Given this lack of success, chemotherapy has remained a last-ditch option. However, more recently there has been increased interest in small molecule agents, notably tyrosine kinase inhibitors, and immunotherapies for patients with recurrent or metastatic disease. These agents include erlotinib, sunitinib, lapatinib, imatinib, sorafenib, nivolumab, and ipilimumab. Various combinations of these agents are currently the subject of clinical trials [1]. More detailed discussion of modern systemic therapy and future directions is discussed in Chap. 16.

## Epidemiology of Chordoma

### Population-Level Data

Similar to other primary bone tumors of the spinal column, chordoma is a rare clinical pathology with previous estimates suggesting an overall prevalence of 0.08–0.5 per 100,000 persons worldwide [141]. Estimates vary widely though and little population-level data exist. Of that which is available, the best data come from the Surveillance, Epidemiology, and End Results (SEER) program of the National Cancer Institute (NCI) [142–144]. The SEER registry of the NCI is a prospectively maintained database covering 28% of the US population [143], which has previously been found to be broadly representative of the US cancer population as a whole [145]. The most recent review of these data was published by Zuckerman et al. [143] based upon the data from 1616 patients with chordoma enrolled between 1973 and 2013. They found that the most common location for chordoma was the skull base (41.1%), followed by the sacrum (31.4%) and mobile spine (27.5%). For those with mobile spine lesions, 60% of patients were male, mean age was 57 years, and the majority of patients identified as white (93%) as opposed to black (2%) or other (6%). For sacral lesions, there was also a male predominance (62%) though the age at presentation was slightly older (mean 63 years) and a smaller proportion of patients identified as white (86%) as opposed to black (3%) or other (11%). No geographic biases were noted and the majority of both patients with mobile spine tumors (74%) and sacral tumors (70%) had their disease confined within the periosteum at the time of diagnosis, consistent with the relatively slow-growing nature of chordoma. Few patients had metastatic disease at presentation (8% of mobile spine; 7% of sacrum). Most patients underwent surgical resection (76% of mobile spine lesions; 67% of sacral lesions), and a large minority of both mobile spine (50%) and sacral lesions (37%) were treated with radiation. Analysis of the data by year suggested no trends in the proportion of patients being treated with surgical resection, though there was a significant decrease in the proportion of sacral lesions being irradiated. Median overall survival is relatively good for both mobile spine (median 95 months) and sacral lesions (median 87 months). In both cases, overall survival is notably higher among patients treated with surgical resection (mobile spine: 105 vs 61 months; sacrum: 111 vs 56 months). The data from Zuckerman et al. [143] also suggest that prognoses may be better for more recently diagnosed patients; however, the trend they identified did not meet statistical significance. Older patients have been found to have poorer survival [143], though the effect size is small and it is unclear if this relationship is tied to the primary malignancy. Other small epidemiological series have been published based upon Scandinavian [3, 88], English [146], and Taiwanese populations [147], which are summarized in Table 3.1.

**Table 3.1** Summary of population-based studies of chordoma epidemiology

| Study | *n* | Population details | Epidemiology data |
|---|---|---|---|
| Eriksson et al., 1981 [88] | 979 | *Country*: Sweden<br>*Time Period*: 1958–1970<br>*Recruitment*: Swedish Cancer Registry | *Age*: mean 57 yr<br>*Sex*: 51% M<br>*Incid*: 0.51 per $10^6$ PY<br>*Prev*: n.g.<br>*Loc*: 27% SB, 16% MS, 57% Scrm<br>*Surv*: mean 3.3 yr (SB), 3.5 yr (MS), 4.6 yr (Scrm) |
| Hung et al., 2014 [147] | 1238 | *Country*: Taiwan<br>*Time Period*: 2003–2010<br>*Recruitment*: Taiwan Cancer Registry | *Age*: median >60 yr<br>*Sex*: 67% M<br>*Incid*: 0.40 per $10^6$ PY<br>*Prev*: n.g.<br>*Loc*: n.g.<br>*Surv*: n.g. |
| McMaster et al., 2001 [144] | 400 | *Country*: USA<br>*Time Period*: 1973–1995<br>*Recruitment*: SEER database | *Age*: mean 54.8 yr<br>*Sex*:60% M<br>*Incid*: n.g.<br>*Prev*: 0.8 per $10^6$<br>*Loc*: 32% SB, 33%MS, 29%Scrm<br>*Surv*: median 6.29 yr; 68% @ 5-yr; 40% @ 10-yr |
| Paavolainen and Teppo, 1976 [3] | <700 | *Country*: Finland<br>*Time Period*: 1953–1971<br>*Recruitment*: Finnish Cancer Registry | *Age*: mean 55.5 yr<br>*Sex*: 60% M<br>*Incid*: M = 0.30 per $10^6$ PY; F = 0.18 per $10^6$ PY<br>*Prev*: per $10^6$<br>*Loc*: 10% SB, 15% MS, 75% Scrm<br>*Surv*: n.g. |
| Smoll et al., 2013 [142] | 623 | *Country*: USA<br>*Time Period*: 1973–2009<br>*Recruitment*: SEER database | *Age*: median 58 yr<br>*Sex*: 59% M<br>*Incid*: n.g.<br>*Prev*: 0.84 per $10^6$<br>*Loc*: n.g.<br>*Surv*: median 7.7 yr; 72% @ 5-yr; 49% @ 10-yr |

**Table 3.1** (continued)

| Study | *n* | Population details | Epidemiology data |
|---|---|---|---|
| Stiller et al., 2013 [153] | 45,568 | *Country*: Europe (EU27 countries)<br>*Time Period*: 1995–2002<br>*Recruitment*: | *Age*: n.g.<br>*Sex*: n.g.<br>*Incid*: <1 per $10^6$ PY<br>*Prev*: 4 per $10^6$<br>*Loc*: n.g.<br>*Surv*: ≈75% @ 5-yr |
| Whelan et al., 2012 [146] | 11,002 | *Country*: England<br>*Time Period*: 1979–2007<br>*Recruitment*: National Cancer Data Repository; Office of National Statistics | *Age*: 75% >50 yr old<br>*Sex*: n.g.<br>*Incid*: 0.03–0.04 per $10^6$ PY<br>*Prev*: 0.3–0.4 per $10^6$<br>*Loc*: 26% SB, 23% MS, 45% Scrm<br>*Surv*: 49–59% @ 5-yr |
| Zuckerman et al., 2018 [143] | 1616 | *Country*: USA<br>*Time period*: 1973–2013<br>*Recruitment*: SEER database | *Age*: mean 54.8 yr<br>*Sex*:58% M<br>*Incid*: n.g.<br>*Prev*: n.g.<br>*Loc*: 41% SB, 27% MS, 32% Scrm<br>*Surv*: median 162mo (SB), 95mo (MS), 87mo (Scrm) |

*Key*: *F* female, *incid* incidence, *loc* location, *M* male, *mo* month, *MS* mobile spine, *n* number, *n.g.* not given, *prev* prevalence, *PY* person-year, *SB* skull base, *Scrm* sacrum, *SEER* surveillance, epidemiology, and end results, *Surv* survival, *yr* year

## Multicenter Cohort Data

Within the mobile spine, lumbar tumors appear to be most common [4]. In a retrospective review of the AOSpine Knowledge Forum Tumor prospective database [148], Gokaslan et al. [4] reported treatment outcomes of 166 patients with mobile spine chordomas who underwent surgical resection. Similar to the findings of Zuckerman et al., mean age was 59 years and two-thirds of patients were male. Half of all lesions localized to the lumbar spine, with the cervical spine being the second most common region (35%). Multilevel involvement is relatively common. Forty-two percent of lesions involve 2 or more consecutive vertebrae. Lesions are also large at diagnosis, with an average lesion size of 4.9 × 4.1 × 4.3 cm (anterior-posterior × transverse × craniocaudal) or 87.7 $cm^3$. The majority of tumors are low grade (63%) at presentation and there is a tendency to locally recur. This is reduced by *en bloc* resection tough, as 5-year local recurrence is 20% for tumors receiving *en bloc* resection with negative margins (Enneking-appropriate) compared to 65% for tumors receiving Enneking-inappropriate resection. To this end, Gokaslan et al. [4] found *en bloc* resection with negative margins to be the strongest protective factor against local recurrence.

Using this same prospective registry, Varga et al. [5] published a description of the AOSpine experience with surgically treated sacral chordomas. Among the 167 included patients, mean age was 57 years and 58% of patients were male, similar to the numbers from the SEER database. Perhaps unsurprisingly, mean tumor size is much larger for sacral lesions (mean 588.1 $cm^3$) and nearly all tumors (98%) had extracompartmental extension at the time of diagnosis. Multilevel disease is also common and 6% of lesions extend into the mobile spine. As with mobile spine lesions, local recurrence is common, even though 80% of lesions are low grade at the time of treatment. Median local recurrence-free survival is roughly 4 years, but this is significantly improved by *en bloc* resection with negative margins [5]. Varga et al. did not find Enneking-appropriate resection to improve overall survival, though the authors attributed this to short overall follow-up and the current consensus is that the best-available data support Enneking-appropriate resection as a means of improving survival in chordoma [133, 149, 150].

## Clinical Presentation

Owing to the slow-growing nature of chordoma, patients commonly have an insidious symptom onset and some are even asymptomatic at the time of radiographic diagnosis [1]. The clinical picture varies depending upon the location of the lesion, but generally stem from mass effect or erosion of adjacent bony structures leading to compromise of the vertebral column's load-bearing capacity. The first attempt to summarize the literature on the clinical presentation of chordoma was performed by Mabrey in 1935, who summarized the data for 150 chordomas described in the literature to date [25]. Of the 86 sacrococcygeal tumors included, the most common symptoms were pain (69%) with (43%) or without (26%) an accompanying palpable mass. Seventeen percent of the identified patients had presented with a tumor without clinical symptoms. Among the 46 skull base lesions, 33% had presented with headache. Localized pain was also common among the 14 mobile spine lesions, occurring in 9 patients (64%). Consistent with the slow-growing nature of chordoma, Mabrey reported an average time between symptom onset and clinical presentation of 41 months for skull base chordomas and 36 months for sacrococcygeal chordomas.

### Data from Multicenter Cohorts

In their multicenter review of 166 patients surgically treated for mobile spine chordomas, Gokaslan and colleagues found that the majority of patients (89%) presented with pain [4]. Only a minority of patients (18%) had evidence of pathological fracture though. Similarly, Varga et al. [5] found nearly all patients with sacral chordoma present with tumor-related pain (96%). Pathologic fracture was again uncommon, being seen in only 4% of patients. A significant minority also present with neurological deficits though. In the Varga et al. study, 24% had motor weakness at the time of presentation and 27% had symptoms consistent with cauda equina syndrome [5].

A smaller, population-based study of Swedish patients by Eriksson et al. [88] found 52% of patients with sacrococcygeal chordoma present with local pain, 31% present with bowel or urinary complaints, and 10% present with asymptomatic masses; 21% of patients presented with sensory deficits and 7% presented with concomitant motor deficits. They reported a median time from symptom onset to diagnosis of roughly 1 year, consistent with the slow-growing nature of chordomas. The authors [88] endorsed a distinct presentation for mobile spine lesions, with only 38% of patients having local pain and 25% having motor deficits at the time of diagnosis. In a second Scandinavian population, Paavolainen and Teppo [3] reported that 73% of sacral chordomas present with pain and 60% noted a palpable mass at the time of presentation; only 13% of patients had urinary complaints at presentation. Tumors of the other locations were too uncommon to derive conclusions about clinical presentation owing to the small population at risk. Median time from symptom onset to diagnosis was 6 months with a mean of 12.7 months [3]. Collectively, these data suggest that patients most commonly present with insidious-onset, localized, non-mechanical pain that in a minority of cases will be accompanied by neurological deficits.

## Conclusion

As relayed in this chapter, chordomas are an extremely uncommon clinical entity, oftentimes known as a "one in a million" disease. Though first described more than 150 years ago, the continuous investigation into the origins and molecular genetics of chordoma (Chap. 2) has identified it as a malignant derivative of the embryonic notochord. Lesions of the spine and sacrum most commonly present with local pain, though neurological symptoms occur in a nontrivial proportion of patients secondary to tumor mass effect. While their overall rarity of chordoma makes it an unlikely cause of spine-related complaints, clinicians should have increased clinical suspicion in patients in the sixth or seventh decade of life with insidious onset, non-mechanical pain. Lesions are easily detected on diagnostic imaging (Chap. 4) and patients with these lesions benefit from earlier detection and referral to high-volume centers of excellence [151, 152].

## References


1. Pennington Z, Ehresman J, McCarthy EF, Ahmed AK, Pittman PD, Lubelski D, Goodwin CR, Sciubba DM. Chordoma of the sacrum and mobile spine: a narrative review. Spine J. 2020;21(3):500–17. https://doi.org/10.1016/j.spinee.2020.10.009.
2. Virchow RLK. Untersuchungen über die entwickelung des schädelgrundes im gesunden und krankhaften zustande, und über den einfluss derselben auf schädelform, gesichtsbildung und gehirnbau. 1st ed. Berlin: G. Reimer; 1857.
3. Paavolainen P, Teppo L. Chordoma in Finland. Acta Orthop Scand. 1976;47:46–51.
4. Gokaslan ZL, Zadnik PL, Sciubba DM, et al. Mobile spine chordoma: results of 166 patients from the AOSpine Knowledge Forum Tumor database. J Neurosurg Spine. 2016;24:644–51.

5. Varga PP, Szövérfi Z, Fisher CG, et al. Surgical treatment of sacral chordoma: prognostic variables for local recurrence and overall survival. Eur Spine J. 2015;24:1092–101.
6. Luschka H. Über gallertartige auswüchse am clivus blumenbachii. Virchows Arch. 1857;11:8–12.
7. Hirsch EF, Ingals M. Sacrococcygeal chordoma. J Am Med Assoc. 1923;80:1369–70.
8. Sahyouni R, Goshtasbi K, Mahmoodi A, Chen JW. A historical recount of chordoma. J Neurosurg Spine. 2018;28:422–8.
9. Müller JP. Ueber das Vorkommen von Resten der Chorda dorsalis bei Menschen nach der Geburt, und über ihr Verhältnis zu den Gallertgeschwulsten der Clivus. Zeitschrift für Ration Med. 1858;2:202–29.
10. Leboucq H. Recherches sur la mode de disparition de la corde dorsale chez les vertébrés supérieurs. Arch Biol (Liege). 1880;1:718–36.
11. Williams LW. The later development of the notochord in mammals. Am J Anat. 1908;8:251–84.
12. Kölliker A. Über die Beziehungen der Chorda dorsalis zur Bildung der Wirbel der Selachier und einiger anderer Fische. In: Verhandlungen der Phys. Gesellschaft zur Würzbg. Würzburg. Würzburg: A. Stuber; 1860. p. 193.
13. Löwe L. Zur Kenntniss der säugethierchorda. Arch für Mikroskopische Anat. 1879;16:597–612.
14. Steiner H. Ueber die ecchondrosis physalifora spheno-occipitalis. Cent für Allg Pathol und Pathol Anat. 1894;5:457.
15. Ribbert MWH. Über die experimentelle Erzeugung einer Ecchondrosis physalifora. Verhandlungen der Kong f inn Med. 1895;13:455–64.
16. Ribbert H. Geschwulstlehre für Ärzte und Studierende. 1st ed. Bonn: Friedrich Coehn; 1904.
17. Congdon CC. Proliferative lesions resembling chordoma following puncture of the nucleus pulposus in rabbits. J Natl Cancer Inst. 1952;12:893–907.
18. Stewart MJ, Burrow JF. Ecchordosis physaliphora spheno-occipitalis. J Neurol Psychopathol. 1923;4:218–20.
19. Bailey P, Bagdasar D. Intracranial chordoblastoma. Am J Pathol. 1929;5:439–450.5.
20. Fischer B, Steiner H. Über ein malignes chordom der schädel-rückgratshöhle. Beiträge zur Pathol Anat und zer Allg Pathol. 1907;40:109–19.
21. Stewart MJ, Morin JE. Chordoma: a review, with report of a new sacrococcygeal case. J Pathol Bacteriol. 1926;29:41–60.
22. Yamaguchi T, Suzuki S, Ishiiwa H, Shimizu K, Ueda Y. Benign notochordal cell tumors: a comparative histological study of benign notochordal cell tumors, classic chordomas, and notochordal vestiges of fetal intervertebral discs. Am J Surg Pathol. 2004;28:756–61.
23. Klebs E. Ein fall von ecchondrosis spheno-occipitalis amylacea. Arch für Pathol Anat und Physiol und für Klin Med. 1864;31:396–9.
24. Hass GM. Chordomas of the cranium and cervical portion of the spine: a review of the literature with report of a case. Arch Neurol Psychiatr. 1934;32:300–27.
25. Mabrey RE. Chordoma: a study of 150 cases. Am J Cancer. 1935;25:501–17.
26. Klebs E. Die allgemeine Pathologie oder die Lehre von den Ursachen und dem Wesen der Krankheitsprocesse: Ein handbuch für studierende und aerzte. 1st ed. Jena: Verlag Von Gustav Fischer; 1889.
27. Henning L. Über congenitale echte Sakraltumoren. Beiträge zur Pathol Anat und zer Allg Pathol. 1900;28:593.
28. Burrow JF, Stewart MJ. Malignant spheno-occipital chordoma. J Neurol Neurosurg Psychiatry. 1923;4:205–17.
29. Grahl O. Eine Ecchondrosis physalifora spheno-occipitalis (Chordom des Türkensattels) ungewöhnlichen Umfangs mit interessanten klinischen. Inaugural-Dissertation 1903.
30. Seiffer. Ein Fall von seltenen Geschwulstbildung der Schädelbasis. Neurol Cent. 1905;24:469.
31. Frenkel H, Bassal L. Sur un cas de chordome malin sphéno-occipital. Arch médecine expérimentale d'anatomie Pathol. 1910;22:703.
32. Eitel W. Ein Beitrag zur Kasuistik der Chordome. Inaugural-Dissertation 1911.

33. Wegelin K. Über ein malignes chordom des clivus blumenbachii. Atti del Congr internazionale dei Patol. 1912;1:70.
34. Linck A. Chordoma malignum, ein Beitrag zur Kenntnis der Geschwülste an der Schädelbasis. Beiträge zur Pathol Anat und zer Allg Pathol. 1909;46:573–85.
35. Feldmann I. Chordoma ossis sacri. Beiträge zur Pathol Anat und zer Allg Pathol. 1910;48:630–4.
36. Mazzia O. Chordom der Sakralgegend. Zentralbl Allg Pathol. 1910;21:769–72.
37. Curtis F, Le Fort R. Tumeur de la région sacro-coccygienne chez un adulte: angio-sarcome a type périthélial développé aux dépens de la glande de Luschka. Rev Chir. 1911;43:1.
38. Stewart MJ. Malignant sacrococcygeal chordoma. J Pathol Bacteriol. 1922;25:40–62.
39. Alézais H, Peyron F. Contribution à l'étude des chordomes. Chordome de la région occipitale. Bull Assoc Fr Etud Cancer. 1914;7:194.
40. Albert H. Chordoma, with the report of a malignant case from the sacrococcygeal region. Surg Gynecol Obstet. 1915;21:766.
41. Daland EM. Chordoma. Bost Med Surg J. 1919;180:571–6.
42. Potoschnig G. Ein Fall von malignem chordom mit metastasen. Beiträge zur Pathol Anat und zer Allg Pathol. 1919;65:356–62.
43. Coenen H. Das chordom. Beitr Klin Chir. 1925;83:1–77.
44. Corsy F, Surmont J. Sur l'histogénèse, l'évolution des tumeurs de la notochorde. Bull Assoc Fr Etud Cancer. 1927;16:316–76.
45. Koritzki GE. Histiogenesis and localization of chordomata. Cent für Allg Pathol und Pathol Anat. 1914;25:638.
46. Rubaschow S. Zur onkologischen Kasuistik: Chordom mit ungewöhnlichem Sitz. Zentralbl Chir. 1929;56:137.
47. Hirsch C. Zur Frage des malignen chordoms. Zeitschrift für Hals-, Nasen-, und Ohren-heilkd. 1931;28:140.
48. Higinbotham NL, Phillips RF, Farr HW, Hustu HO. Chordoma. Thirty-five-year study at memorial hospital. Cancer. 1967;20:1841–50.
49. Rotter J, Mueller K, MacConnell A, McGowan J, Spitz S. Isolated cervical extraosseous intradural chordoma attached to the C5 nerve root: a case report. Chinese Neurosurg J. 2019;5:22.
50. Tomlinson FH, Scheithauer BW, Miller GM, Onofrio BM. Extraosseous spinal chordoma. Case report. J Neurosurg. 1991;75:980–4.
51. Pierre-Khan A, Sarkis A, Lellouch-Tubiana A, Sebag G, Finidori G, Hirsch JF. Epidural chordoma without bone involvement. A propos of a case in a child. Review of the literature. Neurochirurgie. 1991;37:258–63.
52. Kalish G, Rubin BP, Chew FS, Richardson ML. Epidural Chordoma of the cervical spine with secondary bone involvement. Radiol Case Rep. 2006;1:128–33.
53. Jallo J, Nathan D, Bierbrauer K, Farber E. Chordoma: a case report. Surg Neurol. 1997;48:46–8.
54. Katayama Y, Tsubokawa T, Hirasawa T, Takahata T, Nemoto N. Intradural extraosseous chordoma in the foramen magnum region. J Neurosurg. 1991;75:976–9.
55. Vinke RS, Lamers EC, Kusters B, van Lindert EJ. Intradural prepontine chordoma in an 11-year-old boy. A case report. Childs Nerv Syst. 2016;32:169–73.
56. Chang SW, Gore PA, Nakaji P, Rekate HL. Juvenile intradural chordoma: case report. Neurosurgery. 2008;62:E525–7.
57. Fabricius-Möller J. Chordoma of retropharyngeal region. Hospitalstid. 1919;62:849–57.
58. Argaud R. Chordome Malin. Arch médecine expérimentale d'anatomie Pathol. 1918;28:364–74.
59. Argaud R, Clermont D. Chordome primitif malin de la poche de Luschka. Ann Anat Pathol (Paris). 1928;5:145–52.
60. Loebell H. Zur Therapie der bösartigen Clivus- und Nasenrachenchordome. Zeitschrift für Hals-, Nasen-, und Ohren-heilkd. 1928;21:337–48.
61. Congdon CC. Benign and malignant chordomas; a clinico-anatomical study of twenty-two cases. Am J Pathol. 1952;28:793–821.

62. Zoltán L, Fényes I. Stereotactic diagnosis and radioactive treatment in a case of spheno-occipital chordoma. J Neurosurg. 1960;17:888–900.
63. Forsyth PA, Cascino TL, Shaw EG, Scheithauer BW, O'Fallon JR, Dozier JC, Piepgras DG. Intracranial chordomas: a clinicopathological and prognostic study of 51 cases. J Neurosurg. 1993;78:741–7.
64. Sen CN, Sekhar LN, Schramm VL, Janecka IP. Chordoma and chondrosarcoma of the cranial base. Neurosurgery. 1989;25:931–40. discussion 940–941
65. Atkins LW, Khudados ES, Kaleoglu M, Revesz T, Sacares P, Crockard HA. Skull base chordomas: a review of 38 patients, 1958–88. Br J Neurosurg. 1993;7:241–8.
66. Al-Mefty O, Borba LAB. Skull base chordomas: a management challenge. J Neurosurg. 1997;86:182–9.
67. Colli BO, Al-Mefty O. Chordomas of the skull base: follow-up review and prognostic factors. Neurosurg Focus. 2001;10:1–11.
68. Gay E, Sekhar LN, Rubinstein E, Wright DC, Sen C, Janecka IP, Snyderman CH. Chordomas and chondrosarcomas of the cranial base. Neurosurgery. 1995;36:887–97.
69. Lalwani AK, Kaplan MJ, Gutin PH. The transsphenoethmoid approach to the sphenoid sinus and clivus. Neurosurgery. 1992;31:1008–14.
70. Maira G, Pallini R, Anile C, Fernandez E, Salvinelli F, La Rocca LM, Rossi GF. Surgical treatment of clival chordomas: the transsphenoidal approach revisited. J Neurosurg. 1996;85:784–92.
71. Raffel C, Wright DC, Gutin PH, Wilson CB. Cranial chordomas: clinical presentation and results of operative and radiation therapy in twenty-six patients. Neurosurgery. 1985;17:703–10.
72. Laws ER. Transsphenoidal surgery for tumors of the clivus. Otolaryngol Neck Surg. 1984;92:100–1.
73. Frank G, Sciarretta V, Calbucci F, Farneti G, Mazzatenta D, Pasquini E. The endoscopic transnasal transsphenoidal approach for the treatment of cranial base chordomas and chondrosarcomas. Oper Neurosurg. 2006;59:ONS-50–7.
74. Jho H-D, Carrau RL, McLaughlin ML, Somaza SC. Endoscopic transsphenoidal resection of a large chordoma in the posterior fossa. Neurosurg Focus. 1996;1:E5.
75. Jho H-D. Endoscopic transsphenoidal surgery. J Neuro-Oncol. 2001;54:187–95.
76. Cannizzaro D, Tropeano MP, Milani D, Spaggiari R, Zaed I, Mancarella C, Lasio GB, Fornari M, Servadei F, Cardia A. Microsurgical versus endoscopic trans-sphenoidal approaches for clivus chordoma: a pooled and meta-analysis. Neurosurg Rev. 2020; https://doi.org/10.1007/s10143-020-01318-y.
77. Zoli M, Milanese L, Bonfatti R, et al. Clival chordomas: considerations after 16 years of endoscopic endonasal surgery. J Neurosurg. 2018;128:329–38.
78. Syme WS, Cappell DF. A case of chordoma of the cervical vertebræ with involement of the pharynx. J Laryngol Otol. 1926;41:209–22.
79. Raul P, Diss A. Chordome malin de la colonne vertebrale lambaire. Bull la Soc Anat. 1924;94:395–402.
80. Cameron JAM. Case of sacro-coccygeal chordoma. Glasgow Med J. 1926;106:38–43.
81. Cappell DF. Chordoma of the vertebral column with three new cases. J Pathol Bacteriol. 1928;31:797–814.
82. Jones RB. Chordoma of the third lumbar vertebra simulating carcinoma of the prostate with vertebral metastasis. Report of a case. Br J Surg. 1960;48:162–5.
83. Rosenqvist H, Saltzman G-F. Sacrococcygeal and vertebral chordomas and their treatment. Acta Radiol. 1959;52:177–93.
84. Dahlin DC, Maccarty CS. Chordoma. A study of fifty-nine cases. Cancer. 1952;5:1170–8.
85. Azzarelli A, Quagliuolo V, Cerasoli S, Zucali R, Bignami P, Mazzaferro V, Dossena G, Gennari L. Chordoma: natural history and treatment results in 33 cases. J Surg Oncol. 1988;37:185–91.
86. Sundaresan N, Galicich JH, Chu FCH, Huvos AG. Spinal chordomas. J Neurosurg. 1979;50:312–9.

87. Stener B. Complete removal of vertebrae for extirpation of tumors. A 20-year experience. Clin Orthop Relat Res. 1989;245:72–82.
88. Eriksson B, Gunterberg B, Kindblom L-G. Chordoma: a clinicopathologic and prognostic study of a Swedish National Series. Acta Orthop Scand. 1981;52:49–58.
89. Sundaresan N, Huvos AG, Krol G, Lane JM, Brennan M. Surgical treatment of spinal chordomas. Arch Surg. 1987;122:1479–82.
90. Sundaresan N, Steinberger AA, Moore F, Sachdev VP, Krol G, Hough L, Kelliher K. Indications and results of combined anterior—posterior approaches for spine tumor surgery. J Neurosurg. 1996;85:438–46.
91. Heary RF, Vaccaro AR, Benevenia J, Cotler JM. "En-bloc" vertebrectomy in the mobile lumbar spine. Surg Neurol. 1998;50:548–56.
92. Bas T, Bas P, Prieto M, Ramose V, Bas JL, Espinosa C. A lumbar chordoma treated with a wide resection. Eur Spine J. 1994;3:115–7.
93. Boriani S, Bandiera S, Biagini R, Bacchini P, Boriani L, Cappuccio M, Chevalley F, Gasbarrini A, Picci P, Weinstein JN. Chordoma of the mobile spine: fifty years of experience. Spine (Phila Pa 1976). 2006;31:493–503.
94. Mixter CG, Mixter WJ. Surgical management of sacrococcygeal and vertebral chordoma. Arch Surg. 1940;41:408–21.
95. Shackelford RT, Rhode CM. Sacrococcygeal chordoma: its surgical treatment. Ann Surg. 1955;141:952–66.
96. Boriani S, Chevalley F, Weinstein JN, Biagini R, Campanacci L, De Iure F, Piccill P. Chordoma of the spine above the sacrum. Treatment and outcome in 21 cases. Spine. 1996;21:1569–77.
97. Fujiwara T, Tsuda Y, Stevenson J, Parry M, Jeys L. Sacral chordoma: do the width of surgical margin and the use of photon/proton radiotherapy affect local disease control? Int Orthop. 2020;44:381–9.
98. Colangeli S, Muratori F, Bettini L, et al. Surgical treatment of sacral chordoma: En bloc resection with negative margins is a determinant of the long-term outcome. Surg Technol Int. 2018;33:343–8.
99. Kaiser TE, Pritchard DJ, Unni KK. Clinicopathologic study of sacrococcygeal chordoma. Cancer. 1984;53:2574–8.
100. Pearlman AW, Friedman M. Radical radiation therapy of chordoma. Am J Roentgenol. 1970;108:333–41.
101. Enneking WF. A system of staging musculoskeletal neoplasms. Clin Orthop Relat Res. 1986;204:9–4.
102. Enneking WF, Spanier SS, Goodman MA. A system for the surgical staging of musculoskeletal sarcoma. Clin Orthop Relat Res. 1980;153:106–20.
103. Fuchs B, Dickey ID, Yaszemski MJ, Inwards CY, Sim FH. Operative management of sacral chordoma. J Bone Joint Surg Am. 2005;87:2211–6.
104. Radaelli S, Stacchiotti S, Ruggieri P, et al. Sacral chordoma: long-term outcome of a large series of patients surgically treated at two reference centers. Spine (Phila Pa 1976). 2016;41:1049–57.
105. Akiyama T, Ogura K, Gokita T, et al. Analysis of the infiltrative features of chordoma: the relationship between micro-skip metastasis and postoperative outcomes. Ann Surg Oncol. 2018;25:912–9.
106. van Wulfften Palthe ODR, Tromp I, Ferreira A, Fiore A, Bramer JAM, van Dijk NC, DeLaney TF, Schwab JH, Hornicek FJ. Sacral chordoma: a clinical review of 101 cases with 30-year experience in a single institution. Spine J. 2019;19:869–79.
107. Greenwald CM, Meaney TF, Hughes CR. Chordoma – uncommon destructive lesion of cerebrospinal axis. J Am Med Assoc. 1957;163:1240–4.
108. Wood EH, Himadi GM. Chordomas: a roentgenologic study of sixteen cases previously unreported. Radiology. 1950;54:706–16.
109. Kamrin RP, Potanos JN, Pool JL. An evaluation of the diagnosis and treatment of chordoma. J Neurol Neurosurg Psychiatry. 1964;27:157–65.

110. Tewfik HH, McGinnis WL, Nordstrom DG, Latourette HB. Chordoma. Evaluation of clinical behavior and treatment modalities. Int J Radiat Oncol. 1977;2:959–62.
111. Amendola BE, Amendola MA, Oliver E, McClatchey KD. Chordoma: role of radiation therapy. Radiology. 1986;158:839–43.
112. Reddy EK, Mansfield CM, Hartman GV. Chordoma. Int J Radiat Oncol. 1981;7:1709–11.
113. Suit HD, Goitein M, Munzenrider J, Verhey L, Davis KR, Koehler A, Linggood R, Ojemann RG. Definitive radiation therapy for chordoma and chondrosarcoma of base of skull and cervical spine. J Neurosurg. 1982;56:377–85.
114. Fagundes MA, Hug EB, Liebsch NJ, Daly W, Efird J, Munzenrider JE. Radiation therapy for chordomas of the base of skull and cervical spine: patterns of failure and outcome after relapse. Int J Radiat Oncol. 1995;33:579–84.
115. Castro JR, Linstadt DE, Bahary J-P, Petti PL, Daftari I, Collier JM, Gutin PH, Gauger G, Phillips TL. Experience in charged particle irradiation of tumors of the skull base: 1977–1992. Int J Radiat Oncol. 1994;29:647–55.
116. Hug EB, Loredo LN, Slater JDJM, Devries A, Grove RI, Schaefer RA, Rosenberg AE, Slater JDJM. Proton radiation therapy for chordomas and chondrosarcomas of the skull base. J Neurosurg. 1999;91:432–9.
117. Dial BL, Kerr DL, Lazarides AL, et al. The role of radiotherapy for chordoma patients managed with surgery. Spine (Phila Pa 1976). 2020;45:E742–51.
118. Rotondo RL, Folkert W, Liebsch NJ, et al. High-dose proton-based radiation therapy in the management of spine chordomas: outcomes and clinicopathological prognostic factors. J Neurosurg Spine. 2015;23:788–97.
119. Yasuda M, Bresson D, Chibbaro S, Cornelius JF, Polivka M, Feuvret L, Takayasu M, George B. Chordomas of the skull base and cervical spine: clinical outcomes associated with a multimodal surgical resection combined with proton-beam radiation in 40 patients. Neurosurg Rev. 2012;35:171–83.
120. Cavallo LM, Mazzatenta D, D'Avella E, et al. The management of clival chordomas: an Italian multicentric study. J Neurosurg. 2020;4:1–10.
121. Iannalfi A, D'Ippolito E, Riva G, et al. Proton and carbon ion radiotherapy in skull base chordomas: a prospective study based on a dual particle and a patient-customized treatment strategy. Neuro-Oncology. 2020;22:1348–58.
122. Demizu Y, Imai R, Kiyohara H, et al. Carbon ion radiotherapy for sacral chordoma: a retrospective nationwide multicentre study in Japan. Radiother Oncol. 2021;154:1–5.
123. Bostel T, Mattke M, Nicolay NH, Welzel T, Wollschläger D, Akbaba S, Mayer A, Sprave T, Debus J, Uhl M. High-dose carbon-ion based radiotherapy of primary and recurrent sacrococcygeal chordomas: long-term clinical results of a single particle therapy center. Radiat Oncol. 2020;15:206.
124. Uhl M, Welzel T, Jensen A, Ellerbrock M, Haberer T, Jäkel O, Herfarth K, Debus J. Carbon ion beam treatment in patients with primary and recurrent sacrococcygeal chordoma. Strahlentherapie und Onkol. 2015;191:597–603.
125. Imai R, Kamada T, Araki N, et al. Carbon ion radiation therapy for Unresectable sacral chordoma: an analysis of 188 cases. Int J Radiat Oncol. 2016;95:322–7.
126. Debus J, Schulz-Ertner D, Schad L, Essig M, Rhein B, Thillmann CO, Wannenmacher M. Stereotactic fractionated radiotherapy for chordomas and chondrosarcomas of the skull base. Int J Radiat Oncol. 2000;47:591–6.
127. Kondziolka D, Lunsford LD, Flickinger JC. The role of radiosurgery in the management of chordoma and chondrosarcoma of the cranial base. Neurosurgery. 1991;29:38.
128. Muthukumar N, Kondziolka D, Lunsford LD, Flickinger JC. Stereotactic radiosurgery for chordoma and chondrosarcoma: further experiences. Int J Radiat Oncol. 1998;41:387–92.
129. Tanaka T, Kobayashi T, Kida Y, Oyama H, Niwa M. The results of gamma knife radiosurgery for malignant skull base tumors. No Shinkei Geka. 1996;24:235–9.

130. Miller RC, Foote RL, Coffey RJ, Gorman DA, Earle JD, Schomberg PJ, Kline RW. The role of stereotactic radiosurgery in the treatment of malignant skull base tumors. Int J Radiat Oncol. 1997;39:977–81.
131. Kocher M, Voges J, Staar S, Treuer H, Sturm V, Mueller R-P. Linear accelerator radiosurgery for recurrent malignant tumors of the skull base. Am J Clin Oncol. 1998;21:18–22.
132. Stacchiotti S, Gronchi A, Fossati P, et al. Best practices for the management of local-regional recurrent chordoma: a position paper by the Chordoma Global Consensus Group. Ann Oncol. 2017;28:1230–42.
133. Stacchiotti S, Sommer J, Chordoma Global Consensus Group. Building a global consensus approach to chordoma: a position paper from the medical and patient community. Lancet Oncol. 2015;16:e71–83.
134. McSweeney AJ, Sholl PR. Metastatic chordoma. Use of mechlorethamine (nitrogen mustard) in chordoma therapy. AMA Arch Surg. 1959;79:152–5.
135. Rissanen PM, Holsti LR. Sacrococcygeal chordomas and their treatment. Radiol Clin Biol. 1967;36:153–64.
136. Pearlman AW, Singh RK, Hoppenstein R, Wilder J. Chordoma: combined therapy with radiation and surgery: case report and new operative approach. Bull Hosp Joint Dis. 1972;33:47–57.
137. Razis DV, Tsatsaronis A, Kyriazides I, Triantafyllou D. Chordoma of the cervical spine treated with vincristine sulfate. J Med. 1974;5:274–7.
138. Harwick RD, Miller AS. Craniocervical chordomas. Am J Surg. 1979;138:512–6.
139. Spratt JS, Martin AE, McKeown J. Sacral chordoma: a case study and review. J Surg Oncol. 1981;18:101–3.
140. Jacob HE. Chemotherapy for cranial base tumors. J Neuro-Oncol. 1994;20:327–35.
141. Passias PG, Pierce KE, Lafage V, et al. At what point should the thoracolumbar region be addressed in patients undergoing corrective cervical deformity surgery? Spine J. 2020;20:S2–3.
142. Smoll NR, Gautschi OP, Radovanovic I, Schaller K, Weber DC. Incidence and relative survival of chordomas: the standardized mortality ratio and the impact of chordomas on a population. Cancer. 2013;119:2029–37.
143. Zuckerman SL, Bilsky MH, Laufer I. Chordomas of the skull base, mobile spine, and sacrum: an epidemiologic investigation of presentation, treatment, and survival. World Neurosurg. 2018;113:e618–27.
144. McMaster ML, Goldstein AM, Bromley CM, Ishibe N, Parry DM. Chordoma: incidence and survival patterns in the United States, 1973–1995. Cancer Causes Control. 2001;12:1–11.
145. Kuo T-M, Mobley LR. How generalizable are the SEER registries to the cancer populations of the USA? Cancer Causes Control. 2016;27:1117–26.
146. Whelan J, McTiernan A, Cooper N, Wong YK, Francis M, Vernon S, Strauss SJ. Incidence and survival of malignant bone sarcomas in England 1979–2007. Int J Cancer. 2012;131:E508–17.
147. Hung G-Y, Horng J-L, Yen H-J, Yen C-C, Chen W-M, Chen PC-H, Wu H-TH, Chiou H-J. Incidence patterns of primary bone cancer in Taiwan (2003–2010): a population-based study. Ann Surg Oncol. 2014;21:2490–8.
148. Fisher CG, Goldschlager T, Boriani S, et al. An evidence-based medicine model for rare and often neglected neoplastic conditions. J Neurosurg Spine. 2014;21:704–10.
149. Dea N, Fisher CG, Reynolds JJ, et al. Current treatment strategy for newly diagnosed chordoma of the mobile spine and sacrum: results of an international survey. J Neurosurg Spine. 2019;30:119–25.
150. Radaelli S, Fossati P, Stacchiotti S, et al. The sacral chordoma margin. Eur J Surg Oncol. 2020;46:1415–22.
151. Malik AT, Alexander JH, Khan SN, Scharschmidt TJ. Is treatment at a high-volume center associated with an improved survival for primary malignant bone tumors? Clin Orthop Relat Res. 2020;478:631–42.

152. Ogura K, Yasunaga H, Horiguchi H, Ohe K, Shinoda Y, Tanaka S, Kawano H. Impact of hospital volume on postoperative complications and in-hospital mortality after musculoskeletal tumor surgery: analysis of a national administrative database. J Bone Joint Surg Am. 2013;95:1684–91.
153. Stiller CA, Trama A, Serraino D, Rossi S, Navarro C, Chirlaque MD, Casali PG, Group TRW. Descriptive epidemiology of sarcomas in Europe: report from the RARECARE project. Eur J Cancer. 2013;49:684–95.

# Clinical Work-Up, Diagnostic Imaging, and Biopsy

4

Daniel Ryan, John M. Gross, Zach Pennington, and Majid Khan

## Abbreviations

| | |
|---|---|
| ADC | Apparent diffusion coefficient |
| CK | Cytokeratin |
| CT | Computed tomography |
| EMA | Epithelial membrane antigen |
| MRI | Magnetic resonance imaging |
| MUC1 | Polymorphic epithelial mucin/Mucin 1 |
| S-100 | Low molecular weight protein soluble in 100% ammonium sulfate at neutral pH |
| SHH | Sonic hedgehog |

D. Ryan (✉)
Russel H. Morgan Department of Radiology and Radiological Science, Johns Hopkins Hospital, Baltimore, MD, USA
e-mail: dryan21@jhmi.edu

J. M. Gross
Department of Orthopaedic Pathology, Johns Hopkins Hospital, Baltimore, MD, USA

Z. Pennington
Department of Neurosurgery, Johns Hopkins University School of Medicine, Baltimore, MD, USA

M. Khan
Division of Nonvascular Interventional Neuroradiology, Thomas Jefferson University Hospital, Philadelphia, PA, USA



D. M. Sciubba, J. H. Schwab (eds.), *Chordoma of the Spine*,
https://doi.org/10.1007/978-3-030-76201-8_4

## Introduction

The notochord, a primitive cartilage-like rod of mesoderm, is crucial to the patterning and development of the vertebral column and neuraxis [1]. It is born from the dorsal organizer, a glycoprotein-rich structure within the blastopore that involutes at the onset of gastrulation to create the primitive gut (archenteron) and chordamesoderm [2–6]. The chordamesoderm cells subsequently differentiate and take on a notochordal phenotype, creating a rod of notochordal tissue running along the longitudinal axis of the embryo [3, 7, 8]. Consequently, notochord derivatives can appear anywhere along the axial skeleton, stretching from the dorsum sella to the coccyx.

## Notochord Location and Development as an Informant for Workup and Diagnosis

A brief consideration of the development of the notochord (described in depth in Chap. 1) helps to highlight those radiographic and histologic features that can aid in: (1) the diagnosis of notochordal lesions, and (2) the differentiation of notochordal tumors from other lesions of the axial skeleton.

The T-box (TBX) transcription factor T (TBXT) gene *brachyury* is often seen as a pathognomic marker of notochordal tumors [9]. In vitro and in vivo work has demonstrated that *brachyury*, along with a specific set of other tool-kit genes, is crucial to proper notochord development. Experiments in mice have demonstrated that selective deactivation of *brachyury* and other toolkit genes leads to in utero demise secondary to deficient mesoderm development. Additionally, single copy deletions appear to have a significant impact on axial skeletal patterning. Heterozygote mice are viable, but develop a short tail, leading to the name of this gene – brachyury [8].

After the formation of the neural tube, the mesoderm surrounding the notochord differentiates into sclerotomes and myotomes. The sclerotome differentiates into the osseocartilaginous portions of the vertebral column [10]. These tissues, specifically cartilage, share many radiographic and histologic features with notochordal tissue and notochordal tumors. This includes similar imaging characteristics as well as the expression of multiple shared genes, including aggrecan, Sox9, chondromodulin, and both types II and IX collagen. Nevertheless, several key histological distinctions are noted between cartilaginous and notochordal tissue. One of the most important is that chondrocytes secrete a water-rich extracellular matrix that contributes to the structure of cartilage. By contrast, notochordal cells produce a thick basement membrane sheath and have large intracellular vacuoles rich in hydrated materials. These vacuoles exert outward pressure on the thick basement membrane ensheathing the notochordal cells, giving structure to the tissue [2, 11–15].

The development of the notochord and surrounding mesoderm also provides insight into the localization of notochordal lesions versus other pathologies of the axial skeleton. At roughly 6 weeks gestation, several chondrification centers arise within the sclerotomes surrounding the neural tube that lies immediately dorsal to the notochord. Then beginning in the seventh gestational week, the sclerotomes expand and envelop the notochord; they then begin to undergo primary ossification, which ultimately gives rise to the vertebral bodies [16, 17].

As the sclerotomal tissues proliferate and develop, they displace the notochordal tissues, which begin to regress. Ultimately, the tissues undergo such extensive involution that the only notochordal remnants remaining in the postpartum human are small remnants comprising the nuclei pulposi of the intervertebral disks [18]. Failure of the aforementioned involution, which may occur secondary to mutations in the no tail (NTL) or doc (DOC) protein-coding genes, results in the persistence of chordamesodermic cells. These cells remain undifferentiated and persist as a notochordal rest [3, 19]. As a failure of differentiation can occur at any of several points along the developmental pathway, notochordal tumors exist along a continuum of differentiation ranging from the benign notochordal cell tumor (BNCT) to the malignant, undifferentiated chordoma [20, 21]. The latter, while rare (2–8% of all chordomas) [22], are associated with a particularly poor prognosis. Additionally, benign lesions have been reported to undergo degeneration into malignant chordoma [23], though this appears to be an exceptionally rare phenomenon.

## Differential Diagnosis of Chordoma

As alluded to in the prior section, the close proximity of the notochord to sclerotomal mesoderm in the developing embryo means that the differential diagnosis of chordoma includes other primary malignant bone tumors [22]. Additionally included within the differential are BNCTs, vertebral column metastases, and infectious or inflammatory processes, such as osteomyelitis.

Of the entities on the differential, BNCTs are the most difficult to differentiate from chordomas, owing to the common histological origin of these tissues. BNCTs, originally named *ecchordosis physaliphora* by Virchow [24], are thought to be far more common than their malignant counterparts. Based upon the skull base literature, it is suggested that BNCTs are present in nearly 2% of the population [25]. A cadaveric study by Yamaguchi et al. [26] however suggested that intraosseous BNCTs may be even more common than this though. In a series of 100 vertebral columns and 61 skull base samples, the authors found that 11.5% of clivus sample and 19% of vertebral column samples possess BNCTs; spinal lesions were most common in the sacrococcygeal (12%) and cervical regions (5%).

Given this proposed frequency, BNCTs are in many cases the primary alternative diagnosis in patients being worked up for chordoma. In many respects, BNCTs resemble chordoma radiographically; they generally are T1-hypointense, T2-hyperintense with subtle bony sclerosis surrounding the lesion [27, 28]. However, whereas chordomas may erode through cortical bone and into the epidural or paraspinal space, BNCTs (also known as notochordal hamartoma, or giant vertebral notochordal rest) are confined within the vertebral bodies (Fig. 4.1) [21].

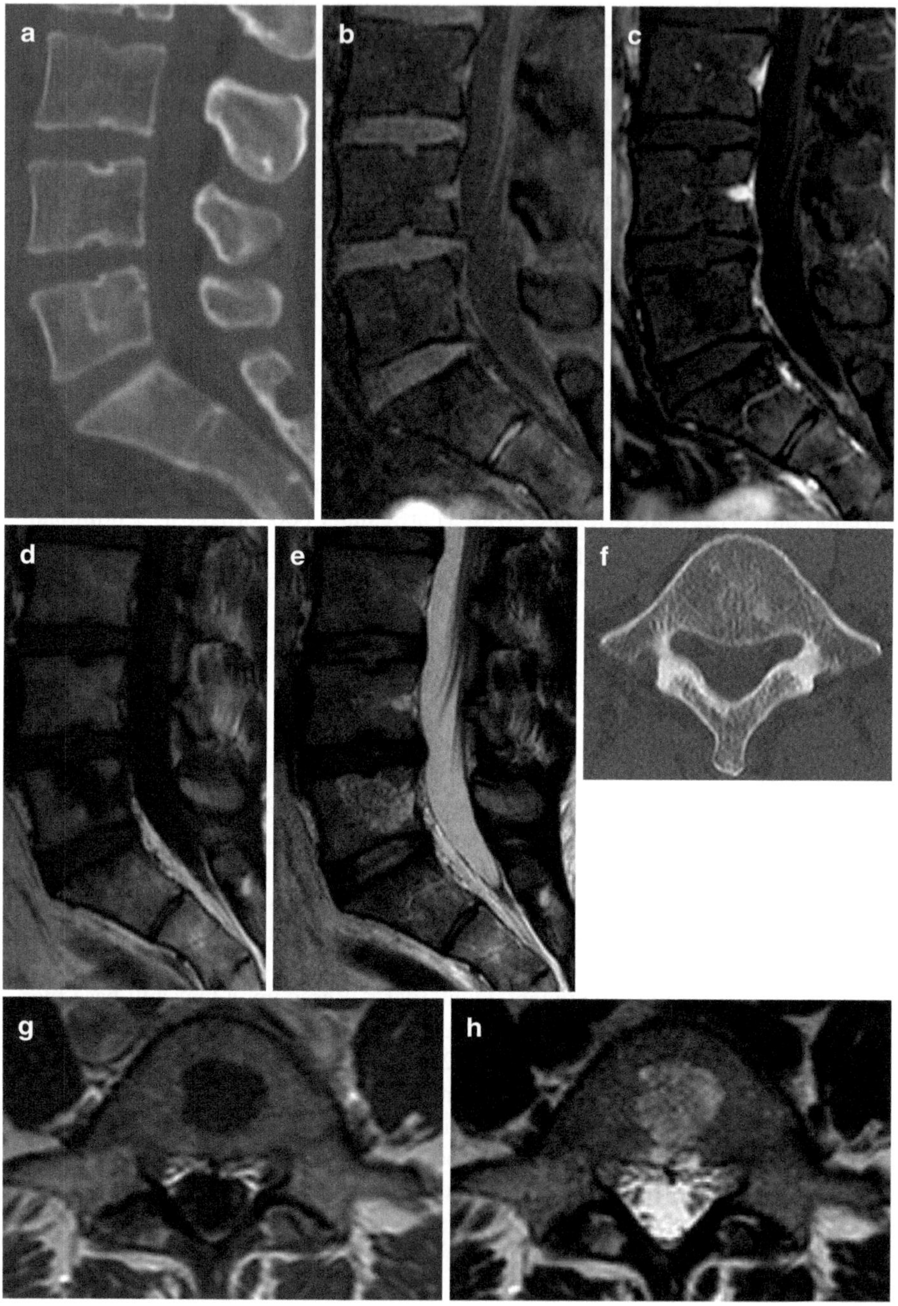


**Fig. 4.1** Giant vertebral notochordal rest or benign notochordal cell tumor. Computed tomographic images demonstrate sclerotic margins of a lesion that extends to the endplates but does not destroy the cortex of the vertebral body. On magnetic resonance images, there is no extra-osseous extension of the lesion or evidence of enhancement of the lesion, compatible with a notochordal rest

Additionally, BNCTs have a quiescent and indolent clinical course and consequently may remain asymptomatic and undetected for years. A recent series from Memorial Sloan Kettering including 13 patients with biopsy-proven BNCTs of the spine found that none of the lesions showed radiographic or symptomatic progression at a median radiographic follow-up of 21.6 months [21]. Based upon series such as this, the previous name for BNCTs – intraosseous chordomas – is now considered archaic and not reflective of the expected natural history of BNCTs [26].

Before discussing other items in the differential, we note that the above-described features of chordoma are for the conventional or classic subtype, which comprises the majority of cases. Chondroid and dedifferentiated lesions have unique histologic features [29, 30] that may lead them to have distinct imaging characteristics. Similar to chondrosarcomas, chondroid chordomas may have intralesional, granular calcification that are apparent on CT [31]. Additionally, some case reports have noted them to be isointense on T2-weighted imaging [32, 33], as compared to the hyperintense signal of most conventional (classic) chordoma. However, this is inconsistent and cannot be used as a means of differentiating the lesions [32]. Dedifferentiated lesions may similarly have low T2-weighted signal [34] with some authors suggesting that the transition from T2-hyperintense to T2-hypointense signal may indicate lesion dedifferentiation [35, 36]. For tumors with paraspinal extension, the soft tissue mass often demonstrates signal inhomogeneity secondary to internal necrosis or hemorrhage [37].

The second highest item on the differential of chordoma are non-chordoma primary neoplasms of the vertebral column, notably chondrosarcoma and osteosarcoma [38]. Chondrosarcomas can be particularly difficult to differentiate from chordoma, as they also have low-to-intermediate T1-weighted signal and high T2-weighted signal owing to the high water content of the hyaline cartilage [39, 40]. However, unlike chordoma, which arise from the vertebral bodies in most cases, chondrosarcomas are isolated to the posterior elements (40%) or involve both the body and posterior elements (45%) in the vast majority of cases [39]. Lesions also commonly have areas of calcification that can be visualized on computed tomography (CT). Chondrosarcomas additionally demonstrate ring and arc enhancement on gadolinium contrast-enhanced MRI sequences, whereas chordomas more commonly demonstrate heterogeneous enhancement [39]. Ring-and-arc enhancement is seen in some chordomas though, notably in the phenotypically similar chondroid chordoma [29], preventing CT imaging from being used for definitive diagnosis. Finally, more recent work from the skull base literature suggests that diffusion-weighted imaging (DWI) may be useful in distinguishing chordomas and chondrosarcomas. In a study of 19 pathologically confirmed skull base lesions, Yeom et al. [34] found that chondrosarcomas had significantly higher apparent diffusion coefficient (ADC) values when compared to classical chordoma ($2051 \pm 261 \times 10^{-6}$ mm$^2$/s vs $1474 \pm 117 \times 10^{-6}$ mm$^2$/s) and dedifferentiated chordoma ($2051 \pm 261 \times 10^{-6}$ mm$^2$/s vs $875 \pm 100 \times 10^{-6}$ mm$^2$/s). The authors argued that this difference is likely due to the mucoid/myxoid stroma of chordomas, which likely limits extracellular free water motion relative to that seen in chondrosarcomas. Additionally, they noted that the use of ADC for differentiation of chordoma from chondrosarcoma is impractical for lesions with intratumoral hemorrhage, which they observed in 10% of their identified samples.

The other two most common primary vertebral column malignancies – osteosarcoma and Ewing sarcoma [41] – share fewer radiographic features with chordoma. Osteosarcomas are more common in the thoracolumbar spine and arise from the posterior elements in nearly 80% of cases [39]. They similarly show matrix mineralization on CT in the majority of cases (≈80%) and generally have intermediate signal on both T1- and T2-weighted sequences. Ewing sarcomas are generally easiest to distinguish based upon patient age. Unlike the other primary vertebral column malignancies, Ewing sarcomas have a median onset in the second or third decade of life [42, 43]. Like chondrosarcomas and osteosarcomas, they most commonly affect the posterior elements (60% of cases in the mobile spine). In the sacrum, they most commonly involve the alae (69%) and seldom involve multiple levels [39]. Lesions are highly lytic and generally demonstrate isointense signal on T1-weighted imaging and hyperintense signal on T2-weighted imaging [38]. A review by Rodallec et al. [39] provides a good overview of the imaging characteristics of the various types of benign and malignant vertebral column tumors.

Metastatic lesions are uncommon in the sacral spine, accounting for only 5% of cases in large series [44]. The imaging characteristics of these lesions are variable and depend upon the primary pathology. However, progressive osteolysis of the involved segment is common. Clinical history can be very informative for these lesions, as the metastatic disease is far more common in patients with a known history of malignancy. Clinical history is similarly useful in distinguishing infectious or inflammatory processes from primary vertebral column lesions. A known history of immunosuppression, prior corticosteroid use, prior surgery at the affected level, renal failure, septicemia, foreign body retention, and intravenous drug use are risk factors for vertebral osteomyelitis [45, 46]. Imaging of spondylodiskitis also commonly demonstrates multilevel involvement with the infective process bridging and obliterating the intervening disk spaces [47, 48]. By comparison, malignancies generally respect disk spaces [39]. Therefore, absent a clinical history of risk factors for vertebral column infection or imaging features suggestive of infection, this item in the differential can generally be eliminated.

## Clinical Workup

Diagnostic workup for a lesion suspicious for chordoma should include an evaluation of the patient's clinical symptoms, biopsy to provide definitive pathological diagnosis, and radiographic staging to assess the potential merits of surgical intervention. As highlighted in Chap. 3, chordomas are exceptionally rare lesions (0.08–0.5 per 100,000 persons) [49]. Based upon data from the Surveillance Epidemiology and End Results database of the National Cancer Institute, suspicion should be highest in whites (83–93% of all cases), males (54–62% of all cases), and patients in the fifth decade of life or beyond. Patients with skull base lesions tend to present at a younger age, potentially due to the small anatomic space in which the lesion is able to grow prior to producing clinical symptoms. At all loci, however, symptom is usually quite gradual given the slow-growing nature of chordoma. In many cases, patients will present with axial pain that has been progressive over months to years. For lesions of the spinal column and sacrum, the mean duration of symptoms prior to presentation has been reported between 4 and 24 months [50, 51].

## Lesions of the Skull Base and Craniocervical Junction

Intracranial chordomas – most commonly arising from the clivus – demonstrate the greatest propensity for significant morbidity and mortality, which occurs secondary to compression of the brainstem and exiting cranial nerves [52]. In these lesions, the most common presenting symptoms include diplopia and occipital or retro-orbital headache. Diplopia is generally secondary due to dysfunction of the abducens nerves, which have the longest intracranial course and run dorsally along the clivus. This is frequently localized to Dorello's canal, as infiltration of clival chordomas between the periosteal and parietal dural layers can result in basilar venous plexus compression and a local compartment syndrome of Dorello's canal [53]. Headaches are thought to occur secondary to distention of the meninges and/or alteration of the cerebrospinal fluid flow dynamics [54].

Other common neuropathies include palsies of the third and fourth nerves, which occur secondary to cavernous sinus invasion [55]. Cavernous sinus invasion is more common for chondrosarcomas [33]. These lesions arise from the petroclival synchondrosis and are typically eccentrically located, whereas chordomas generally arise from the midline (Fig. 4.2) [56].

Dorsal expansion of clival chordomas can directly compress the brainstem, which may present as a combination of gait ataxia, hemiparesis, and dysphagia. Progressive dorsal expansion may also lead to intradural extension in up to 50% of cases, [53] theoretically seeding the subarachnoid space and limiting the ability to achieve long-term disease-free survival. Ventral lesion extension through the sphenoid sinus may result in nasal obstruction and ventrolateral expansion may lead to eustachian tube occlusion [53]. Consequently, preoperative evaluation should include examination of the nasopharynx and a thorough neurological examination that includes cranial nerve testing, gait testing, and evaluation of the motor and sensory function of the extremities. Question about bowel and bladder dysfunction (e.g., urinary incontinence) should also be considered.

## Mobile Spine Lesions

As with lesions of the skull base, pain and neurological dysfunction secondary to mass effect are the two primary presenting features of mobile spine lesions. Early in the disease course, patients are likely asymptomatic, which can be used to explain the often large size of mobile spine chordomas at presentation [57]. As the lesion erodes through the overlying cortex, it distends the overlying periosteum. This

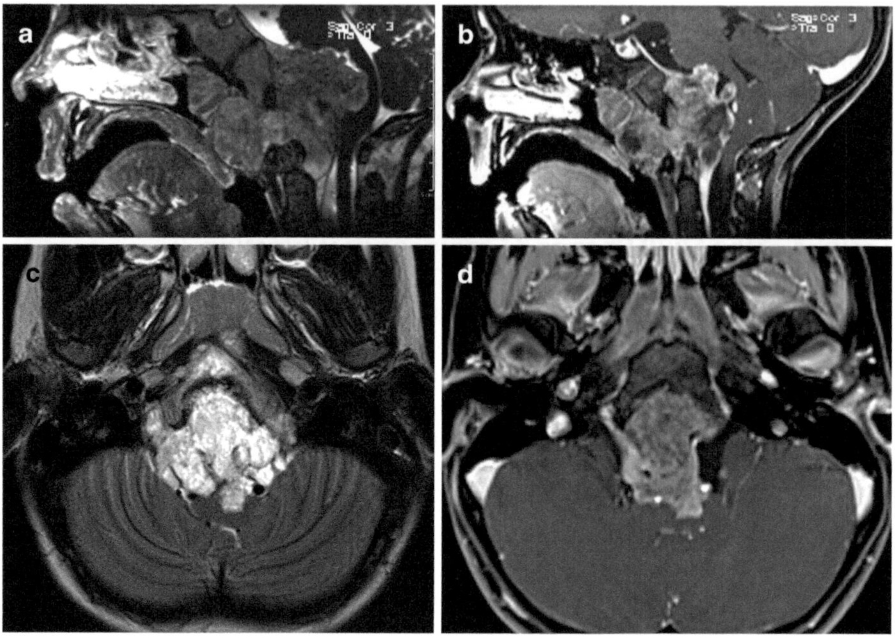

**Fig. 4.2** Clival chordoma. Magnetic resonance images demonstrate a T2-hyperintense multiseptated mass with honeycomb-like enhancement when erodes through and remodels the clivus extending into the nasopharynx

stretching activates nociceptive fiber afferents [58] innervating the periosteum, leading to oncologic pain that is generally localizable to the level of the lesion. Further expansion and compromise of the cortical bone can destabilize the spinal column, causing mechanical axial and/or radicular back pain. Extension posterior into the foramina and epidural space results in compression of the neural elements, which may present as radicular pain, motor or sensory dysfunction, gait impairment, or bowel/bladder dysfunction [50]. The epidural tumor component may allow the tumor to secondarily involve adjacent vertebral levels while sparing the intervertebral disk [59]. Alternatively, this secondary involvement may be mediated by extension of the lesion anterior and laterally into the paraspinal space. Such extension is common [59].

Given these growth characteristics, it is clear that the clinical presentation will be dictated by the level of lesion origination. For all patients, workup should include an assessment of the motor and sensory function of the lower extremities, along with interrogation of gait, and questions about bowel and bladder dysfunction. For patients with lesions arising in the cervical spine (Fig. 4.3) and cervicothoracic junction, the examination should also include motor and sensory testing of the upper extremities. Patients with these upper spine lesions seem more likely to have neurological deficits at the time of presentation, as: (1) there is relatively less space in the spinal canal relative to the diameter of the cord at this level result, and (2) the

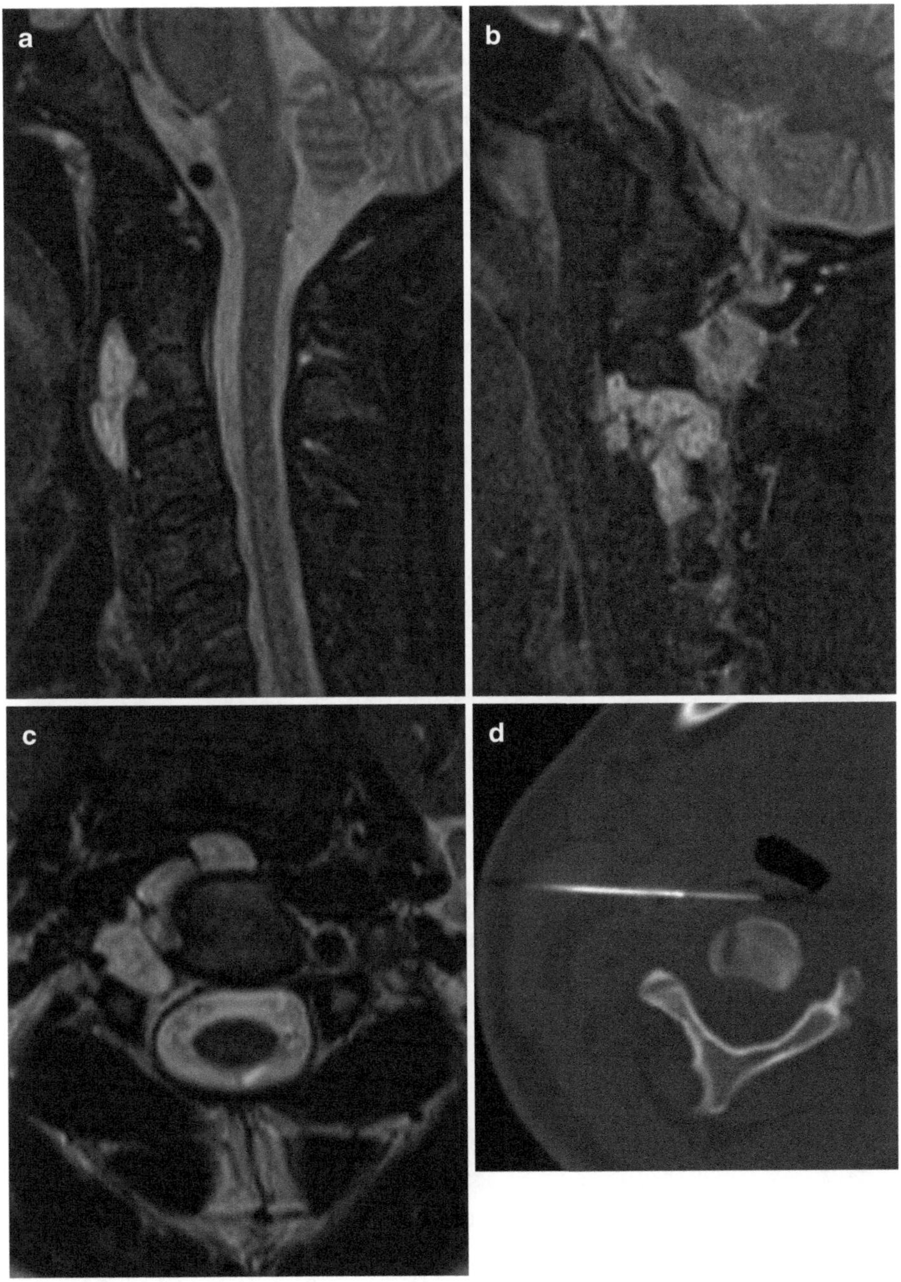

**Fig. 4.3** Cervical chordoma. Magnetic resonance images demonstrate a small amount of scalloping of the right lateral portion of the C2 vertebral body with a right anterolateral extraosseous soft tissue component demonstrating a multilobulated multiseptated appearance

vertebral bodies are smaller and therefore are capable of accommodating less neoplastic growth prior to the invasion of the epidural space [50]. Though a thorough neurological examination may include assessment of the upper extremities for lesions of the thoracic (Fig. 4.4) or lumbar spine (Fig. 4.5), this is not routinely necessary as such deficits are not localizable to the lesion.

## Sacrococcygeal Lesions

Owing to the relatively capacious spinal canal and minimal contribution of the sacral roots to lower extremity function, sacrococcygeal lesions are generally able

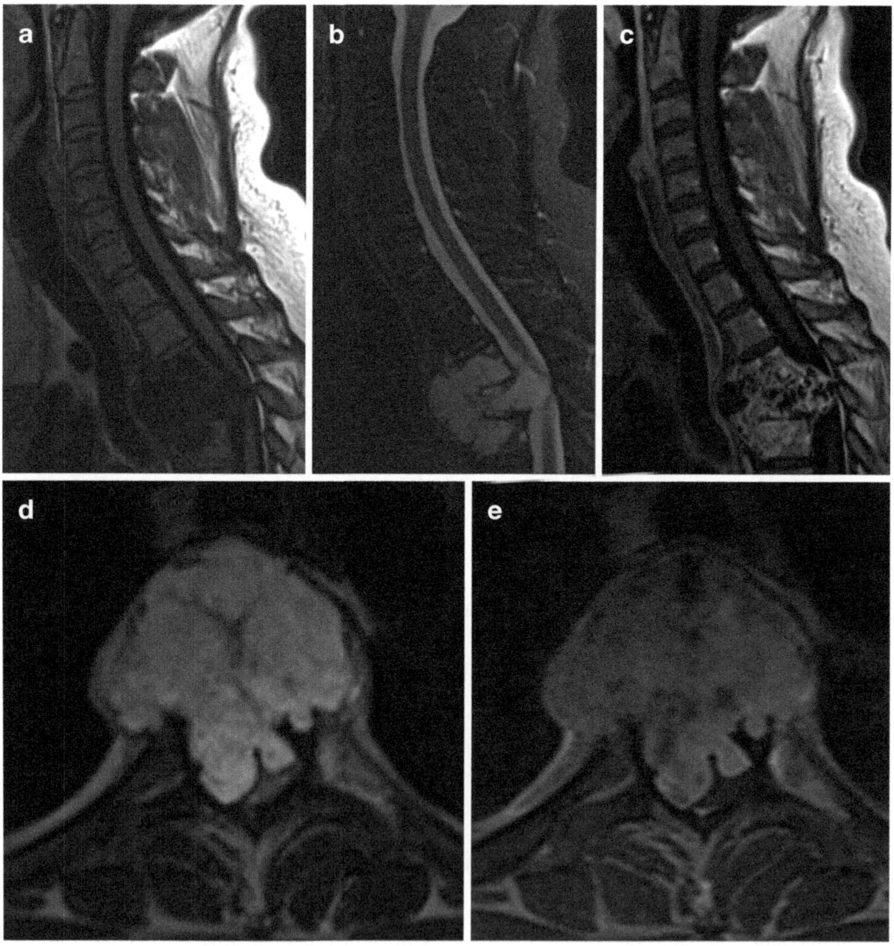


**Fig. 4.4** Thoracic chordoma. Magnetic resonance images demonstrate a multilobulated multiseptated mass which replaces the vertebral body and extends into the surrounding spinal canal and paraspinal soft tissues

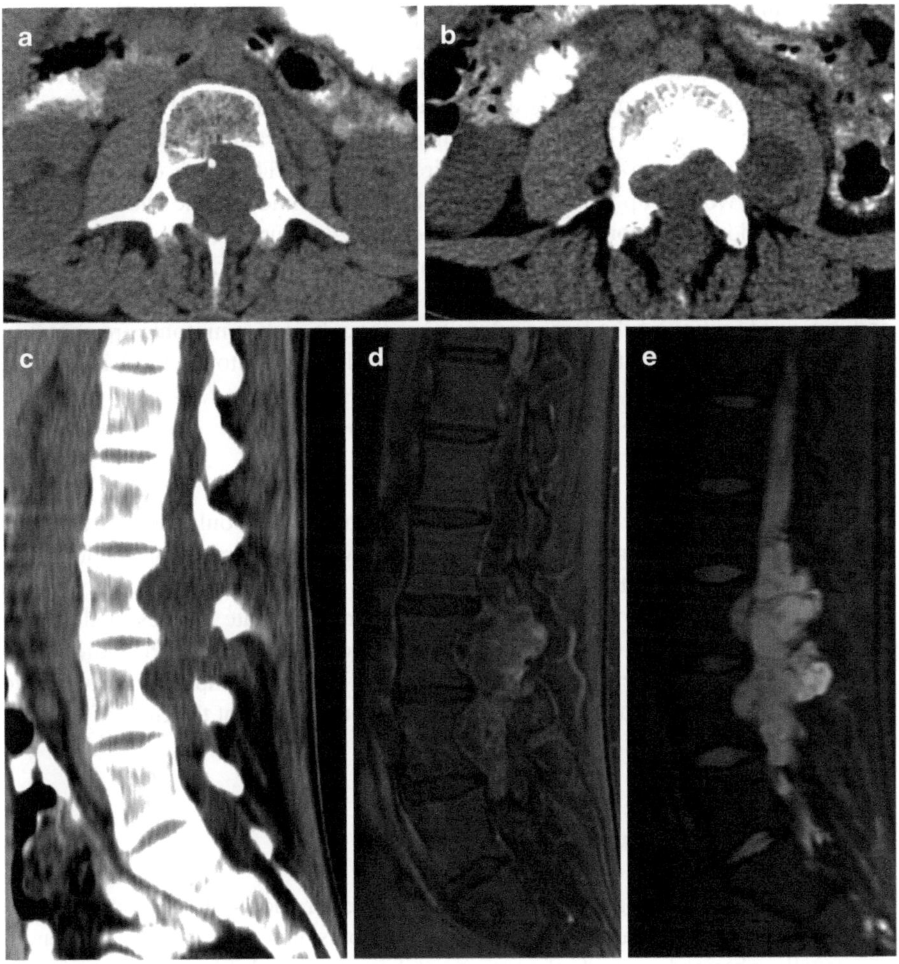


**Fig. 4.5** Lumbar chordoma. Computed tomographic images demonstrate a relatively small amount of posterior scalloping of the vertebral body which could be radiographically occult in earlier stages. Additionally, the included images demonstrate a bulky epidural component of the mass which contributes a significant mass effect upon the thecal sac, impinging the cauda equina. Magnetic resonance images demonstrate the honeycomb-like enhancement with a multiseptated T2-hyperintense soft tissue lesion extending into the spinal canal

to grow the largest prior to presenting clinically [60, 61]. The most common presenting symptom for lesions at this level is low back pain, with a large multi-institutional series finding that tumor-associated pain was present in 96% of patients at presentation [62]. Neurological symptoms are significantly less common, though 1/4–1/3 of patients may have signs of lumbosacral trunk compression at baseline [62]. Bowel and bladder symptoms are also common, with 1/3 presenting with urinary tract symptoms, and 10–27% presenting with cauda equina syndrome [29, 61, 62].

Large tumors may also expand into the pelvis and secondarily involve the rectum, bladder, or presacral neurovascular structures. This may result in constipation, urinary frequency, tenesmus, or feelings of pelvic fullness. True invasion of the presacral viscera is uncommon though, as the sacral periosteum and presacral fascia serve as an anatomic barrier [63]. Large masses with dorsal extension may be palpable and/or cause pain with sitting or direct pressure. Thorough examination of patients being worked up for sacrococcygeal lesions should include questions about bowel or bladder symptoms (e.g., incontinence, tenesmus, constipation), perineal anesthesia, and mechanical sacropelvic pain (which could identify the need for post-resection stabilization). Examination should include evaluation of the motor and sensory function of the lower extremities, though such symptoms are common only with the superior extension of sacrococcygeal lesions into the lumbar spine.

## Diagnostic Imaging

While chordomas may be discovered incidentally, most commonly they are detected as part of a workup for one of the symptoms outlined in the preceding section [29]. Plain radiographs are seldom employed and are of minimal clinical utility in the diagnosis of chordomas, which only infrequently demonstrate intralesional calcification. Rather, CT scans and MRI are of the greatest utility. However, radiographs may play a role in surgical planning for lesions of the mobile spine and sacrum to help establish the need for concomitant deformity correction at the time of surgical resection [64].

### MRI Characteristics and Use

MRI is generally the imaging of modality of choice for chordoma. As most patients present with refractory pain or neurological symptoms, non-contrast MRI sequences are usually obtained as part of routine workup. Standard T1- and T2-weighted sequences will highlight the tumor pseudocapsule, the presence of cortical bone compromise, the presence of paraspinal soft tissue expansion, and the presence of epidural extension. T2-weighted sequences additionally facilitate the identification of dural transgression [33]. Lesions generally have low-to-intermediate signal on T1-weighted imaging and high signal on T2-weighted imaging [29], with the exceptions noted in the previous sections for chondroid and dedifferentiated chordoma. In the minority of cases, skull base lesions may have high signal intensity on T1-weighted sequences secondary to high protein content within their myxoid matrix [65].

Once the lesion is recognized, contrast-enhanced sequences should be acquired to characterize the lesion and outline the soft tissue extension [37]. Contrast-enhanced sequences generally demonstrate a heterogeneous honeycomb-like pattern of enhancement on venous phase T1-weighted post-contrast sequences, reflecting the intratumoral fibrous septations and pseudocapsule [37]. Some investigators have suggested that greater homogeneity of enhancement of these lesions is associated with a poorer prognosis [66]. Contrast-enhanced sequences may also help to identify locoregional metastases, though systemic imaging, e.g., PET/CT, is generally preferred as it also allows for oncological staging. Diffusion-weighted imaging may also be obtained to aid in the differentiation of chordoma from chondrosarcoma, as the latter have significantly higher ADCs [34]. By contrast, dedifferentiated chordomas have the lowest ADC values. Given this, low ADC values may indicate a more aggressive or dedifferentiated lesion as low ADC values are known to correlate well with increased tumor cellularity [67]. However, the evidence supporting DWI use in diagnosis is limited and does not eliminate the need for biopsy to achieve a definitive diagnosis. Susceptibility-weighted imaging (SWI) may also be obtained, but this is not routinely done as it does not eliminate the need for biopsy. If obtained though, SWI may show intralesional hypointensity consistent with hemorrhage; this is most common in larger chordomas [37].

For skull base lesions, T2-weighted imaging can be used to aid in the assessment of dural transgression. If there is dural involvement, then the affected dura must be resected to achieve oncologic resection. This may be associated with high or unacceptable neurological morbidity though, depending upon the proximity of the tumor and affected dura to the cranial nerves. High-resolution sequences, such as constructive interference in steady state (CISS) or fast imaging employing steady-state acquisition cycled phases (FIESTA-C) sequences, can be added to the imaging protocol where there is a concern for cranial nerve involvement. These high-resolution anatomic sequences help to effectively delineate the courses of the cranial nerves [68] and to identify any potential involvement by the tumor [33]. Magnetic resonance angiogram may also be considered for lesions of the skull base and cervical spine to map the courses of the carotid and vertebral arteries. Involvement of these structures by the tumor may necessitate the sacrifice of these vascular structures [69]; vessel imaging therefore helps the treating surgeon determine whether this is feasible. Conventional angiography or CT angiography are potential alternatives.

For mobile spine and sacral lesions, a basic battery of non-contrast-enhanced T1-weighted and T2-weighted images, along with a post-contrast fat-suppressed T1-weighted sequence, is generally adequate for preoperative evaluation. Of note, sacral lesions, it has been suggested that MRI may play a role in prognostication. In a series of 41 patients who underwent *en bloc* resection of sacral chordoma, Zuckerman et al. [70] found that extension into the subcutaneous fat was independently predictive of poorer overall survival. These data are limited, but nevertheless merit further investigation in an attempt to improve individualized patient counseling.

## CT Characteristics and Use

Computed tomography is also considered to be a standard part of the preoperative evaluation of chordoma. High-resolution CT can help to delineate the extent of vertebral column or sacral bone compromise and assist with osteotomy planning.

CT also helps to demonstrate intratumoral calcifications, which have been shown in up to 90% of sacrococcygeal lesions [71] and 30% of mobile spine lesions [72]. Said calcifications are reported as predominately localizing to the periphery of the lesion [72]. They may adopt either the ring-and-arc appearance that is classical in chondrosarcoma, or they can present as randomly arranged punctate foci. Because of this, while the pattern of calcification on CT may favor chondrosarcoma or chordoma, it cannot distinguish between the two lesions. For skull base lesions, contrast-enhanced CT volumes are useful for evaluating the involvement of the intracranial vasculature. CT with thin cuts can also aid the assessment of tumor invasion through the anterior clivus into the posterior pharynx or the sphenoid sinus.

For sacral lesions, CT helps to evaluate the involvement of the sacroiliac joints [72, 73]. Destabilization of the SI joints is used as an indication for intraoperative reconstruction of the pelvic ring. Standard axial cuts may be adequate for assessing SI joint involvement. However, we also regularly obtain coronal oblique cuts, which can further aid in assessing the degree of SI joint compromise. Additionally, oblique cuts are useful for assessing the involvement of the ventral neural foramina.

## Nuclear Imaging for Staging Purposes

Metastatic spread from chordoma is relatively uncommon. Nevertheless, it is not so uncommon to eliminate the utility of staging imaging. For example, a recent bi-institutional series pooling patients from the Massachusetts General Hospital and University of Miami [74] found that roughly 18% of patients developed metastatic spread at a median of 130 months. Spread was most common for thoracic lesions (31%) though rates appeared statistically similar for lesions of the mobile spine and sacrum. The most common site of metastasis was the lungs (54% of metastases), though metastatic spread to the distal bone (21%), soft tissue (15%), and liver (8%) were also relatively common. Based upon the results of this series, staging appears most important for young patients, as they found that rates of metastatic spread were highest in those under 24 years of age at diagnosis. Younger patients are also likely the best surgical candidates ceteris paribus due to the absence of medical comorbidities. The combination of the nontrivial rate of metastatic spread along with the disproportionate burden of metastatic spread within the best surgical patients underlies the importance of obtaining radiographic staging in all potential surgical candidates.

In addition to determining surgical candidacy, radiographic evaluation for metastatic spread is important for survival prognostication. Those with metastatic spread have significantly poorer overall survival than those with isolated disease [74]. Multiple strategies can be employed for radiographic staging, including bone scintigraphy, CT with windows of the chest, abdomen, and pelvis, and PET/CT. However, our preferred strategy is to stage with PET/CT. As a rule, we generally avoid $^{99m}$Tc bone scintigraphy. While $^{99m}$Tc scintigraphy can be used to look for osseous metastatic spread, it is prone to high false-positive rates. Herzog and colleagues [75] recently reported a series of 32 patients treated for biopsy-proven vertebral chordoma at the Mayo Clinic. They found that five of these patients had potentially metastatic foci with increased $^{99m}$Tc-MDP uptake concerning for metastatic spread. Follow-up imaging demonstrated all potential metastases to be consistent with a benign etiology. Additionally, they found there to be no association between $^{99m}$Tc-MDP uptake and lesion size or pattern of osseous involvement. This is consistent with prior examinations of sacral chordoma, which have reported varying levels of radiotracer uptake [71, 76, 77], suggesting that $^{99m}$Tc-MDP bone scintigraphy may be of limited utility of chordoma.

For these reasons, we prefer to stage with PET/CT images. This is consistent with the strategy employed by others [78]. Multiple radiotracers have been described, including the ubiquitous [18], FDG-PET/CT [79, 80], and the less commonly employed $^{68}$Ga-DOTA-TATE PET/CT technique. Derlin et al. [81] found both to demonstrate increased uptake in a patient treated for a previously resected metastatic sacral chordoma. They argued that given the nature of 68Ga-DOTA-TATE as a somatostatin receptor agonist, it may provide additional utility by identifying a druggable target in patients with metastatic chordoma. Nevertheless, the support for this is minimal outside of the primitive neuroendocrine tumor literature. Another strategy, employed by Cheney and colleagues at the Massachusetts General Hospital, employs $^{18}$F-fluoromisonidazole (FMISO) PET/CT. The FMISO-PET/CT technique allows teams to identify targetable hypoxic subvolumes within chordomas [82]. This may improve radiotherapy planning in both surgical and nonsurgical patients, particularly in patients at high risk for local recurrence. A second group in France has espoused a similar strategy for skull base lesions [83]. Additionally, they note that [18]FDG-PET/CT signal and FMISO-PET/CT signal do not correlate and so FMISO-PET/CT may facilitate superior boosted volume definition during radiotherapy planning.

## Biopsy

Despite the various radiographic properties proposed to help distinguish chordoma from other lesions of the axial skeleton, definitive diagnosis relies upon biopsy and pathologic confirmation. The first stage in biopsy involves choosing a path for which sensitive structures are least likely to be injured in the process of obtaining core and fine needle specimens [84]. This frequently involves traversing the least amount of tissue possible as well as avoiding structures likely to cause significant disability as a result of their violation. Planning, therefore, relies on a thorough review of cross-sectional imaging obtained prior to biopsy [85]. The choice to extend one's biopsy tract through an osseous channel, such as the pedicle, largely depends upon the extent of tumoral posterolateral expansion [86]. If a soft tissue trajectory is possible with a relatively low chance of injury to adjacent or deep vital structures, CT-guided paraspinal posterolateral or transcostovertebral soft tissue biopsy is recommended [87]. If the lesion is relatively confined to the vertebral body with little extra-canalicular, extra-osseous extension, then either biplanar fluoroscopic or computed of tissue possible as well as avoiding structures likely to cause significant disability as a tomographic guidance may be useful to direct a biopsy cannula through the bone to the level of the neoplasm [88]. Through either approach, the selection of an appropriately sized cannulas and needles in both length and width should precede the sample gathering [89]. Additionally, regardless of lesion location or approach, biopsy should be done with a core needle [90, 91], as fine needle aspiration has lower diagnostic accuracy [92–94].

Frequently, a vertebral transpedicular approach is warranted [95]. To avoid seeding the bone with skin flora or other pathogens, a strict sterile technique must be observed. This includes observing aseptic precautions, donning sterile gloves and gown, employing multiple concentric applications of an iodine-based cleaning solution at the planned skin entry site (which should be allowed to dry), and then extending drapes beyond the region of cleaned skin to maximize the size of the sterile field [96]. After this process and safety checks, a local anesthetic is injected at both the level of the skin and periosteum. The remainder of the procedure is similar to the placement of percutaneous screws. First, a skin incision is created at the planned entry point. A guide pin is then advanced through the paraspinal muscles to the level of the bone [88]. The pin is driven 1.5–2 cm into the vertebral body [97]. The ideal entry point for biopsy is similar to that for a pedicle screw – the junction of the midportion of the facet and the mid-transverse process. Once the guide pin is docked, a sleeve is advanced over it and docked on the pedicle entry point. A bone-cutting biopsy needle is then advanced over the guide pin and through the sleeve. A mallet is then used to gently advance the cannula through the pedicle [98]. This biopsy cannula is then advanced under CT-based navigation or fluoroscopic guidance until it has entered the lesion within the vertebral body. When fluoroscopy is used, repeated pulses should be acquired during cannula passing to confirm positioning [88]. After penetrating the lesion, the needle is rotated in an alternating clockwise and counterclockwise fashion to free sample tissue from the surrounding tissue. A syringe is then connected to the proximal end of the needle to apply suction while the cannula is withdrawn [88]. The specimens are then submitted for histologic evaluation through cell smear and cell block [99]. Of note, the biopsy tract should lie within the planned surgical incision site, as chordoma may seed along the biopsy site; transrectal biopsy of sacral lesions is to be avoided despite the shorter anatomic path [38].

Histology specimens should demonstrate lobulated grey-to-dark colored tissue. The tumor is overall soft in consistency, but can have firm and grainy regions due to fibrous septations and intratumoral calcification. The latter is more common in chondrosarcoma though [53]. Even with the best planning and technique, the overall diagnostic accuracy of percutaneous biopsy is highly variable, with rates between 61% and 100% [100].

Microscopically, samples will show a highly cellular lesion composed of typical physaliphorous cells with a "bubbly" or vacuolated cytoplasm and round nuclei, surrounded by a myxoid supportive cytoarchitecture upon light microscopy [101]. Pleomorphism, bi- or multinucleation, mitotic figures, and nuclear inclusions of the physaliphorous cells are indicative of de-differentiation [99]. Characteristically, these tumors' cell blocks immunohistologically stain positive for S-100, epithelial membrane antigen (EMA) or polymorphic epithelial mucin/Mucin 1 (MUC1), cytokeratins (with the monoclonal antibody CAM5.2 reacting with CK8, CK18, CK19 and the monoclonal antibody AE1/AE3 reacting with CKs 1–8, CK10, CKs 14–16, and CK19), and vimentin [102, 103]. Additionally, genetic analysis reveals an abnormal karyotype in approximately 29% of newly diagnosed chordomas, 69% of recurrent chordoma cases. Lesions almost uniformly stain positive for brachyury, a developmental transcription factor which has a high sensitivity and specificity for chordoma [29]. The aforementioned biomarkers, especially the cytokeratins and EMA positivity, help to distinguish chordoma from low-grade chondrosarcoma, which may otherwise be histologically and radiologically indistinguishable [53]. However, it should be noted that dedifferentiated subvarieties of chordoma often lose expression of cytokeratins, which may make histological differentiation from chondrosarcoma difficult [101].

## Conclusion

Radiographic and histological evaluation of chordoma is crucial to both diagnosis and prognostication. MRI and CT are considered standard aspects of radiographic workup and are used to define the lesion anatomy, assess the amenability of the lesion to surgical resection, and facilitate surgical planning. Nuclear imaging studies, notably PET/CT, are employed for oncologic staging, which dictates the patient's surgical candidacy. Despite previous descriptions of unique imaging characteristics of chordoma, as of present no pathognomonic radiographic signs have been identified. Consequently, the biopsy is considered standard of care for diagnosis, with core needle biopsy being preferred. Information gleaned from the histological analysis may have prognostic value and, in the future, may play a role in individualized systemic therapy.

## References


1. Ramesh T, Nagula SV, Tardieu GG, et al. Update on the notochord including its embryology, molecular development, and pathology: a primer for the clinician. Cureus. 2017;9(4):e1137.
2. Stemple DL. Structure and function of the notochord: an essential organ for chordate development. Development. 2005;132(11):2503–12.
3. Corallo D, Trapani V, Bonaldo P. The notochord: structure and functions. Cell Mol Life Sci. 2015;72(16):2989–3008.
4. Borycki A-G, Mendham L, Emerson CP. Control of somite patterning by Sonic hedgehog and its downstream signal response genes. Development. 1998;125(4):777–90.
5. Yüksel KZ, Adams MS, Chamberlain RH, et al. Pullout resistance of thoracic extrapedicular screws used as a salvage procedure. Spine J. 2007;7(3):286–91.
6. Choi K-S, Lee C, Harfe BD. Sonic hedgehog in the notochord is sufficient for patterning of the intervertebral discs. Mech Dev. 2012;129(9–12):255–62.
7. de Bree K, de Bakker BS, Oostra R-J. The development of the human notochord. Klymkowsky M, ed. PLoS One. 2018;13(10):e0205752.
8. Satoh N, Tagawa K, Takahashi H. How was the notochord born? Evol Dev. 2012;14(1):56–75.

9. Chen M, Wu Y, Zhang H, Li S, Zhou J, Shen J. The roles of embryonic transcription factor brachyury in tumorigenesis and progression. Front Oncol. 2020;10:961.
10. Stern CD, Keynes RJ. Interactions between somite cells: the formation and maintenance of segment boundaries in the chick embryo. Development. 1987;99(2):261–72.
11. Domowicz M, Li H, Hennig A, Henry J, Vertel BM, Schwartz NB. The biochemically and immunologically distinct CSPG of notochord is a product of the aggrecan gene. Dev Biol. 1995;171(2):655–64.
12. Sachdev SW, Dietz UH, Oshima Y, et al. Sequence analysis of zebrafish chondromodulin-1 and expression profile in the notochord and chondrogenic regions during cartilage morphogenesis. Mech Dev. 2001;105(1–2):157–62.
13. Knudson CB, Knudson W. Cartilage proteoglycans. Semin Cell Dev Biol. 2001;12(2):69–78.
14. Koehl MAR, Quillin KJ, Pell CA. Mechanical design of fiber-wound hydraulic skeletons: the stiffening and straightening of embryonic notochords. Am Zool. 2000;40(1):28–041.
15. Adams DS, Keller R, Koehl MAR. The mechanics of notochord elongation, straightening and stiffening in the embryo of Xenopus laevis. Development. 1990;110(1):115–30.
16. Kaplan KM, Spivak JM, Bendo JA. Embryology of the spine and associated congenital abnormalities. Spine J. 2005;5(5):564–76.
17. Babic MS. Development of the notochord in normal and malformed human embryos and fetuses. Int J Dev Biol. 1991;35(3):345–52.
18. Urban JPG, Ralph JR. The nucleus of the intervertebral disc from development to degeneration. Am Zool. 2000;40(1):53–61.
19. Odenthal J, Haffter P, Vogelsang E, et al. Mutations affecting the formation of the notochord in the zebrafish, Danio rerio. Development. 1996;123(1):103–15.
20. Bakker SH, Jacobs WCH, Pondaag W, et al. Chordoma: a systematic review of the epidemiology and clinical prognostic factors predicting progression-free and overall survival. Eur Spine J. 2018;27(12):3043–58.
21. Iorgulescu JB, Laufer I, Hameed M, et al. Benign notochordal cell tumors of the spine. Neurosurgery. 2013;73(3):411–6.
22. Chugh R, Tawbi H, Lucas DR, Biermann JS, Schuetze SM, Baker LH. Chordoma: the nonsarcoma primary bone tumor. Oncologist. 2007;12(11):1344–50.
23. Yamaguchi T, Yamato M, Saotome K. First histologically confirmed case of a classic chordoma arising in a precursor benign notochordal lesion: differential diagnosis of benign and malignant notochordal lesions. Skelet Radiol. 2002;31(7):413–8.
24. Virchow RLK. Untersuchungen Über Die Entwickelung Des Schädelgrundes Im Gesunden Und Krankhaften Zustande, Und Über Den Einfluss Derselben Auf Schädelform, Gesichtsbildung Und Gehirnbau. 1st ed. G. Reimer; 1857.
25. Park HH, Lee K-S, Ahn SJ, Suh SH, Hong C-K. Ecchordosis physaliphora: typical and atypical radiologic features. Neurosurg Rev. 2017;40(1):87–94.
26. Yamaguchi T, Suzuki S, Ishiiwa H, Ueda Y. Intraosseous benign notochordal cell tumours: overlooked precursors of classic chordomas? Histopathology. 2004;44(6):597–602.
27. Yamaguchi T, Iwata J, Sugihara S, et al. Distinguishing benign notochordal cell tumors from vertebral chordoma. Skelet Radiol. 2008;37(4):291–9.
28. Sung MS, Lee GK, Kang HS, et al. Sacrococcygeal chordoma: MR imaging in 30 patients. Skelet Radiol. 2005;34(2):87–94.
29. Kshettry VR, Yu JS, Venur VA, Ahluwalia MS, Recinos PF. Comprehensive management of chordoma. In: Raghavan D, Ahluwalia MS, Blanke CD, et al., editors. Textbook of uncommon cancer. 5th ed. Wiley; 2017. p. 847–55.
30. Mohyeldin A, Vaz-Guimaraes F, Carrau RL, Prevedello DM. Molecular drivers in chordoma. In: Harsh GR, Vaz-Guimaraes F, editors. Chordomas and chondrosarcomas of the skull base and spine. 2nd ed. Academic Press; 2017. p. 23–9.
31. Demireli P, Ovali GY, Yegen G, Temiz C, Tarhan S. Chondroid chordoma of the thoracic spine: case report. Pathology. 2007;39(2):280–2.

32. Fernández Carballal C, González Rodrigalvarez R, López De La Riva M, Ares C. Dumbbell-shaped thoracic chondroid chordoma mimicking a neurinoma. Acta Neurochir. 2010;152(2):325–6.
33. Zamora C, Castillo M. Sellar and parasellar imaging. Neurosurgery. 2017;80(1):17–38.
34. Yeom KW, Lober RM, Mobley BC, et al. Diffusion-weighted MRI: distinction of skull base chordoma from chondrosarcoma. Am J Neuroradiol. 2013;34(5):1056–61.
35. Hanna SA, Tirabosco R, Amin A, et al. Dedifferentiated chordoma: a report of four cases arising "de novo". J Bone Joint Surg Br. 2008;90-B(5):652–6.
36. Kato S, Gasbarrini A, Ghermandi R, Gambarotti M, Bandiera S. Spinal chordomas dedifferentiated to osteosarcoma: a report of two cases and a literature review. Eur Spine J. 2016;25(S1):251–6.
37. Erdem E, Angtuaco EC, Van Hemert R, Park JS, Al-Mefty O. Comprehensive review of intracranial chordoma. Radiographics. 2003;23(4):995–1009.
38. Pennington Z, Ehresman J, McCarthy EF, et al. Chordoma of the sacrum and mobile spine: a narrative review. Spine J. 2021;21(3):500–17.
39. Rodallec MH, Feydy A, Larousserie F, et al. Diagnostic imaging of solitary tumors of the spine: what to do and say. Radiographics. 2008;28(4):1019–41.
40. Almefty K, Pravdenkova S, Colli BO, Al-Mefty O, Gokden M. Chordoma and chondrosarcoma: similar, but quite different, skull base tumors. Cancer. 2007;110(11):2467–77.
41. Mukherjee D, Chaichana KL, Gokaslan ZL, Aaronson OS, Cheng JS, McGirt MJ. Survival of patients with malignant primary osseous spinal neoplasms: results from the surveillance, epidemiology, and end results (SEER) database from 1973 to 2003. J Neurosurg Spine. 2011;14(2):143–50.
42. Ilaslan H, Sundaram M, Unni KK, Dekutoski MB. Primary Ewing's sarcoma of the vertebral column. Skelet Radiol. 2004;33(9):506–13.
43. Charest-Morin R, Dirks MS, Patel S, et al. Ewing sarcoma of the spine: prognostic variables for survival and local control in surgically treated patients. Spine (Phila Pa 1976). 2018;43(9):622–9.
44. Wang F, Zhang H-R, Yang L, et al. Epidemiological characteristics of 1196 patients with spinal metastases: a retrospective study. Orthop Surg. 2019;11(6):1048–53.
45. Bhavan KP, Marschall J, Olsen MA, Fraser VJ, Wright NM, Warren DK. The epidemiology of hematogenous vertebral osteomyelitis: a cohort study in a tertiary care hospital. BMC Infect Dis. 2010;10(1):158.
46. Zadran S, Pedersen PH, Eiskjær S. Vertebral osteomyelitis: a mortality analysis comparing surgical and conservative management. Glob Spine J. 2020;10(4):456–63.
47. Hong SH, Choi J-Y, Lee JW, Kim NR, Choi J-A, Kang HS. MR imaging assessment of the spine: infection or an imitation? Radiographics. 2009;29(2):599–612.
48. Dagirmanjian A, Schils J, McHenry M, Modic MT. MR imaging of vertebral osteomyelitis revisited. Am J Roentgenol. 1996;167(6):1539–43.
49. Passias PG, Pierce KE, Lafage V, et al. At what point should the thoracolumbar region be addressed in patients undergoing corrective cervical deformity surgery? Spine J. 2020;20(9):S2–3.
50. Sciubba DM, Chi JH, Rhines LD, Gokaslan ZL. Chordoma of the spinal column. Neurosurg Clin N Am. 2008;19(1):5–15.
51. Chandawarkar RY. Sacrococcygeal chordoma: review of 50 consecutive patients. World J Surg. 1996;20(6):717–9.
52. Denaro L, Berton A, Ciuffreda M, et al. Surgical management of chordoma: a systematic review. J Spinal Cord Med. 2020;43(6):797–812.
53. Van Gompel JJ, Janus JR. Chordoma and chondrosarcoma. Otolaryngol Clin N Am. 2015;48(3):501–14.
54. Kamrin RP, Potanos JN, Pool JL. An evaluation of the diagnosis and treatment of chordoma. J Neurol Neurosurg Psychiatry. 1964;27(2):157–65.

55. Volpe NJ, Liebsch NJ, Munzenrider JE, Lesseil S. Neuro-ophthalmologic findings in chordoma and chondrosarcoma of the skull base. Am J Ophthalmol. 1993;115(1):97–104.
56. Korchi AM, Cuvinciuc V, Caetano J, Becker M, Lovblad KO, Vargas MI. Imaging of the cavernous sinus lesions. Diagn Interv Imaging. 2014;95(9):849–59.
57. Gokaslan ZL, Zadnik PL, Sciubba DM, et al. Mobile spine chordoma: results of 166 patients from the AOSpine knowledge forum tumor database. J Neurosurg Spine. 2016;24(4):644–51.
58. Pennington Z, Goodwin ML, Westbroek EM, Cottrill E, Ahmed AK, Sciubba DM. Lactate and cancer: spinal metastases and potential therapeutic targets (part 2). Ann Transl Med. 2019;7(10):221.
59. Wippold FJ, Koeller KK, Smirniotopoulos JG. Clinical and imaging features of cervical chordoma. Am J Roentgenol. 1999;172(5):1423–6.
60. Jeys L, Gibbins R, Evans G, Grimer R. Sacral chordoma: a diagnosis not to be sat on? Int Orthop. 2008;32(2):269–72.
61. Pillai S, Govender S. Sacral chordoma: a review of literature. J Orthop. 2018;15(2):679–84.
62. Varga PP, Szövérfi Z, Fisher CG, et al. Surgical treatment of sacral chordoma: prognostic variables for local recurrence and overall survival. Eur Spine J. 2015;24(5):1092–101.
63. Atalar H, Selek H, Yıldız Y, Sağlık Y. Management of sacrococcygeal chordomas. Int Orthop. 2006;30(6):514–8.
64. Sankey EW, Park C, Howell EP, et al. Importance of spinal alignment in primary and metastatic spine tumors. World Neurosurg. 2019;132:118–28.
65. Mechri M, Riahi H, Sboui I, Bouaziz M, Vanhoenacker F, Ladeb M. Imaging of malignant primitive tumors of the spine. J Belgian Soc Radiol. 2018;102(1):56.
66. Lin E, Scognamiglio T, Zhao Y, Schwartz TH, Phillips CD. Prognostic implications of gadolinium enhancement of skull base chordomas. Am J Neuroradiol. 2018;39(8):1509–14.
67. Malayeri AA, El Khouli RH, Zaheer A, et al. Principles and applications of diffusion-weighted imaging in cancer detection, staging, and treatment follow-up. Radiographics. 2011;31(6):1773–91.
68. Blitz AM, Macedo LL, Chonka ZD, et al. High-resolution CISS MR imaging with and without contrast for evaluation of the upper cranial nerves. Neuroimaging Clin N Am. 2014;24(1):17–34.
69. Westbroek EM, Pennington Z, Ehresman J, Ahmed AK, Gailloud P, Sciubba DM. Vertebral artery sacrifice versus skeletonization in the setting of cervical spine tumor resection: case series. World Neurosurg. 2020;139:e601–7.
70. Zuckerman SL, Amini B, Lee S-H, Rao G, Tatsui CE, Rhines LD. Predictive value of preoperative magnetic resonance imaging findings for survival and local recurrence in patients undergoing En Bloc resection of sacral chordomas. Neurosurgery. 2019;85(6):834–42.
71. Smith J, Ludwig RL, Marcove RC. Sacrococcygeal chordoma: a clinicoradiological study of 60 patients. Skelet Radiol. 1987;16(1):37–44.
72. Murphey MD, Andrews C, Flemming DJ, Temple HT, Smith WS, Smirniotopoulos JG. Primary tumors of the spine: radiologic pathologic correlation. Radiographics. 1996;16(5):1131–58.
73. Gerber S, Ollivier L, Leclere J, et al. Imaging of sacral tumours. Skelet Radiol. 2008;37(4):277–89.
74. Young VA, Curtis KM, Temple HT, Eismont FJ, DeLaney TF, Hornicek FJ. Characteristics and patterns of metastatic disease from chordoma. Sarcoma. 2015;2015:1–7.
75. Herzog L, Gottsacker J, Olson J, Broski S. Role of $^{99m}$Tc-MDP bone scan in staging vertebral chordoma. J Nucl Med. 2020;61(Supplement 1):3051.
76. Rossleigh MA, Smith J, Yeh SD. Scintigraphic features of primary sacral tumors. J Nucl Med. 1986;27(5):627–30.
77. Suga K, Tanaka N, Nakanishi T, Utsumi H, Yamada N. Bone and gallium scintigraphy in sacral chordoma report of four cases. Clin Nucl Med. 1992;17(3):206–12.
78. Santegoeds RGC, Temel Y, Beckervordersandforth JC, Van Overbeeke JJ, Hoeberigs CM. State-of-the-art imaging in human chordoma of the skull base. Curr Radiol Rep. 2018;6(5):16.

79. Ochoa-Figueroa MA, Martínez-Gimeno E, Allende-Riera A, Cabello-García D, Muñoz-Iglesias J, Cárdenas-Negro C. Papel de la 18F-FDG PET-TC en el estudio del cordoma sacrocoxígeo. Rev Esp Med Nucl Imagen Mol. 2012;31(6):359–61.
80. Park S-A, Kim HS. F-18 FDG PET/CT evaluation of sacrococcygeal cordoma. Clin Nucl Med. 2008;33(12):906–8.
81. Derlin T, Sohns JM, Hueper K. 68Ga-DOTA-TATE PET/CT for molecular imaging of somatostatin receptor expression in metastasizing chordoma. Clin Nucl Med. 2017;42(4):e210–1.
82. Cheney MD, Chen Y-L, Lim R, et al. [18F]-Fluoromisonidazole positron emission tomography/computed tomography visualization of tumor hypoxia in patients with chordoma of the mobile and sacrococcygeal spine. Int J Radiat Oncol. 2014;90(5):1030–6.
83. Mammar H, Kerrou K, Nataf V, et al. Positron emission tomography/computed tomography imaging of residual skull base chordoma before radiotherapy using fluoromisonidazole and fluorodeoxyglucose: potential consequences for dose painting. Int J Radiat Oncol. 2012;84(3):681–7.
84. Yang SY, Oh E, Kwon JW, Kim HS. Percutaneous image-guided spinal lesion biopsies: factors affecting higher diagnostic yield. Am J Roentgenol. 2018;211(5):1068–74.
85. Tehranzadeh J, Tao C, Browning CA. Percutaneous needle biopsy of the spine. Acta Radiol. 2007;48(8):860–8.
86. Peh W. CT-guided percutaneous biopsy of spinal lesions. Biomed Imaging Interv J. 2006;2(3):e25.
87. Yaffe D, Greenberg G, Leitner J, Gipstein R, Shapiro M, Bachar GN. CT-guided percutaneous biopsy of thoracic and lumbar spine: a new coaxial technique. Am J Neuroradiol. 2003;24(10):2111–3.
88. Dave BR, Nanda A, Anandjiwala JV. Transpedicular percutaneous biopsy of vertebral body lesions: a series of 71 cases. Spinal Cord. 2009;47(5):384–9.
89. Ali N. Percutaneous spine biopsy: a literature review. Int J Radiol Radiat Oncol. 2015;1(1):023–8.
90. Stacchiotti S, Sommer J. Building a global consensus approach to chordoma: a position paper from the medical and patient community. Lancet Oncol. 2015;16(2):e71–83.
91. Stacchiotti S, Gronchi A, Fossati P, et al. Best practices for the management of local-regional recurrent chordoma: a position paper by the chordoma global consensus group. Ann Oncol. 2017;28(6):1230–42.
92. Laurent F, Latrabe V, Vergier B, Michel P. Percutaneous CT-guided biopsy of the lung: comparison between aspiration and automated cutting needles using a coaxial technique. Cardiovasc Intervent Radiol. 2000;23(4):266–72.
93. Yao X, Gomes MM, Tsao MS, Allen CJ, Geddie W, Sekhon H. Fine-needle aspiration biopsy versus core-needle biopsy in diagnosing lung cancer: a systematic review. Curr Oncol. 2012;19(1):e16–27.
94. Wolinski K, Stangierski A, Ruchala M. Comparison of diagnostic yield of core-needle and fine-needle aspiration biopsies of thyroid lesions: systematic review and meta-analysis. Eur Radiol. 2017;27(1):431–6.
95. Pierot L, Boulin A. Percutaneous biopsy of the thoracic and lumbar spine: transpedicular approach under fluoroscopic guidance. Am J Neuroradiol. 1999;20(1):23–5.
96. Baines S. Surgical asepsis: principles and protocols. In Pract. 1996;18(1):23–33.
97. Stringham DR, Hadjipavlou A, Dzioba RB, Lander P. Percutaneous Transpedicular Biops of the spine. Spine (Phila Pa 1976). 1994;19(17):1985–91.
98. Chooi YS, Kamil OIM, Fazir M, Kob SC. Percutaneous transpedicular biopsy of the spine. Med J Malaysia. 2007;62(1):46–8.
99. Crapanzano JP, Ali SZ, Ginsberg MS, Zakowski MF. Chordoma: a cytologic study with histologic and radiologic correlation. Cancer. 2001;93(1):40–51.
100. Garg V, Kosmas C, Josan ES, et al. Computed tomography–guided percutaneous biopsy for vertebral neoplasms: a department's experience and hybrid biopsy technique to improve yield. Neurosurg Focus. 2016;41(2):E17.

101. Kerr DA, Rosenberg AE. Pathology of chordoma and chondrosarcoma of the axial skeleton. In: Harsh GR, Vaz-Guimaraes F, editors. Chordomas and chondrosarcomas of the skull base and spine. 2nd ed. Academic Press; 2017. p. 11–21.
102. Naka T, Iwamoto Y, Shinohara N, Chuman H, Fukui M, Tsuneyoshi M. Cytokeratin subtyping in chordomas and the fetal notochord: an immunohistochemical analysis of aberrant expression. Mod Pathol. 1997;10(6):545–51.
103. Diaz RJ, Luck A, Bondoc A, et al. Characterization of a clival chordoma xenograft model reveals tumor genomic instability. Am J Pathol. 2018;188(12):2902–11.

# Histopathologic Classification of Spinal Chordoma

# 5

John M. Gross and Edward F. McCarthy

## Abbreviations

| | |
|---|---|
| BNCT | Benign notochordal cell tumor |
| cm | Centimeter |
| CT | Computed tomography |
| FISH | Fluorescence in situ hybridization |
| IHC | Immunohistochemistry |
| MRI | Magnetic resonance imaging |

## Introduction

Chordomas represent one of several members of the family of notochord-derived tumors, which also includes benign notochordal cell tumors (BNCTs). As indicated in Chap. 4, imaging alone is insufficient for diagnosis, which depends upon biopsy and tissue examination. The results of biopsy in turn have significant implications for treatment, as BNCTs may be observed, whereas the various chordoma subtypes generally benefit from aggressive surgical resection. Formulation of the optimal treatment plan is then contingent upon knowing the characteristic histopathologic and immunohistochemical features that distinguish BNCTs from chordoma and that differentiate the various chordoma subtypes.

Table 5.1 contains a concise summary of the various chordoma subtypes including pertinent diagnostic features. It must be noted that given the common origin, there are some shared features between the immunophenotypes of the varying

J. M. Gross (✉) · E. F. McCarthy
Department of Orthopaedic Pathology, Johns Hopkins Hospital, Baltimore, MD, USA
e-mail: jgross28@jhmi.edu



D. M. Sciubba, J. H. Schwab (eds.), *Chordoma of the Spine*,
https://doi.org/10.1007/978-3-030-76201-8_5

**Table 5.1** Overview of the distinct clinical and histopathological features of the various chordoma subtypes

| Subtype | Age | Site | Clinical | Histology | Immunophenotype |
|---|---|---|---|---|---|
| BNCT | Mostly adults | Intraosseous, vertebral bodies | Asymptomatic; generally an incidental finding | Adipocyte-like cells with lightly eosinophilic to clear cytoplasm and bland round nuclei. Non-infiltrative growth | Brachyury, keratin, EMA, variable S100 |
| Conventional | Mostly adults | Bone (rare soft tissue) Sacrococcygeal most common, then skull base and mobile spine | Pain, neurologic symptoms of compression | Lobular infiltrative growth of cords and chains of epithelioid cells with eosinophilic cytoplasm and prominent cell borders within abundant myxoid stroma. Scattered bubbly mutlivacuolated "physaliphorous" cells | Brachyury, keratin, EMA, variable S100 |
| Dedifferentiated | Exclusively adults | Bone almost exclusively sacrococcygeal | Pain, neurologic symptoms of compression | Destructive large mass showing a biphasic tumor with a conventional chordoma juxtaposed with a high-grade pleomorphic spindle cell sarcoma | Brachyury, keratin, EMA, variable S100 in conventional; all IHC antigens lost in high-grade sarcomatous component which may show heterologous rhabdomyoblastic or osteosarcomatous differentiation |
| Poorly differentiated | Children and young adults | Skull base (clivus) most common followed by cervical spine | Headache, pain, cranial nerve symptoms | High-grade epithelioid cells with rhabdoid morphology, geographic necrosis, scant myxoid stroma | Brachyury, keratin, EMA, variable S100, loss of INI1 (SMARCB1) |

*Key*: *BNCT* benign notochordal tumor, *EMA* epithelial membrane antigen, *IHC* immunohistochemistry, *SMARCB1* SWI/SNF-related matrix-associated actin-dependent regulator of chromatin subfamily B member 1

notochord-derived tumors. This includes strong and diffuse nuclear expression of brachyury, a transcription factor required for notochordal differentiation [1, 2]. In addition, cytokeratin and EMA are positive whereas expression of S100 is more variable. To this end, benign notochordal tumor and conventional chordomas are nearly indistinguishable from an immunohistochemical standpoint. However, dedifferentiated chordoma can be distinguished from the former two by the loss of brachyury expression. Dedifferentiated chordoma may also downregulate other antigens within the high-grade pleomorphic sarcomatous component. Poorly differentiated chordoma similarly shows downregulation of specific markers seen in immunohistochemical staining of BNCT and conventional chordoma, notably abnormal loss of INI1 (SMARCB1). In this chapter, we elaborate on the unique histopathological and immunohistochemical fingerprints of the varying notochord-derived tumors. Where appropriate, we also present evidence regarding the prognostic significance of specific genetic mutations.

## Benign Notochordal Tumor

A BNCT is a benign tumor showing notochordal differentiation. BNCTs are usually found in the skull base, vertebral bodies, and sacrococcygeal spine [3, 4]. Rare examples of extraosseous BNCTs have been reported in various sites including the lung [5]. Benign notochordal cell tumors are usually found in adults with rare reports in children. Most BNCTs are found incidentally with imaging although they may be associated with pain. Radiographs and CT may show a radiodensity with mild sclerosis surrounding the tumor without any bone destruction or extraosseous tumor extension, although they may fail to show any abnormality whatsoever. MRI reveals homogenously enhancing high-signal intensity on T2-weighted imaging, homogeneously low signal intensity on T1-weighted imaging, and no contrast enhancement on gadolinium (Gd)-enhanced T1-weighted imaging, respectively [6, 7]. Occasionally, chordomas may arise in the setting of a BNCT [8–10].

On gross macroscopic examination, BNCTs often show a well-demarcated, dense tan-white abnormality with a sclerotic rim corresponding to the reactive sclerotic bone. Consistent with radiographic findings, macroscopic evaluation of a BNCT shows a lack of bone destruction, an absence of gelatinous areas, and a lack of a lobular architecture (Fig. 5.1).

BNCTs consist of well-delineated sheet of large, polyhedral epithelioid cells with well-defined cytoplasmic membranes which is sharply demarcated from and surrounded by a rim of sclerotic bone. On close inspection, the cells of interest contain adipocyte-like vacuolated cells with bland, condensed nuclear chromatin without mitotic activity or myxoid stroma (Fig. 5.2). Unlike chordoma, BNCTs lack a lobular growth pattern, fibrous septa and thin fibrous pseudocapsule, extracellular myxoid matrix, or tumor vasculature. Ancillary studies are not diagnostically helpful in distinguishing a BNCT from a chordoma as both are immunoreactive to brachyury (Fig. 5.2), cytokeratin, EMA, and (variably) S100.

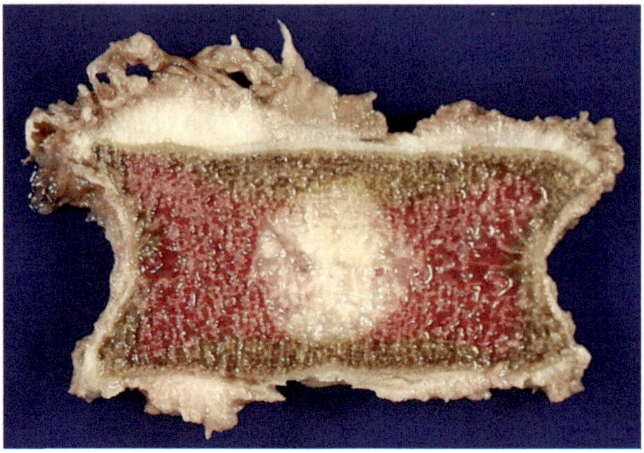

**Fig. 5.1** Gross cut section of a vertebral body show a benign notochordal tumor as a well-demarcated, dense, ivory tumor without any bone destruction

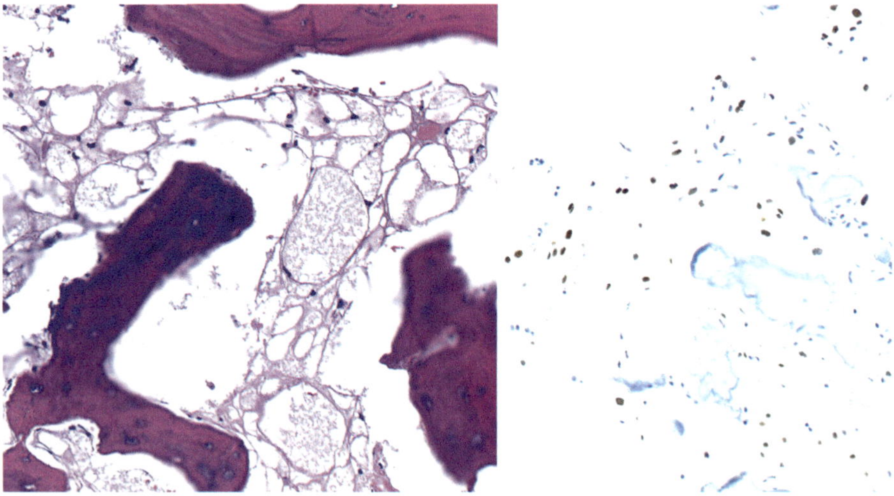

**Fig. 5.2** (Left) Benign notochordal tumor consists of adipocyte-like vacuolated cells with lightly eosinophilic cytoplasm and bland, round nuclei. (Right) Nuclear immunoreactivity is seen with brachyury

## Conventional Chordoma

Chordoma is an uncommon malignant tumor of bone (or rarely soft tissue) with a phenotype recapitulating notochordal differentiation. Chordomas can arise from all levels of the axial skeleton, with a recent review of the Surveillance Epidemiology and End Results dataset showing 41.1% arise from the skull base, 31.5% from the sacrum, and 27.4% from the mobile spine [11]. Chordomas are usually diagnosed in the 4th to 8th decades with a slight male predominance. By imaging, chordoma is generally a lytic, destructive neoplasm arising in the midline. It tends to grow slowly by expanding the bone and is frequently associated with a large destructive mass (Figs. 5.3 and 5.4). Chordomas are not mineralized but bone fragments may be seen near the periphery of the mass. On MRI, similar to BNCTs, chordomas are hyperintense on T2-weighted imaging and have low signal on T1-weighted images. Gadolinium enhancement pattern is heterogenous and often septal with myxoid areas showing poor enhancement [12–15].

The gross macroscopic examination of chordomas depends somewhat on the site. In general, chordomas are soft, tan-gray, gelatinous, and lobulated tumors that are well-delineated from the surrounding tissues even though they grow in a bone destructive pattern (Fig. 5.3). Sacrococcygeal tumors tend to be larger than those at other sites, most likely related to a longer symptom-free interval (Fig. 5.4).

The histologic features of chordomas are unique. At low power, chordomas grow in a lobular pattern separated by fibrous septa within abundant extracellular myxoid matrix. The cells of interest grow in cords, chains, and nests. On close inspection, two types of cells are identified with similar nuclei. One cell type is chiefly polygonal and containing a round centrally located nucleus with dense, eosinophilic cytoplasm and prominent cell borders (Fig. 5.5). The other cell type shows a similar nucleus but instead contains bubbly multivacuolated cytoplasm ("physaliphorous cell") (Fig. 5.6). Note the corded, linear arrangement of the cells (Fig. 5.7) which can also be appreciated with brachyury immunohistochemistry (Fig. 5.8). In general, chordomas show minimal nuclear enlargement; however, some degenerative so-called "ancient change" can be seen. Mitotic activity is rare.

Chordomas often show a substantial degree of intratumoral cytologic heterogeneity, with features including nuclear atypia and pleomorphism ranging from minimal to severe, occasionally showing bizarre or spindling nuclei.

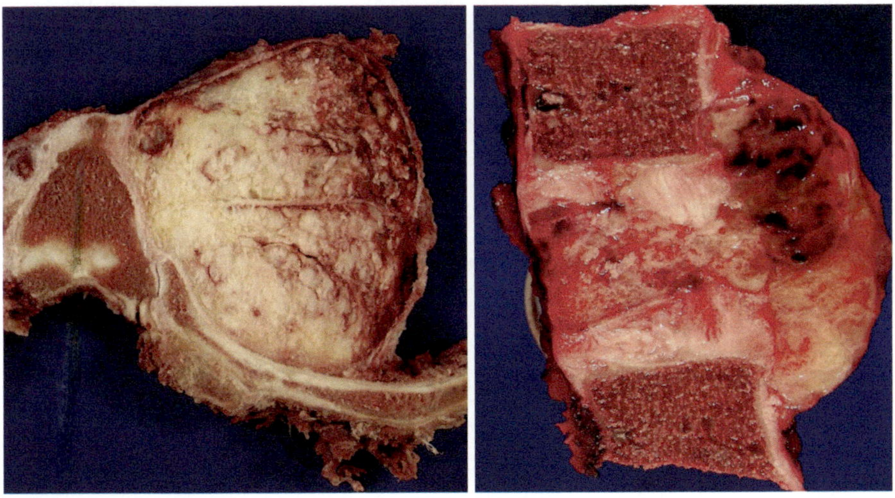

**Fig. 5.3** (Left) A large chordoma is seen extending from the vertebrae and involving the adjacent ribs. (Right) A chordoma is seen destroying the vertebrae with soft tissue extension

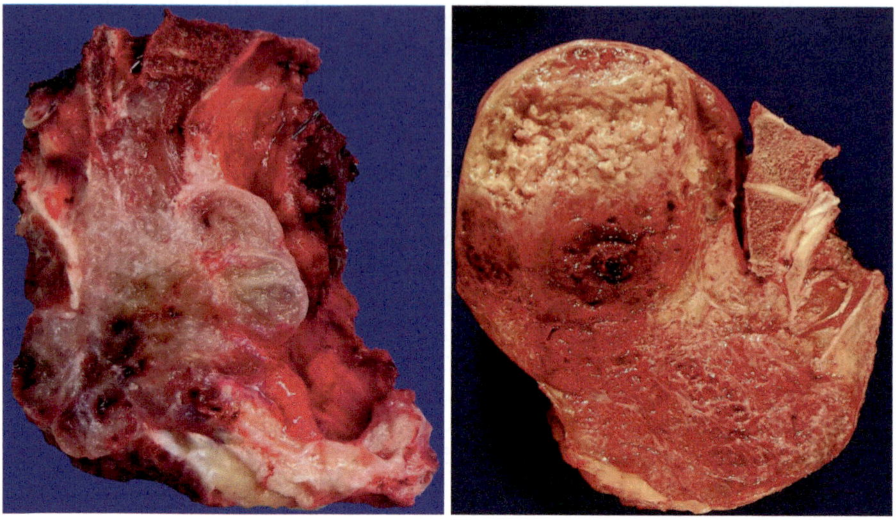

**Fig. 5.4** (Left) Sacrectomy specimen on the left shows a conventional chordoma destroying the sacrum as a heterogenous, lobulated, and gelatinous mass. (Right) Large destructive chordoma with hemorrhage and a fleshy solid area

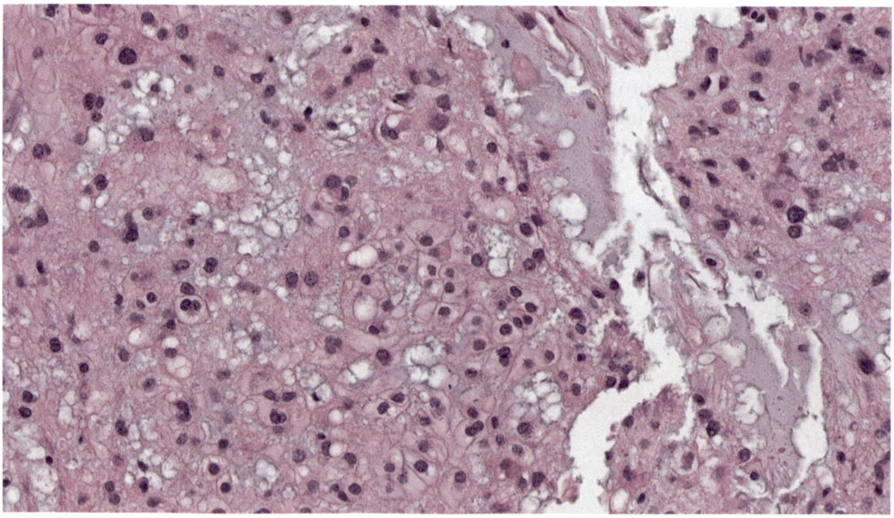

**Fig. 5.5** Classic appearance of chordoma showing epithelioid cells with eosinophilic cytoplasm and prominent cell membranes containing round nuclei

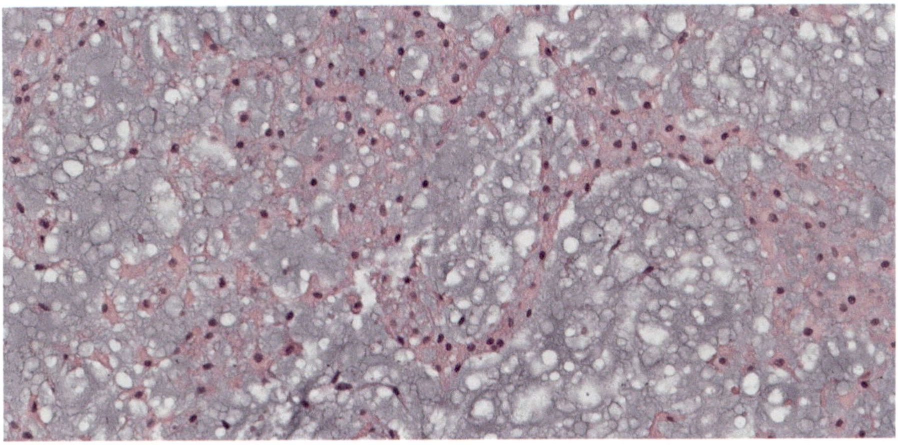

**Fig. 5.6** Tumor cells are arranged in linear cords within a typical light basophilic appearance to the myxoid matrix

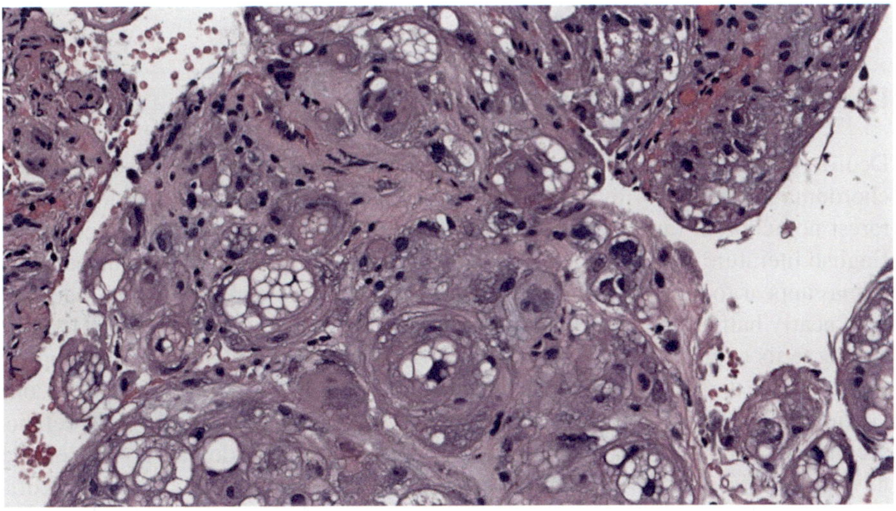

**Fig. 5.7** Note the cells with bubbly cytoplasm (physaliphorous cells) in conventional chordoma

Rarely, extra-axial chordomas may develop but are histologically identical to their osseous counterparts [16]. The term "chondroid chordoma" is a morphologic description in which a conventional chordoma shows areas of hyaline matrix mimicking cartilage. It is unclear whether chondroid chordoma is a specific subtype of chordoma after more than four decades of debate. Previous literature on this topic is no longer reliable because data were derived from the pre-brachyury era and therefore some cases coded as "chondroid chordoma" may have been in fact low-grade conventional chondrosarcoma [17].

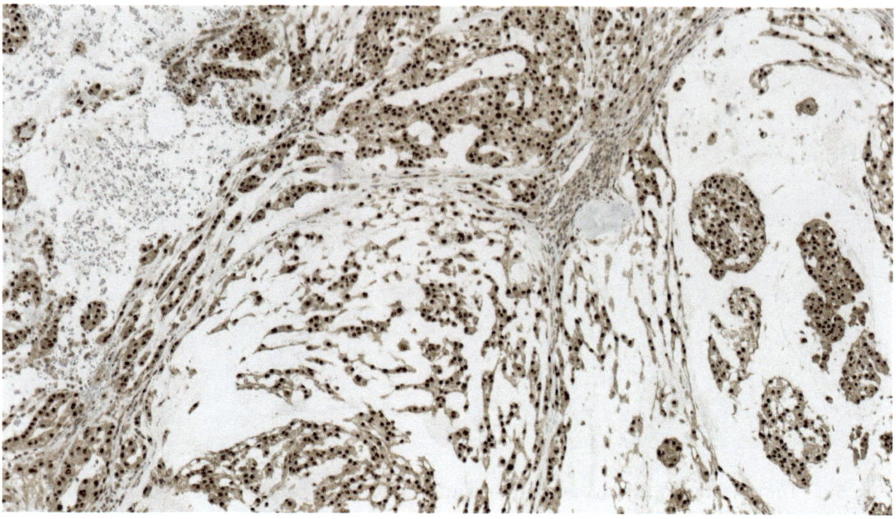

**Fig. 5.8** Chordoma showing strong nuclear immunoreactivity to brachyury. Note the linear cords and nested growth pattern

## Dedifferentiated Chordoma

Dedifferentiated chordoma is a biphasic tumor characterized by a conventional chordoma juxtaposed with a high-grade sarcoma. Dedifferentiated chordoma is the rarest notochordal tumor with only case reports and small series published in the English literature [18, 19]. Based upon these limited reports, dedifferentiated chordomas appear to have an anatomic distribution similar to conventional chordomas, with nearly half of described cases arising from the sacrococcygeal region [18, 19]. Owing to its aggressive nature of these lesions, clinical symptoms may develop far more rapidly than in patients with conventional chordoma. However, as with conventional chordoma, the most common symptoms are pain and neurologic deficits secondary to local tumor mass effect. Dedifferentiated chordoma may present de novo or arise from a previously resected conventional chordoma. By imaging, dedifferentiated chordoma shows a morphology like that of conventional chordomas by radiographs and CT. A biphasic appearance may be appreciated on MRI with the dedifferentiated component suggested by areas of tumor that are relatively hypointense on T2-weighted imaging [20].

On macroscopic examination, the tumor presents as a large mass with a biphasic appearance. The dedifferentiated component resembles a high-grade sarcoma with a fleshy solid surface which is generally juxtaposed to a gelatinous and myxoid conventional chordoma.

Histologic sections show conventional chordoma juxtaposed with an undifferentiated pleomorphic spindle cell sarcoma (Fig. 5.9). The high-grade component may develop after multiple interventions of a conventional chordoma or may occur de

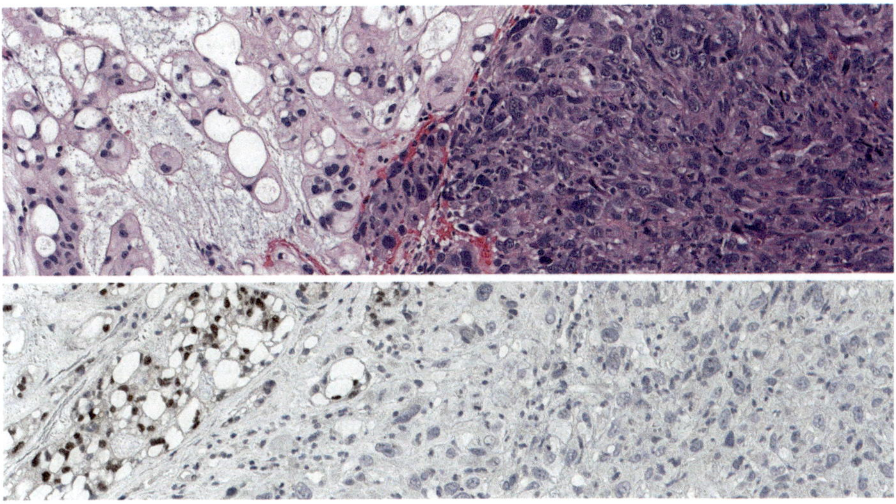

**Fig. 5.9** (Top) Dedifferentiated chordoma showing a biphasic appearance with conventional chordoma on the left and an abrupt change to a high-grade anaplastic sarcoma on the right. (Below) Note the expression of brachyury is positive in the conventional chordoma on the left but lost (negative) in the dedifferentiated component

novo [18, 19]. The high-grade spindle cell sarcoma may show rhabdomyoblastic or osteosarcomatous differentiation [21]. The two components are usually abruptly separated and juxtaposed without mixing; however, given the loose and myxoid gelatinous consistency of conventional chordoma, some intermingling can be seen.

In the conventional chordoma component, expression of brachyury, keratin, EMA, and variable S100 will be seen; however, the high-grade pleomorphic spindle cell sarcoma will often lose expression of these antigens. The dedifferentiated component may show focal cytokeratin expression but does not express brachyury (Fig. 5.9). Specific lineages, such as rhabdomyoblastic, should be supported by immunohistochemical expression of desmin and myogenin [21]. INI1 (SMARCB1) is retained (normal).

Molecular mechanisms that account for the dedifferentiation remain unclear, though tumor suppressor genes such as p53 have been implicated analogous to the role p53 in dedifferentiated chondrosarcoma. While aberrant p53 expression has been used as a surrogate for *TP53* mutations status in various tumors, how p53 expression correlates with *TP53* mutation in chordoma is unclear [19, 22].

## Poorly Differentiated Chordoma

Poorly differentiated chordoma is a high-grade neoplasm with notochordal differentiation, usually arising in the axial skeleton, and characterized by loss of *SMARCB1* (INI1) expression. Poorly differentiated chordoma is extremely rare with approximately 60 cases reported in the English language literature [23–27]. Tumors typically arise in children, though occasionally this diagnosis is made in young adults. Unlike conventional chordoma, poorly differentiated chordomas disproportionately burden females, who are roughly twice as likely to be affected as their male counterparts. In the largest series to date, the age range was 1–29 years with a median age of 11 [24]. The most common site of disease origin is the clivus, followed by the cervical spine. Unlike other chordoma subtypes, lesions in the sacrococcygeal region are rare. Patients typically present with non-specific symptoms such as headache, pain, and cranial nerve disturbances. By imaging, these tumors are destructive and arise in bone with common extension into the adjacent soft tissues. CT shows lytic masses that are heterogeneous on T1- and T2-weighted MRI [24].

Macroscopically, poorly differentiated chordomas may vary in size from less than 2.0 cm to greater than 10.0 cm, although the majority are approximately 5.0 cm at the time of clinical presentation. Due to the rarity of these tumors, there is little data regarding the gross cut surface, but they may be well-demarcated, multilobulated, and destructive [24].

Histologic sections of poorly differentiated chordoma are composed of cohesive sheets and nests of epithelioid cells often with variably rhabdoid morphology

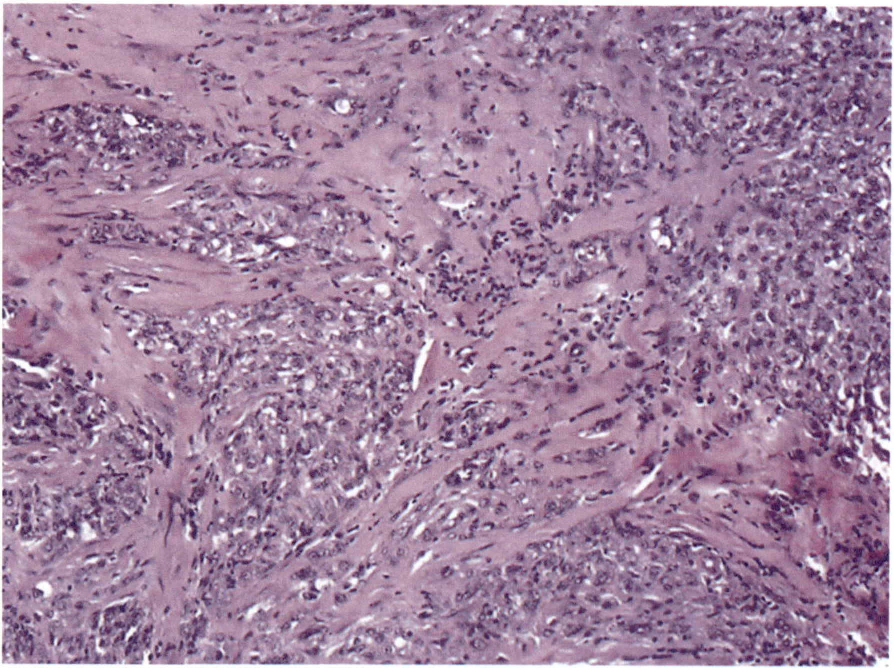

**Fig. 5.10** Poorly differentiated chordoma showing sheets of high-grade epithelioid to rhabdoid tumor cells. INI1 (*SMARCB1*) is abnormally lost in this rare subtype but, characteristic of all tumors of notochordal differentiation, this tumor will express brachyury (not shown)

(Fig. 5.10). The cells of interest contain ample eosinophilic cytoplasm with scattered cytoplasmic vacuoles. On close inspection, the chromatin is vesicular with mild to moderate cytologic atypia, mitotic activity, and tumor necrosis. Most poorly differentiated chordomas will show prominent nucleoli and geographic necrosis is often extensive. In contrast to conventional chordomas, poorly differentiated chordomas seldom possess a myxoid stroma or cords of epithelioid cells. If this architecture is present, it accounts for only a fraction of the total neoplasm. Owing to the absence of these histologic features, poorly-differentated chordoma is often a challenging diagnosis without immunohistochemistry.

Like other tumors of notochordal differentiation, poorly differentiated chordoma will express brachyury, keratins, EMA, and show variable expression of S100. Unique to this subtype, however, is the loss of *SMARCB1* (INI1) expression. This can be detected by routine immunohistochemistry or fluorescence in situ hybridization (FISH) to identify deletions in the *SMARCB1* locus. An important pitfall, however, is that FISH for *EWSR1* may also be co-deleted along with *SMARCB1*; therefore, FISH must be interpreted with caution in the appropriate morphologic and immunophenotypic context [27].

## Conclusion

Chordomas are uncommon, malignant, bone (or rarely soft tissue) tumors. Chordomas most commonly affect adults with a subset showing a propensity for children (poorly differentiated chordoma). Histologically, tumors of notochordal differentiation are linked by their common expression of the brachyury antigen which can be identified by immunohistochemistry. Conventional chordomas grow in a lobulated pattern and contain linear cords or nests of epithelioid cells with scattered cells containing cytoplasmic vacuolization (physaliphorous cells). While all chordomas are malignant, rare subtypes of dedifferentiated chordoma and poorly differentiated chordoma assume a more aggressive clinical course emphasizing the value of proper histologic classification. Due to their rarity and unpredictable behavior, chordomas should be treated with a multidisciplinary approach for optimal patient outcomes.

## References

1. Vujovic S, Henderson S, Presneau N, Odell E, Jacques T, Tirabosco R, Boshoff C, Flanagan A. Brachyury, a crucial regulator of notochordal development, is a novel biomarker for chordomas. J Pathol. 2006;209:157–65.
2. Tirabosco R, Mangham DC, Rosenberg AE, et al. Brachyury expression in extra-axial skeletal and soft tissue chordomas: a marker that distinguishes chordoma from mixed tumor/myoepithelioma/parachordoma in soft tissue. Am J Surg Pathol. 2008;32:572–80.
3. Yamaguchi T, Suzuki S, Ishiiwa H, Ueda Y. Intraosseous benign notochordal cell tumours: overlooked precursors of classic chordomas? Histopathology. 2004;44:597–602.

4. Yamaguchi T, Suzuki S, Ishiiwa H, Shimizu K, Ueda Y. Benign notochordal cell tumors: a comparative histological study of benign notochordal cell tumors, classic chordomas, and notochordal vestiges of fetal intervertebral discs. Am J Surg Pathol. 2004;28:756–61.
5. Kikuchi Y, Yamaguchi T, Kishi H, Azuhata K, Kimizuka G, Hiroshima K, Nakatani Y. Pulmonary tumor with notochordal differentiation: report of 2 cases suggestive of benign notochordal cell tumor of extraosseous origin. Am J Surg Pathol. 2011;35:1158–64.
6. Kyriakos M. Benign notochordal lesions of the axial skeleton: a review and current appraisal. Skelet Radiol. 2011;40:1141–52.
7. Nishiguchi T, Mochizuki K, Ohsawa M, Inoue T, Kageyama K, Suzuki A, Takami T, Miki Y. Differentiating benign notochordal cell tumors from chordomas: radiographic features on MRI, CT, and tomography. Am J Roentgenol. 2011;196:644–50.
8. Arain A, Hornicek FJ, Schwab JH, Chebib I, Damron TA. Chordoma arising from benign multifocal notochordal tumors. Skelet Radiol. 2017;46:1745–52.
9. Deshpande V, Petur Nielsen G, Rosenthal DI, Rosenberg AE. Intraosseous Benign Notochord Cell tumors (BNCT): further evidence supporting a relationship to chordoma. Am J Surg Pathol. 2007;31:1573–7.
10. Yamaguchi T, Watanabe-Ishiiwa H, Suzuki S, Igarashi Y, Ueda Y. Incipient chordoma: a report of two cases of early-stage chordoma arising from benign notochordal cell tumors. Mod Pathol. 2005;18:1005–10.
11. Zuckerman SL, Bilsky MH, Laufer I. Chordomas of the skull base, mobile spine, and sacrum: an epidemiologic investigation of presentation, treatment, and survival. World Neurosurg. 2018;113:e618–27.
12. Golden L, Pendharkar A, Fischbein N. Imaging chordoma and chondrosarcoma of the vertebrae and sacrum. In: Harsh GR, Vaz-Guimaraes F, editors. Chordomas chondrosarcomas skull base spine. 2nd ed. Elsevier; 2018. p. 79–86.
13. Rosenthal D, Scott J, Mankin H, Wismer G, Brady T. Sacrococcygeal chordoma: magnetic resonance imaging and computed tomography. Am J Roentgenol. 1985;145:143–7.
14. Sung MS, Lee GK, Kang HS, Kwon ST, Park JG, Suh JS, Cho GH, Lee SM, Chung MH, Resnick D. Sacrococcygeal chordoma: MR imaging in 30 patients. Skelet Radiol. 2005;34:87–94.
15. Wippold FJ, Koeller KK, Smirniotopoulos JG. Clinical and imaging features of cervical chordoma. Am J Roentgenol. 1999;172:1423–6.
16. Evans S, Khan Z, Jeys L, Grimer R. Extra-axial chordomas. Ann R Coll Surg Engl. 2016;98:324–8.
17. Wojno KJ, Hruban RH, Garin-Chesa P, Huvos AG. Chondroid chordomas and low-grade chondrosarcomas of the craniospinal axis. Am J Surg Pathol. 1992;16:1144–52.
18. Meis JM, Raymond AK, Evans HL, Charles RE, Giraldo AA. "Dedifferentiated" chordoma. A clinicopathologic and immunohistochemical study of three cases. Am J Surg Pathol. 1987;11:516–25.
19. Hung YP, Diaz-Perez JA, Cote GM, et al. Dedifferentiated chordoma: clinicopathologic and molecular characteristics with integrative analysis. Am J Surg Pathol. 2020;44:1213–23.
20. Hanna SA, Tirabosco R, Amin A, Pollock RC, Skinner JA, Cannon SR, Saifuddin A, Briggs TWR. Dedifferentiated chordoma: a report of four cases arising "de novo". J Bone Joint Surg Br. 2008;90-B:652–6.
21. Chak Lam Chan A, Yick Woon Tsang W, Pak To Chan G, Lee Lam Y, Kwong Chan M. Dedifferentiated chordoma with rhabdomyoblastic differentiation. Pathology. 2007;39:277–80.
22. Bovée JVMG, Cleton-Jansen A-M, Rosenberg C, Taminiau AHM, Cornelisse CJ, Hogendoorn PCW. Molecular genetic characterization of both components of a dedifferentiated chondrosarcoma, with implications for its histogenesis. J Pathol. 1999;189:454–62.
23. Curcio C, Cimera R, Aryeequaye R, Rao M, Fabbri N, Zhang Y, Hameed M. Poorly differentiated chordoma with whole-genome doubling evolving from a SMARCB1-deficient conventional chordoma: a case report. Genes Chromosom Cancer. 2021;60:43–8.
24. Shih AR, Cote GM, Chebib I, et al. Clinicopathologic characteristics of poorly differentiated chordoma. Mod Pathol. 2018;31:1237–45.

25. Yeter HG, Kosemehmetoglu K, Soylemezoglu F. Poorly differentiated chordoma: review of 53 cases. APMIS. 2019;127:607–15.
26. Hasselblatt M, Thomas C, Hovestadt V, et al. Poorly differentiated chordoma with SMARCB1/INI1 loss: a distinct molecular entity with dismal prognosis. Acta Neuropathol. 2016;132:149–51.
27. Huang S-C, Zhang L, Sung Y-S, Chen C-L, Kao Y-C, Agaram NP, Antonescu CR. Secondary EWSR1 gene abnormalities in SMARCB1 -deficient tumors with 22q11-12 regional deletions: potential pitfalls in interpreting EWSR1 FISH results. Genes Chromosom Cancer. 2016;55:767–76.

# Multidisciplinary Planning for Treatment of Chordoma

6

Nicholas A. Shepard and Matthew W. Colman

## Abbreviations

| | |
|---|---|
| CT | Computed tomography |
| CTV | Clinical target volume |
| GyRBE | Gray-equivalent relative biologic effectiveness |
| ICA | Internal carotid artery |
| LC | Local control |
| LR | Local recurrence |
| MRI | Magnetic resonance imaging |
| OS | Overall survival |
| PFS | Progression-free survival |
| RT | Radiation therapy |
| SBRT | Stereotactic body radiation therapy |
| SRS | Stereotactic radiosurgery |

## Introduction

Chordoma is a rare, locally aggressive neoplasm derived from notochordal remnants that affects the axial skeleton. With an annual age-adjusted incidence of 0.08 per 100,000 individuals and prevalence of less than one per 100,000 people, chordomas account for approximately 1–4% of all primary bone tumors [1, 2]. Traditionally thought of as predominantly affecting the sacrum (55%), skull base

N. A. Shepard · M. W. Colman (✉)
Department of Orthopedic Surgery, Midwest Orthopaedics at Rush University Medical Center, Chicago, IL, USA
e-mail: matthew.colman@rushortho.com





D. M. Sciubba, J. H. Schwab (eds.), *Chordoma of the Spine*,
https://doi.org/10.1007/978-3-030-76201-8_6

(35%), and mobile spine (10%), recent evidence suggests a more equal distribution throughout the axial skeleton [2, 3]. However, chordomas are the most common primary bone tumor affecting the sacrum and disproportionately account for more than 50% of primary sacral neoplasms [4].

Chordomas are characterized by insidious growth that can make timely diagnosis difficult. Depending on location, symptoms are often vague and consist of gastrointestinal, neurologic, or urinary complaints that result from mass effect or local invasion of surrounding neurologic structures. The locally aggressive and destructive nature combined with a propensity for local tumor recurrence has equated to morbidity and poor survival rates of approximately 60% at 5 years and 40% at 10 years [5].

## Basis for a Multidisciplinary Approach

The diagnosis and management of chordomas is complex due to tumor location, significant tumor burden involving critical neurovascular structures, tumor radio- and chemoresistance, and poor margination. As such, there is significant variability in the treatment of chordoma even among high-volume centers [6]. This discordance highlights the need for multidisciplinary involvement in specialized referral centers with access to the necessary resources in order to ensure optimum care and outcomes. This multidisciplinary approach is similar to best practices for other types of musculoskeletal neoplasms [7]. The management of chordomas requires multispecialty coordination between pathology, oncology (medical, radiation, surgical), radiology (radiation therapy, interventional, diagnostic), surgical subspecialties (orthopedics, neurosurgery, urology, otolaryngology, plastic and reconstructive), and palliative care or patient support infrastructure.

While critical, the extent and type of multispecialty involvement in chordoma is often driven by individual tumor characteristics. For example, if the location and tumor extent in the cervical spine or skull-base chordomas precludes en-bloc resection, alternative options focused on radiation or chemotherapy may take higher priority. This is particularly true in skull-base chordomas where the treatment goal of obtaining wide margins must be weighed against patient morbidity, preservation of neurologic function, and maintaining the quality of life [8, 9]. Similarly, if tumor extension into the spinal canal limits the ability to obtain wide margins, additional treatment modalities should be initiated to improve morbidity and decrease recurrence.

The literature regarding the management of chordomas is limited due to the rarity of the condition and is largely composed of lower quality observational data and case series. In December 2013, the Chordoma Global Census Group held a meeting involving international multispecialty providers that highlighted the need for a multidisciplinary approach for treating primary chordomas [10]. This was followed by a second consensus meeting in January 2015 that further reinforced the importance of multispecialty involvement in cases of chordoma recurrence

[11]. In the remainder of the chapter, we will highlight the importance of multidisciplinary involvement from the initial diagnosis to definitive treatment and follow-up.

## Diagnosis and Staging

### Diagnostic Radiology and Interventional Radiology

Advanced imaging is essential in the initial workup for chordomas for both diagnostic and staging purposes. While plain radiographs and computed tomography (CT) are helpful, especially for surgical planning, magnetic resonance imaging (MRI) of the entire spinal axis remains the mainstay of diagnostic imaging [12, 13]. With the help of an experienced radiologist, it may be possible to use these imaging modalities to differentiate between chordomas and other neoplasms of the sacrum, spine, and skull base including benign notochordal cell tumors, giant cell tumors, schwannoma, or chondrosarcoma (Fig. 6.1). Additionally, at the time of diagnosis, it is critical to identify synchronous foci of tumor in distant spinal axis locations, as these may require further interrogation or treatment.

Additional diagnostic imaging with the assistance of interventional radiology may also be necessary, particularly in cases of skull-base or mobile spine chordoma that may require vertebral or key segmental vessel sacrifice. Given tumor proximity to essential structures within the neck including the internal carotid artery (ICA) and vertebral artery, angiography with MR-angiogram or CT-angiogram is occasionally encouraged to better assess vessel patency, artery dominance, and delineate the intracranial vascular anatomy in preparation for surgical resection. In cases of vertebral artery or ICA involvement, formal angiography helps to determine whether the artery can be sacrificed during surgical tumor resection. Other interventions such as temporary balloon occlusion under direct neuromonitoring, coiling, or stenting can be considered depending on the oncologic goals of the multidisciplinary team [11]. Angiography is also helpful in defining the vascular supply to the spinal cord and key radiculomedullary vessel involvement in cases of planned thoracic segmental resection.

Coordination with interventional radiology is also useful in helping to establish a tissue diagnosis via image-guided needle biopsy. As in other settings, a biopsy in suspected cases of chordoma is essential to establish an accurate diagnosis and to delineate treatment options. Biopsy is highly recommended with the exception of rare cases of chordomas where biopsy would inflict significant morbidity or tumor contamination [10]. Indeed, chordoma remains one of the most fastidious and "seedable" tumors, and so the biopsy must be done with clean technique in a meticulously planned manner at the treating center. Communication between the surgical team and interventionalist is paramount in order to appropriately plan the biopsy in the setting of eventual surgical resection that allows tract resection and minimizes the risk of tumor seeding.

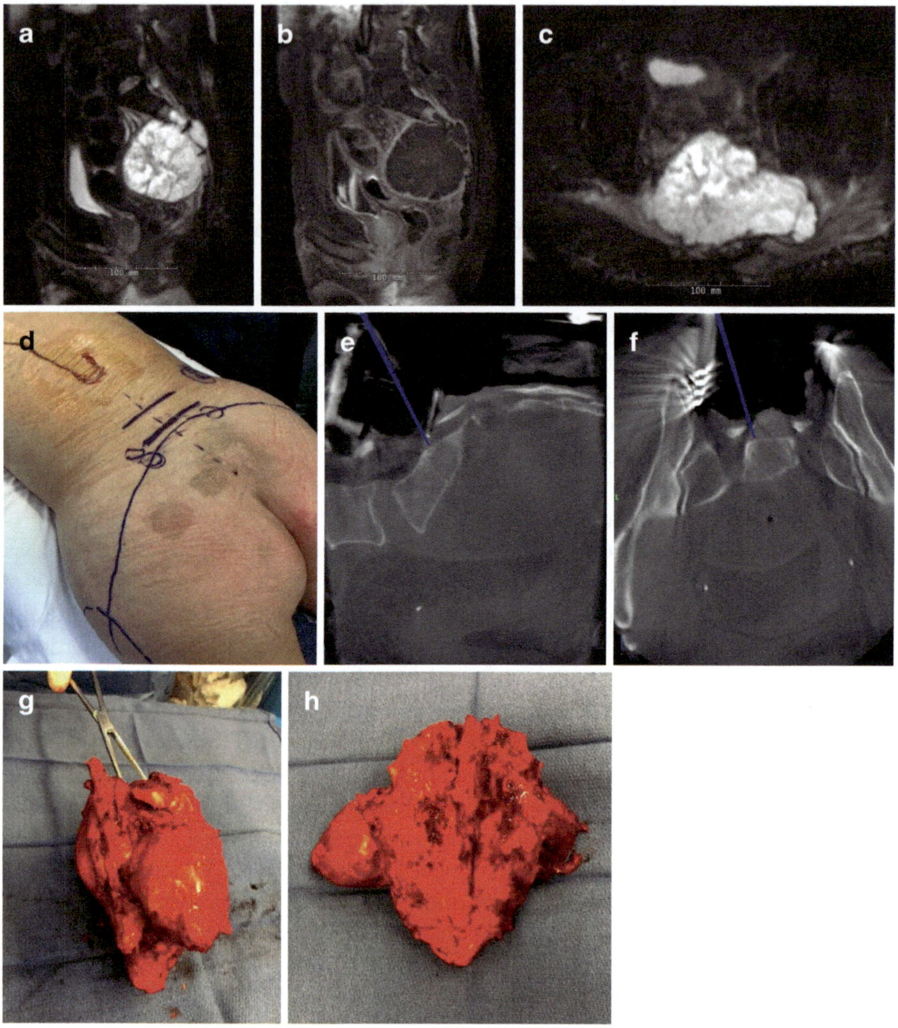

**Fig. 6.1** T2- and T1-weighted sagittal (**a**, **b**) and axial (**c**) MRI demonstrating the diagnostic complexity when considering chordoma as a diagnosis, and highlights the importance of multidisciplinary discussions in establishing the correct diagnosis. Despite the characteristic lobular T2 bright appearance with local invasion along the piriformis (**a**–**c**), an image-guided needle biopsy (**d**–**f**) demonstrated a chondroid pattern without physalipherous cells and negative staining for CK8/18, S100, and brachyury. Final pathology specimen was consistent with high-grade chondrosarcoma requiring wide surgical resection (**g**, **h**), and brachyury staining remained negative

## Pathology

Once a tissue sample is obtained, coordination with an experienced pathologist with access to the necessary immunostaining is critical to a prompt and accurate diagnosis. This includes staining for cytokeratin, epithelial membrane antigen, and S100

[14]. In addition, recent evidence has demonstrated the importance of brachyury (TBXT, T-Box Transcription Factor T), a transcription factor essential for notochord differentiation that is specific to notochord tumors and has prognostic implications [15, 16]. Combined positivity for brachyury and cytokeratin has shown very high sensitivity and specificity and is pathognomonic for chordomas [17].

Histiopathologic classification of chordomas further helps to direct management and prognosis. Subtypes include conventional, chondroid, dedifferentiated, and undifferentiated [18]. Conventional chordoma is the most frequently occurring subtype, while dedifferentiated chordomas account for 2–5% of all chordomas and are particularly concerning given their aggressive nature and high metastatic potential [19, 20]. While rare, treatment of dedifferentiated chordomas poses a challenge to traditional treatment paradigms and may benefit from systemic chemotherapy. These tumors must also be differentiated from benign notochordal cell tumors (BNTCs), which may be related to chordomas [21].

## Neoadjuvant and Adjuvant Treatments

### Radiation Oncology

Historically, radiation therapy (RT) as either a primary or adjuvant treatment for chordoma has been controversial due to the tumor's low-grade nature and slow growth which impart resistance to conventional fractional RT. However, advances in RT technology and improved RT protocols have led to increased use of RT in the treatment of skull-base, mobile spine, and sacral chordomas with the goal of eliminating microscopic disease, decreasing tumor burden, and decreasing local recurrence after surgery [22]. Although the gold standard for protocol, dosing, and timing remains undefined, modern indications for the use of radiation therapy in the treatment of chordoma include neoadjuvant or adjuvant use in primary resectable tumors, definitive treatment for unresectable tumors, adjuvant use with intentional or unintentional surgical margin contamination, and in cases of tumor recurrence [23]. Recent systematic analyses have demonstrated the clinical benefit of perioperative RT with improved survival and decreased recurrence [23–25]. This is particularly evident following surgical resection with positive margins, where adjuvant RT has been shown to increase OS [26].

Early use of photon radiotherapy was limited to doses less than 60 GyE due to its deleterious effects on adjacent structures. These limitations equated to recurrence rates ranging from 50% to 100% and five-year progression-free survival (PFS) less than 25% [27]. Specifically, multiple studies have noted standard photon RT at doses less than 70 Gy following surgical resection was not associated with improved OS or LC [28, 29]. Modern photon-based RT technology includes alternative means of radiation delivery including intensity modulated radiation therapy (IMRT) and stereotactic imaging guidance. These modalities achieve high doses of radiation while minimizing damage to surrounding tissue [30, 31]. One benefit to IMRT used in conjunction with imaging guidance is the ability to deliver significantly higher doses of RT in a single or hypofractionated manner. Hypofractionation of RT in a short time period has the potential benefit of overcoming the tumor cell's radioresistance by inducing higher degrees of apoptosis and DNA damage [32].

Another advancement in RT is the use of particle beam modalities (e.g., proton radiation) that deliver smaller doses of radiation to normal tissue and have a less exit-dose effect, thereby decreasing the risk of toxicity to critical structures [33]. One landmark study by the Delaney group analyzed the use of proton/photon RT in primary spinal and sacral tumors including chordomas. Their protocol included high-dose RT administered perioperatively with additional rounds based on tumor margin for a total median dose of 70.2 GCE for R0 resection (negative margins) and 77.4 GCE for R1/R2 resection (positive margins). In patients with chordoma, the authors noted over 90% local control (LC) rate at 7.3 years follow-up with only one patient developing local recurrence [34]. However, similar studies have failed to reproduce these benefits, which underscores the importance of multidisciplinary planning and recognition of center-specific capabilities [35].

Carbon ions are another particle beam RT that has gained increasing use in the treatment of chordomas. Compared to photons and proton RT, carbon ions deliver a greater amount of energy per unit length, or linear energy transfer (LET) [23]. When used in conjunction with surgical resection for primary chordoma, carbon ions have an 85% local control rate at 2 years follow-up [36]. In cases of inoperable or recurrent sacral chordoma, or in patients who cannot undergo surgery due to comorbidities, carbon ion RT has also been shown to have an LC rate of 53–77% and overall survival of 74–81.1% at 5 years with a relatively safe side effect profile [35, 37]. A limitation of this modality is widespread availability with carbon ion RT being performed at a limited number of international tertiary centers compared to the more common proton and photon RT modalities.

One other important multidisciplinary discussion between the surgical and radiation oncology teams surrounds implant selection for reconstruction. In addition to impairment of postoperative surveillance imaging, metal artifact including that from titanium-based implants impairs imaging and perturbs ion delivery within the clinical target volume (CTV), thereby decreasing the ability to achieve adequate dose delivery [38]. This was noted by Staub et al., who reported significantly lower LC rates in patients undergoing RT following surgical stabilization versus those with resection alone (100% vs 30%, respectively) [35]. Hence, effective communication and planning between the surgeon and radiation oncologist with minimization of metallic hardware and use of allografts or radiolucent implants is ideal for patients undergoing adjuvant RT.

Lastly, close communication and pre/post-resection imaging review between the surgeon and the radiation oncologist helps define high risk areas and the extent of dose delivery.

While adjuvant RT is beneficial for improving LC rates and overall survival, especially in cases with positive margins or recurrent chordoma, its use must be balanced against the potential for toxicity and adverse effects. Importantly, organs at risk include the optic nerves, temporal lobe, brainstem, spinal cord, peripheral nerves, gastrointestinal tract, visceral organs, and skin [10]. Toxic effects will often present late and may complicate the healing and recovery process following surgical intervention. Sacral insufficiency fractures are particularly common in RT treatment of sacral chordoma, with rates up to 47% following RT [39]. Therefore, it is critical to have a shared discussion with the patient, surgeon, and radiation oncologist prior to initiating definitive treatment.

## Medical Oncology

While surgical resection and RT remain the mainstay for treatment of chordoma of the skull base, mobile spine, and sacrum, there is increased interest in adjuvant and neoadjuvant medical therapy. However, there are no standard systemic agents currently approved for treatment of chordoma and their use has been confined to advanced symptomatic recurrent disease, metastases, and dedifferentiated chordoma [40]. Traditional medications such as anthracyclines, cisplatin, and camptothecin have shown minimal clinical benefit [41]. Irinotecan, one of the few drugs tested in a phase 2 trial, demonstrated a median 6-month progression-free survival of only 33%.

On the other hand, there has been recent interest in pathway inhibitors and molecular targeted therapy including vascular endothelial growth factor receptor (VEGFR), EGFR, platelet derived growth factor receptor (PDGFR), and the mammalian target of rapamycin (mTOR) pathway [42]. Imatinib is the most commonly used first-line agent and has been shown to produce moderate improvements in OS and PFS though its use may be complicated by anemia, fatigue, and intraventricular hemorrhage [43, 44]. Second-line treatment includes EGFR inhibitors (e.g., erlotinib, gefitinib, afatinib, and apatinib), which may be indicated following the failure of PDGFR inhibitors [45–47]. Afatinib has shown early success and may also promote degradation of brachyury increasing its application for chordoma [48].

Significant advancements in the understanding of chordoma biology have paralleled efforts to develop mechanism-based therapies. Multiple chromosomal abnormalities have been identified that are contributory in tumor development, though specific oncogenes have yet to be discovered [42]. One of the most promising findings has been the association of brachyury as a critical transcription factor for chordoma progression, making it a potential molecular target for medical therapy [49, 50]. A phase 1 trial studied the potential for a brachyury vaccine in 11 patients and noted two patients with evidence of disease control (one mixed response and one partial response) [51]. Interestingly, both patients had received adjuvant RT highlighting the complex interaction between radiation and immunogenic modulation. Similarly, as improvements in targeted-based therapy continue so will the need for coordination between radiation and medical oncologists.

Despite significant advancements, the role of immunotherapy remains poorly defined with low quality of evidence regarding their use in primary or recurrent chordoma. Multiple clinical trials are being planned or are ongoing dedicated to novel therapeutic targets specific to chordoma and its molecular mechanisms. As part of the initial treatment planning, discussion with a medical oncologist is necessary to provide insight whether targeted systemic therapy can be incorporated into the overall treatment algorithm.

## Surgical Care

### Perioperative Care

Surgical resection remains the mainstay for most primary, nonmetastatic chordomas. Achieving adequate margins while limiting morbidity is a challenge, even for specialized surgical teams, and often requires an extensive approach especially in the mobile spine and sacrum. With evolutions in perioperative care including multidisciplinary coordination, intensive care units, blood banking, and advancements in anesthesia, wide resection is an increasingly feasible and safe procedure [52]. In addition, improved neuromonitoring especially in cases involving cranial and spinal nerves or wide resection at cord level in the mobile spine help to reduce significant morbidity associated with neurologic injury. Given the complexity associated with these procedures and the extensive postoperative care often necessary, these cases should be performed in high-volume tertiary centers with access to multispecialty involvement.

### Establishing Surgical Goals

A critical question in the surgical management of chordoma is defining and achieving adequate margins. Surgical margins have been identified as one of the most important prognostic factors in chordoma treatment with the goal of obtaining wide resection with negative microscopic margins [53–56]. This is complicated by the tendency for loco-regional spread and the presence of skip-lesions that can be found up to 2 cm outside of the primary tumor mass in greater than 40% of cases [57]. Particular regions, especially those in skull-base or cervical spine, may not be amenable to wide resection or may have risk and morbidity profiles which outweigh the oncologic benefits of wide resection. In order to best define the surgical margins, it is imperative to have a multidisciplinary approach including pathologists, radiation oncologists, surgical oncologists, and additional primary surgical team members. Coordination with these additional surgical subspecialties (e.g., general surgeons, otolaryngologists, urologists, and thoracic surgeons) is necessitated by the tumor location, involvement of visceral structures, and surgical approach.

While en bloc resection with negative surgical margins remains the mainstay of surgical treatment, lesions not amenable to resection require alternative margin strategies. In these instances, stereotactic radiosurgery (SRS) or stereotactic body radiation therapy (SBRT) may be an alternative treatment method. SRS typically refers to high-dose, image-guided conformal radiation delivered as a single or hypofractionated dose and can be combined with a limited surgical approach, or "separation surgery." The goals of separation surgery include circumferential decompression and tumor removal around the spinal cord, with possible stabilization [58]. However, unlike en bloc resection, separation surgery aims at limited intralesional tumor resection to create a tumor-free zone around the spinal cord and maximize the efficacy and minimize the toxicity of SRS [59]. Separation surgery in combination with SRS has been used for chordoma of the mobile spine and sacrum with high LR and OS rates [60, 61].

Another major consideration in surgical planning that requires coordination between a multidisciplinary team is whether any surgical intervention is the optimal treatment for a specific patient. In some instances, the potential operative risks and postoperative morbidity may outweigh the benefits of either en bloc resection or more limited separation surgery. Factors to consider include tumor location, patient comorbidities, and patient preference (Fig. 6.2). In cases where surgical resection is not viable, SRS has been found to be an acceptable treatment alternative. Jin et al. reported on 35 patients undergoing SRS for mobile spine and sacral chordoma, including 12 treated definitively with SRS. In patients with sacral chordoma, the authors found no difference in LCR between those treated with surgery versus those undergoing SRS alone [60]. Additional studies have also supported the use of definitive SRS and RT in both primary and recurrent chordoma of the skull base, mobile spine, and sacrum [24, 37, 62, 63].

## Surgical Coordination

Achieving the desired surgical margin requires careful consideration of the specific steps required to do so. The spinal surgery oncologist may be best equipped to plan critical technical steps in en bloc resection such as the opening of the spinal ring, protection of neurologic structures, specimen removal, and reconstruction. However,

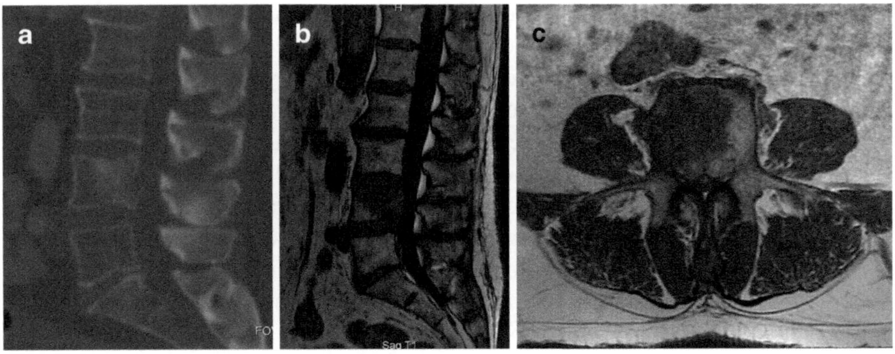


**Fig. 6.2** Sagittal CT (**a**), T1-weighted sagittal (**b**), and axial (**c**) MRI demonstrating a case of an isolated biopsy-proven mobile spine chordoma with feasible and low-morbidity en bloc resection as the standard treatment option. However, after thorough multidisciplinary discussion and ethics consultation, the patient with sound mind and informed consent elected definitive XRT because of family and personal preferences. The patient received definitive SBRT radiation therapy (long-term follow-up not available at the time of this preparation)

multidisciplinary partners including general surgery, urologic surgery, thoracic surgery, ENT, intensive care medicine, and others are just as vital in planning, staging, and order of approaches, surgical management of surrounding viscera, and perioperative physiologic care.

Tumors of the cervical and upper thoracic spine are complicated by tumor location relative to the esophagus, trachea, nerve roots, and essential vascular structures including the vertebral arteries in the cervical spine and great vessels in the thoracic spine. If an anterior cervical approach is necessary, collaboration with an otolaryngologist is helpful in delineating the complex neck anatomy in order to reduce morbidity. As a consequence of this approach, surgical resection or adjuvant RT function of the esophagus and/or trachea may also be compromised necessitating tracheostomy and temporary or permanent percutaneous endoscopic gastrostomy (PEG) tube placement [52]. Similarly, if anterior approaches to the thoracolumbar spine are required it should be done in coordination with a thoracic, general, or vascular surgeon, who can also assist with approach and resection of viscerally or vascularly involved tumor.

Surgical management of sacral chordoma poses unique challenges given the proximity of the tumor mass to intrapelvic viscera and critical neurovascular structures [64]. Coordination with a general surgeon is often helpful for many reasons. First, in cases of neoplastic extension to the mesorectum or posterior abdominal wall, the risk of tumor involvement is particularly high and may require bowel resection and colostomy in order to obtain adequate margins [9]. Soft tissue reconstruction may also be necessary to prevent bowel herniation through the surgical defect behind the rectum. Most importantly, sacral chordomas requiring bone osteotomy above S3 are best managed with a combined approach with anterior exposure, mid-sacral and internal vasculature control, colostomy, rectus abdominus flap harvest, and other viscera management, followed in a staged fashion with posterior tumor resection, removal, and soft tissue reconstruction. General surgery and plastic surgery are key partners in the success of the combined anterior/posterior approach (Fig. 6.3). Coordination with urology may also be needed in cases with tumor encroachment of the ureters or bladder. In our center, every anterior sacral approach is proceeded by bilateral ureteral stent placement preoperatively.

Another difficulty seen with resection of chordoma is coverage and wound issues that result from resection and RT. This is of particular importance in sacral chordoma, where wound dehiscence has been reported in up to 46% of cases [65, 66]. Preoperative and intra-operative consultation with a plastic surgeon regarding the need for various reconstruction options may be necessary. These include local flaps (e.g., gluteal), pedicle flaps (e.g., rectus abdominus or myocutaneous), and free flaps (e.g., latissimus dorsi) depending on the size of the defect and available tissue following wide resection [67, 68]. Occasionally, flap coverage is deferred until confirming adequate histologic margins, so in the interim vacuum-assisted closure can be used to promote granular tissue formation and a clean wound bed.

Surgical management of chordoma has a high risk of complication given the proximity of the tumor to essential structures including the brainstem, spinal cord,

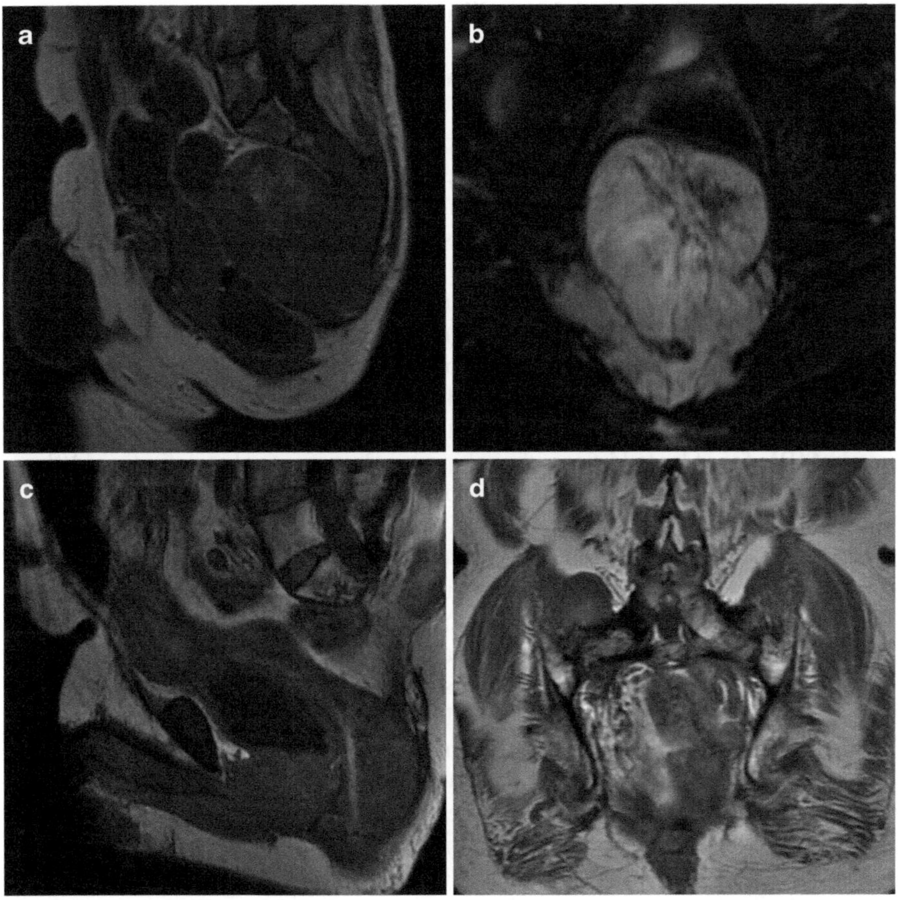


**Fig. 6.3** Sagittal T1- (**a**) and coronal T2 (**b**)-weighted MRI demonstrating a massive sacral chordoma with intracanal extension and spread along the piriformis and mesorectum. The surgical approach consisted of multidisciplinary anterior/posterior en bloc sacrectomy, transection of the thecal sac below the S1 nerve roots, and colostomy (**c**/**d**). A multidisciplinary team including general surgery, urology, orthopedic spine oncology, and plastic surgery was involved

peripheral nerves, and visceral structures. In a series of sacral chordoma treated with surgical resection at Memorial Sloan Kettering, complications included the need for self-catheterization (74%), sexual dysfunction (67%), and permanent colostomy (29%) [64]. Another series helped define the critical sacral nerve root as S3 in preserving bowel, bladder, and sexual function [69]. Functional loss may also occur, especially in cases of intentional nerve root resection in the cervical, lumbar, or sacral spines. This may be ameliorated by an eventual tendon or nerve transfer. Preoperative patient counseling with a multidisciplinary team regarding these outcomes and possible need for prolonged care is necessary prior to surgical intervention and should take patient preferences into consideration as part of shared decision-making.

## Postoperative Care and Surveillance

### Tumor Surveillance and Monitoring

Coordinated efforts between surgical specialties, medical and radiation oncologists to monitor disease progression or recurrence is crucial to the chordoma treatment paradigm. Local or regional recurrence may exceed 50% following surgical resection with or without RT, and often occurs late highlighting the need for long-term follow-up at 5 and 10 years or beyond [10]. Unfortunately, data on long-term recurrence-free survival (RFS) are lacking though estimates for 10-year RFS in skull base (42–71%), mobile spine (32%), and sacral chordoma (43%) point to the high risk of recurrence without a noticeable plateau even at 15-year follow-up [70–72]. Current recommendations include MRI of the primary tumor site and areas at risk for tumor seeding at 3–6-month intervals for the first 5 years, followed by yearly MRIs for at least 15 years though protocols may vary by institution [10].

Continued monitoring for metastatic spread is another important consideration in chordoma surveillance. While chordoma is typically a low-grade, locally aggressive tumor, metastases are noted in 5% of cases at presentation and have been noted in 30–40% of cases in late stages of the disease [73]. Common sites of metastases include the lung or bone. As such, additional imaging including total body CT and full spine MRI may be necessary to evaluate for distant spread during the follow-up period, especially in cases of recurrent disease [11].

Monitoring tumor response following RT and systemic therapies remains a challenge. Two commonly used criteria include Choi's criteria, which assesses tumor size and density based on contrast CT or MRI, and the Response Evaluation Criteria in Solid Tumors (RECIST), which defines a partial response as ≥20% decrease in tumor growth and clinically meaningful response as ≥30% decrease in maximum tumor diameter [74, 75]. Additional radiographic assessment includes evaluation of tumor caliber, density, contrast enhancement, and uptake on PET scan. Clinical parameters indicative of symptomatic improvement include pain relief and patient-reported outcomes, which may supplement radiographic data regarding tumor activity.

## Patient Support and Specialty Services

### Palliative Care

Palliative care plays a key role in providing supportive care to patients with chordoma and is recommended in all stages of disease. As with other serious illnesses, palliative care is part of the comprehensive treatment approach and helps to address psychosocial concerns in addition to clinical symptoms [76]. Importantly, palliative care may be actively involved with analgesia which is complicated in chordoma of the skull, spine, and sacrum. Given the intricate relationship between the tumor and surrounding neurologic structures, significant neuropathic pain often accompanies somatic pain related to the soft tissue burden and active disease process [77]. Delineating the source of pain is crucial to guide appropriate pain management strategies including medical therapy and additional analgesic procedures as needed [78].

Additionally, palliative care can help to coordinate psychosocial support structures to address patient-specific needs. These include chaplain or religious services, family unit and social support, and general well-being. In cases of late-stage or recurrent disease, their role is critical in coordinating goals of care between the patient and treatment teams. By facilitating shared decision-making, decisions can be made regarding short- and long-term prognostication, continued treatment and palliative procedures, advance directives, and end-of-life decision-making [11].

## Future Directions

### Prognostication

Identifying prognostic factors that predict survival and treatment response is beneficial to physicians as they develop individualized treatment algorithms and counsel patients throughout the disease process. Recent research has been geared toward better delineating factors that influence PFS and OS. A systematic review by Bakker et al. noted multiple adverse prognostic factors including female sex, increasing extent of tumor invasion, presence of metastasis, older age, non-total reaction, large tumor size, and dedifferentiated subtypes [79]. The development of a population-based nomogram provides further utility in using these prognostic factors to assess and guide treatment [80, 81]. Additionally, the development of machine learning to predict survival and response to treatment is an emerging area of research that can be used to individualize treatment algorithms and assist in patient counseling [82, 83].

### Genomic Analysis

Improvements in genomic sequencing have led to a greater understanding of novel pathways and biologic markers in chordoma [42, 84, 85]. These include mutations in cell cycle regulation, growth factor signaling pathways, and immune checkpoints that could serve as therapeutic targets [86, 87]. Multiple clinical trials are underway as a result of advances in genomic sequencing; however, enrollment is often limited to advanced, recurrent, or metastatic disease. Additionally, the genomic landscape likely differs based on location between skull-based, mobile spine, and sacral chordoma.

It may also be possible to repurpose existing medications used or developed for other pathologies for the treatment of chordoma. Using a combination of computational drug repositioning strategies, in vitro assessment, and pre-existing drug databases researchers have identified potential compounds that may work synergistically to inhibit chordoma-specific cell lines. Since these medications have already gone through human safety trials, their approval for use in chordoma could be expeditious and less costly versus identifying and developing de novo therapeutic agents [83].

## Conclusion

Chordoma involving the skull base, mobile spine, or sacrum is a complex disease that poses challenges in all stages of care. Multidisciplinary involvement and coordination is required in diagnosing, prognosticating, treating, following, and supporting these patients. Specialist involvement is highly dependent on tumor location, but often involves a team of medical and surgical oncologists, radiologists, and a variety of surgical subspecialties. Coordination between the patient and the multidisciplinary team is critical for the development of an individualized treatment regimen, with the goal or tumor control and optimizing function while limiting patient morbidity.

## References

1. Stiller CA, Trama A, Serraino D, et al. Descriptive epidemiology of sarcomas in Europe: report from the RARECARE project. Eur J Cancer. 2013;49(3):684–95.
2. McMaster ML, Goldstein AM, Bromley CM, Ishibe N, Parry DM. Chordoma: incidence and survival patterns in the United States, 1973–1995. Cancer Causes Control. 2001;12(1):1–11.
3. Chugh R, Tawbi H, Lucas DR, Biermann JS, Schuetze SM, Baker LH. Chordoma: the nonsarcoma primary bone tumor. Oncologist. 2007;12(11):1344–50.
4. Cheng EY, Ozerdemoglu RA, Transfeldt EE, Thompson RC Jr. Lumbosacral chordoma. Prognostic factors and treatment. Spine (Phila Pa 1976). 1999;24(16):1639–45.
5. Lee IJ, Lee RJ, Fahim DK. Prognostic factors and survival outcome in patients with chordoma in the United States: a population-based analysis. World Neurosurg. 2017;104:346–55.
6. Dea N, Fisher CG, Reynolds JJ, et al. Current treatment strategy for newly diagnosed chordoma of the mobile spine and sacrum: results of an international survey. J Neurosurg Spine. 2018;30(1):119–25.
7. Randall RL, Bruckner JD, Papenhausen MD, Thurman T, Conrad EU 3rd. Errors in diagnosis and margin determination of soft-tissue sarcomas initially treated at non-tertiary centers. Orthopedics. 2004;27(2):209–12.
8. Di Maio S, Temkin N, Ramanathan D, Sekhar LN. Current comprehensive management of cranial base chordomas: 10-year meta-analysis of observational studies. J Neurosurg. 2011;115(6):1094–105.
9. Radaelli S, Fossati P, Stacchiotti S, et al. The sacral chordoma margin. Eur J Surg Oncol. 2020;46(8):1415–22.
10. Stacchiotti S, Sommer J, Chordoma Global Consensus Group. Building a global consensus approach to chordoma: a position paper from the medical and patient community. Lancet Oncol. 2015;16(2):e71–83.
11. Stacchiotti S, Gronchi A, Fossati P, et al. Best practices for the management of local-regional recurrent chordoma: a position paper by the Chordoma Global Consensus Group. Ann Oncol. 2017;28(6):1230–42.

12. Smolders D, Wang X, Drevelengas A, Vanhoenacker F, De Schepper AM. Value of MRI in the diagnosis of non-clival, non-sacral chordoma. Skelet Radiol. 2003;32(6):343–50.
13. Llauger J, Palmer J, Amores S, Bague S, Camins A. Primary tumors of the sacrum: diagnostic imaging. AJR Am J Roentgenol. 2000;174(2):417–24.
14. Crapanzano JP, Ali SZ, Ginsberg MS, Zakowski MF. Chordoma: a cytologic study with histologic and radiologic correlation. Cancer. 2001;93(1):40–51.
15. Vujovic S, Henderson S, Presneau N, et al. Brachyury, a crucial regulator of notochordal development, is a novel biomarker for chordomas. J Pathol. 2006;209(2):157–65.
16. Otani R, Mukasa A, Shin M, et al. Brachyury gene copy number gain and activation of the PI3K/Akt pathway: association with upregulation of oncogenic Brachyury expression in skull base chordoma. J Neurosurg. 2018;128(5):1428–37.
17. Oakley GJ, Fuhrer K, Seethala RR. Brachyury, SOX-9, and podoplanin, new markers in the skull base chordoma vs chondrosarcoma differential: a tissue microarray-based comparative analysis. Mod Pathol. 2008;21(12):1461–9.
18. Jo VY, Fletcher CD. WHO classification of soft tissue tumours: an update based on the 2013 (4th) edition. Pathology. 2014;46(2):95–104.
19. Yamada Y, Gounder M, Laufer I. Multidisciplinary management of recurrent chordomas. Curr Treat Options in Oncol. 2013;14(3):442–53.
20. Hanna SA, Tirabosco R, Amin A, et al. Dedifferentiated chordoma: a report of four cases arising 'de novo'. J Bone Joint Surg Br. 2008;90(5):652–6.
21. Deshpande V, Nielsen GP, Rosenthal DI, Rosenberg AE. Intraosseous benign notochord cell tumors (BNCT): further evidence supporting a relationship to chordoma. Am J Surg Pathol. 2007;31(10):1573–7.
22. Rotondo RL, Folkert W, Liebsch NJ, et al. High-dose proton-based radiation therapy in the management of spine chordomas: outcomes and clinicopathological prognostic factors. J Neurosurg Spine. 2015;23(6):788–97.
23. Pennicooke B, Laufer I, Sahgal A, et al. Safety and local control of radiation therapy for chordoma of the spine and sacrum: a systematic review. Spine (Phila Pa 1976). 2016;41(Suppl 20):S186–92.
24. Kabolizadeh P, Chen YL, Liebsch N, et al. Updated outcome and analysis of tumor response in mobile spine and sacral chordoma treated with definitive high-dose photon/proton radiation therapy. Int J Radiat Oncol Biol Phys. 2017;97(2):254–62.
25. Aibe N, Demizu Y, Sulaiman NS, et al. Outcomes of patients with primary sacral chordoma treated with definitive proton beam therapy. Int J Radiat Oncol Biol Phys. 2018;100(4):972–9.
26. Dial BL, Kerr DL, Lazarides AL, et al. The role of radiotherapy for chordoma patients managed with surgery: analysis of the national cancer database. Spine (Phila Pa 1976). 2020;45(12):E742–51.
27. Catton C, O'Sullivan B, Bell R, et al. Chordoma: long-term follow-up after radical photon irradiation. Radiother Oncol. 1996;41(1):67–72.
28. Yolcu Y, Wahood W, Alvi MA, et al. Evaluating the role of adjuvant radiotherapy in the management of sacral and vertebral chordoma: results from a national database. World Neurosurg. 2019;127:e1137–44.
29. Houdek MT, Rose PS, Hevesi M, et al. Low dose radiotherapy is associated with local complications but not disease control in sacral chordoma. J Surg Oncol. 2019;119(7):856–63.
30. Suit HD, Goitein M, Munzenrider J, et al. Definitive radiation therapy for chordoma and chondrosarcoma of base of skull and cervical spine. J Neurosurg. 1982;56(3):377–85.
31. Zabel-du Bois A, Nikoghosyan A, Schwahofer A, et al. Intensity modulated radiotherapy in the management of sacral chordoma in primary versus recurrent disease. Radiother Oncol. 2010;97(3):408–12.
32. Garcia-Barros M, Paris F, Cordon-Cardo C, et al. Tumor response to radiotherapy regulated by endothelial cell apoptosis. Science. 2003;300(5622):1155–9.
33. Hug EB, Slater JD. Proton radiation therapy for chordomas and chondrosarcomas of the skull base. Neurosurg Clin N Am. 2000;11(4):627–38.

34. DeLaney TF, Liebsch NJ, Pedlow FX, et al. Long-term results of Phase II study of high dose photon/proton radiotherapy in the management of spine chordomas, chondrosarcomas, and other sarcomas. J Surg Oncol. 2014;110(2):115–22.
35. Staab A, Rutz HP, Ares C, et al. Spot-scanning-based proton therapy for extracranial chordoma. Int J Radiat Oncol Biol Phys. 2011;81(4):e489–96.
36. Uhl M, Welzel T, Jensen A, et al. Carbon ion beam treatment in patients with primary and recurrent sacrococcygeal chordoma. Strahlenther Onkol. 2015;191(7):597–603.
37. Imai R, Kamada T, Araki N, Working Group for Bone and Soft Tissue Sarcomas. Carbon ion radiation therapy for unresectable sacral chordoma: an analysis of 188 cases. Int J Radiat Oncol Biol Phys. 2016;95(1):322–7.
38. Nevelsky A, Borzov E, Daniel S, Bar-Deroma R. Perturbation effects of the carbon fiber-PEEK screws on radiotherapy dose distribution. J Appl Clin Med Phys. 2017;18(2):62–8.
39. Osler P, Bredella MA, Hess KA, et al. Sacral insufficiency fractures are common after high-dose radiation for sacral chordomas treated with or without surgery. Clin Orthop Relat Res. 2016;474(3):766–72.
40. Fleming GF, Heimann PS, Stephens JK, et al. Dedifferentiated chordoma. Response to aggressive chemotherapy in two cases. Cancer. 1993;72(3):714–8.
41. Walcott BP, Nahed BV, Mohyeldin A, Coumans JV, Kahle KT, Ferreira MJ. Chordoma: current concepts, management, and future directions. Lancet Oncol. 2012;13(2):e69–76.
42. Meng T, Jin J, Jiang C, et al. Molecular targeted therapy in the treatment of chordoma: a systematic review. Front Oncol. 2019;9:30.
43. Casali PG, Messina A, Stacchiotti S, et al. Imatinib mesylate in chordoma. Cancer. 2004;101(9):2086–97.
44. Mercier F, Guiot MC, Bojanowski MW. Treatment of chordoma with imatinib complicated by intracranial hemorrhage: a case showing dissociation between biological effect and therapeutic outcome. J Neuro-Oncol. 2012;107(2):435–7.
45. Launay SG, Chetaille B, Medina F, et al. Efficacy of epidermal growth factor receptor targeting in advanced chordoma: case report and literature review. BMC Cancer. 2011;11:423.
46. Singhal N, Kotasek D, Parnis FX. Response to erlotinib in a patient with treatment refractory chordoma. Anti-Cancer Drugs. 2009;20(10):953–5.
47. Liu C, Jia Q, Wei H, et al. Apatinib in patients with advanced chordoma: a single-arm, single-centre, phase 2 study. Lancet Oncol. 2020;21(9):1244–52.
48. Magnaghi P, Salom B, Cozzi L, et al. Afatinib is a new therapeutic approach in chordoma with a unique ability to target EGFR and brachyury. Mol Cancer Ther. 2018;17(3):603–13.
49. Presneau N, Shalaby A, Ye H, et al. Role of the transcription factor T (brachyury) in the pathogenesis of sporadic chordoma: a genetic and functional-based study. J Pathol. 2011;223(3):327–35.
50. Henderson SR, Guiliano D, Presneau N, et al. A molecular map of mesenchymal tumors. Genome Biol. 2005;6(9):R76.
51. Heery CR, Singh BH, Rauckhorst M, et al. Phase I trial of a yeast-based therapeutic cancer vaccine (GI-6301) targeting the transcription factor brachyury. Cancer Immunol Res. 2015;3(11):1248–56.
52. Bongers MER, Dea N, Ames CP, Schwab JH. Surgical strategies for chordoma. Neurosurg Clin N Am. 2020;31(2):251–61.
53. Bergh P, Kindblom LG, Gunterberg B, Remotti F, Ryd W, Meis-Kindblom JM. Prognostic factors in chordoma of the sacrum and mobile spine: a study of 39 patients. Cancer. 2000;88(9):2122–34.
54. Kayani B, Sewell MD, Tan KA, et al. Prognostic factors in the operative management of sacral chordomas. World Neurosurg. 2015;84(5):1354–61.
55. Angelini A, Pala E, Calabro T, Maraldi M, Ruggieri P. Prognostic factors in surgical resection of sacral chordoma. J Surg Oncol. 2015;112(4):344–51.
56. Varga PP, Szoverfi Z, Fisher CG, et al. Surgical treatment of sacral chordoma: prognostic variables for local recurrence and overall survival. Eur Spine J. 2015;24(5):1092–101.

57. Akiyama T, Ogura K, Gokita T, et al. Analysis of the infiltrative features of chordoma: the relationship between micro-skip metastasis and postoperative outcomes. Ann Surg Oncol. 2018;25(4):912–9.
58. Ibarra-Perez C, Green L. Electric cardiac pacemakers. Prensa Med Mex. 1971;36(1):40–6.
59. Laufer I, Iorgulescu JB, Chapman T, et al. Local disease control for spinal metastases following "separation surgery" and adjuvant hypofractionated or high-dose single-fraction stereotactic radiosurgery: outcome analysis in 186 patients. J Neurosurg Spine. 2013;18(3):207–14.
60. Jin CJ, Berry-Candelario J, Reiner AS, et al. Long-term outcomes of high-dose single-fraction radiosurgery for chordomas of the spine and sacrum. J Neurosurg Spine. 2019:1–10.
61. Lockney DT, Shub T, Hopkins B, et al. Spinal stereotactic body radiotherapy following intralesional curettage with separation surgery for initial or salvage chordoma treatment. Neurosurg Focus. 2017;42(1):E4.
62. Wu S, Li P, Cai X, et al. Carbon ion radiotherapy for patients with extracranial chordoma or chondrosarcoma – initial experience from Shanghai Proton and Heavy Ion Center. J Cancer. 2019;10(15):3315–22.
63. Demizu Y, Jin D, Sulaiman NS, et al. Particle therapy using protons or carbon ions for unresectable or incompletely resected bone and soft tissue sarcomas of the pelvis. Int J Radiat Oncol Biol Phys. 2017;98(2):367–74.
64. Schwab JH, Healey JH, Rose P, Casas-Ganem J, Boland PJ. The surgical management of sacral chordomas. Spine (Phila Pa 1976). 2009;34(24):2700–4.
65. Sciubba DM, Nelson C, Gok B, et al. Evaluation of factors associated with postoperative infection following sacral tumor resection. J Neurosurg Spine. 2008;9(6):593–9.
66. Ruggieri P, Angelini A, Pala E, Mercuri M. Infections in surgery of primary tumors of the sacrum. Spine (Phila Pa 1976). 2012;37(5):420–8.
67. Kim JE, Pang J, Christensen JM, et al. Soft-tissue reconstruction after total en bloc sacrectomy. J Neurosurg Spine. 2015;22(6):571–81.
68. Reynolds JJ, Khundkar R, Boriani S, et al. Soft tissue and bone defect management in total sacrectomy for primary sacral tumors: a systematic review with expert recommendations. Spine (Phila Pa 1976). 2016;41(Suppl 20):S199–204.
69. van Wulfften Palthe OD, Houdek MT, Rose PS, et al. How does the level of nerve root resection in en bloc sacrectomy influence patient-reported outcomes? Clin Orthop Relat Res. 2017;475(3):607–16.
70. Tzortzidis F, Elahi F, Wright D, Natarajan SK, Sekhar LN. Patient outcome at long-term follow-up after aggressive microsurgical resection of cranial base chordomas. Neurosurgery. 2006;59(2):230–7; discussion 230–237.
71. Cloyd JM, Acosta FL Jr, Polley MY, Ames CP. En bloc resection for primary and metastatic tumors of the spine: a systematic review of the literature. Neurosurgery. 2010;67(2):435–44; discussion 444–435.
72. Radaelli S, Stacchiotti S, Ruggieri P, et al. Sacral chordoma: long-term outcome of a large series of patients surgically treated at two reference centers. Spine (Phila Pa 1976). 2016;41(12):1049–57.
73. Bjornsson J, Wold LE, Ebersold MJ, Laws ER. Chordoma of the mobile spine. A clinicopathologic analysis of 40 patients. Cancer. 1993;71(3):735–40.
74. Choi H, Charnsangavej C, Faria SC, et al. Correlation of computed tomography and positron emission tomography in patients with metastatic gastrointestinal stromal tumor treated at a single institution with imatinib mesylate: proposal of new computed tomography response criteria. J Clin Oncol. 2007;25(13):1753–9.
75. Eisenhauer EA, Therasse P, Bogaerts J, et al. New response evaluation criteria in solid tumours: revised RECIST guideline (version 1.1). Eur J Cancer. 2009;45(2):228–47.
76. Tassinari D, Drudi F, Monterubbianesi MC, et al. Early palliative care in advanced oncologic and non-oncologic chronic diseases: a systematic review of literature. Rev Recent Clin Trials. 2016;11(1):63–71.

77. Phimolsarnti R, Waikakul S. Prevalence of neuropathic pain after radical sacral chordoma resection: an observational cohort study with 10-year follow-up. Eur J Orthop Surg Traumatol. 2015;25(Suppl 1):S225–31.
78. Caraceni A, Hanks G, Kaasa S, et al. Use of opioid analgesics in the treatment of cancer pain: evidence-based recommendations from the EAPC. Lancet Oncol. 2012;13(2):e58–68.
79. Bakker SH, Jacobs WCH, Pondaag W, et al. Chordoma: a systematic review of the epidemiology and clinical prognostic factors predicting progression-free and overall survival. Eur Spine J. 2018;27(12):3043–58.
80. Lin K, Song K, Wang S, Jiang L, Wang H, Dong J. Predict overall survival of spinal conventional chordoma: development and assessment of a new predictive nomogram. Clin Neurol Neurosurg. 2020;197:106174.
81. Zheng W, Huang Y, Guan T, et al. Application of nomograms to predict overall and cancer-specific survival in patients with chordoma. J Bone Oncol. 2019;18:100247.
82. Karhade AV, Thio Q, Ogink P, et al. Development of machine learning algorithms for prediction of 5-year spinal chordoma survival. World Neurosurg. 2018;119:e842–7.
83. Anderson E, Havener TM, Zorn KM, et al. Synergistic drug combinations and machine learning for drug repurposing in chordoma. Sci Rep. 2020;10(1):12982.
84. Tarpey PS, Behjati S, Young MD, et al. The driver landscape of sporadic chordoma. Nat Commun. 2017;8(1):890.
85. Frezza AM, Botta L, Trama A, Dei Tos AP, Stacchiotti S. Chordoma: update on disease, epidemiology, biology and medical therapies. Curr Opin Oncol. 2019;31(2):114–20.
86. Hoffman SE, Al Abdulmohsen SA, Gupta S, et al. Translational windows in Chordoma: a target appraisal. Front Neurol. 2020;11:657.
87. Gill CM, Fowkes M, Shrivastava RK. Emerging therapeutic targets in chordomas: a review of the literature in the genomic era. Neurosurgery. 2020;86(2):E118–23.

# Part III

# Surgical Management of Chordoma

# Surgical Management of Chordoma of the Occipitocervical Junction

7

Zach Pennington, Jeff Ehresman, Andrew Schilling, and Daniel M. Sciubba

## Abbreviations

| | |
|---|---|
| ALL | Anterior longitudinal ligament |
| BSSMO | Bilateral-sagittal split mandibular osteotomy |
| CBVA | Chin-brown vertical angle |
| CT | Computed tomography |
| IMRT | Intensity-modulated radiation therapy |
| LMG | Labial-mandibular-glossotomy |
| MRI | Magnetic resonance imaging |
| OC | Occipitocervical |
| SBRT | Stereotactic external beam radiotherapy |
| SVA | Sagittal vertical axis |
| TCR | Transmandibular-circumglossal-retropharyngeal |
| WBB | Weinstein-Boriani-Biagini |
| XRT | X-ray therapy |

## Introduction

Chordoma can occur anywhere along the axial skeleton from the dorsum sella to the sacrum. This includes the occipitocervical junction, defined anatomically by the atlas (C1 vertebra), axis (C2 vertebra), and skull base, along with the associated

Z. Pennington · J. Ehresman · A. Schilling · D. M. Sciubba (✉)
Department of Neurosurgery, Johns Hopkins University School of Medicine, Baltimore, MD, USA
e-mail: dsciubba1@northwell.edu



D. M. Sciubba, J. H. Schwab (eds.), *Chordoma of the Spine*,
https://doi.org/10.1007/978-3-030-76201-8_7

ligaments that maintain the integrity of this highly mobile osseoligamentous complex. Lesions of the occipitocervical junction represent a pathology unique from the well-known skull base lesions, as resection of the former is extremely destabilizing and may require a highly morbid, staged surgical approach in order to achieve *en bloc* R0 resection.

Owing to the relative rarity of chordomas overall and the complex nature of the local anatomy, descriptions of the surgical management of craniocervical chordoma are less common than those of purely clival lesions. The first report of a craniocervical chordoma was made by Fischer and Steiner in 1907 [1], who described the biopsy of a large chordoma extending from the clivus to the axis. However, it was not until 1979 that the surgical management of a craniocervical lesion was described. At that time Wu and colleagues reported treating a C1 chordoma with transoral biopsy followed by an occiput-C4 fusion [2]. Since then, other reports have been published [3–5], with the largest series being published by Shin et al. [5] as part of a larger series of craniovertebral junction tumors. Good data regarding the relative frequency of these lesions are not available, as the Surveillance, Epidemiology, and End Results (SEER) registry does not segregate craniocervical lesions from lesions of the mobile spine or skull bones. However, a recent multi-institutional series published by the AOSpine Tumor Knowledge Forum found less than 25% of mobile spine lesions localized to the cervical vertebrae [6]. Consequently, it seems likely that lesions centered at the craniocervical junction are extremely rare.

In this chapter we describe the operative management of these lesions, focusing on the technical aspects of the different approaches, as well as reconstruction techniques and potential pitfalls/complications of the different surgical options. For a discussion of radiotherapy and chemotherapy for mobile spine chordoma, we refer the reader to Chaps. 14, 15, and 16. Additionally, while we touch on the use of multidisciplinary teams, we refer the reader to Chap. 12 for a more detailed discussion.

## Anatomy of the Craniocervical Junction

The bony components of the craniocervical junction can be biomechanically divided into two components – the central bony pillar and the circumferential double-ringed system. The former comprises the clivus/skull base, odontoid process, and C2 body, whereas the bony rings are the foramen magnum and atlas [7]. Integrated within the rings are the weight-bearing lateral pillars that extend from the occipital condyles through the C1 lateral masses into the lateral masses of the axis. The ligaments connecting the bony pillar to the basioccipital and atlantal circumferential rings restrict movement in flexion-extension and axial rotation [8]. The main points of articulation are: (1) the occipitoatlantal joints formed by the occipital condyles and superior articular surfaces of the C1 lateral masses, (2) the lateral atlantoaxial joints formed by the inferior articular surfaces of the C1 lateral masses and superior articular surfaces of the C2 lateral masses, and (3) the anterior articulation of the odontoid peg with the posterior aspect of the anterior C1 arch (fovea dentis) [8].

## Range of Motion and Biomechanics

The craniocervical junction consists of the atlanto-occipital and atlanto-axial joints, which account for roughly 50% of flexion-extension and axial rotation in the cervical spine, respectively [8]. Craniocervical mobility is of greatest importance in elderly patients, as progressive osteoarthritic changes in the subaxial cervical spine cause a greater proportion of overall neck movement to occur at the O-C1-C2 junction [9].

The main movement of the atlantooccipital joint is flexion-extension; it affords roughly 25° of flexion extension (3.5° flexion, 21° extension), 11° of lateral bending, and 15° of axial rotation [10, 11]. By contrast, axial rotation is the major movement at the C1–2 joint; the flat C1–2 articular surfaces enable the atlas to rotate around a craniocaudally oriented axis running through the odontoid. Biomechanical testing of this segment by Panjabi et al. [10]. found roughly 80° of axial rotation compared to 22° of flexion-extension movement (11° flexion, 11° extension) and 13° of lateral bending. *In vivo* testing using MRI [12] and CT [13, 14] has reported similar findings.

Disruption of the occipital condyle (e.g., secondary to condyle resection) produces gross craniocervical instability. Resecting 50% of the condyle significantly increases flexion-extension (≈150% increase), lateral bending (41%), and axial rotation (28%) [15].

## Ligamentous Structures

There are several key ligaments, the disruption of which has a significant impact on the biomechanics of the craniovertebral junction. These include the alar ligaments, the atlanto-occipital facet capsules, and the cruciate (cruciform) ligament [16]. The cruciate ligament is the strongest of these ligaments and comprises vertical (failure strength ≈450 N) and horizontal limbs (failure strength ≈450 N) [8]. The vertical limb stretches from the posterior body of C2 to the clivus, inserting cephalad to the basion [8]. The horizontal limb of the cruciate ligament is also known as the transverse ligament of the atlas. It maintains close apposition of the C1 anterior arch and the odontoid process [17, 18]. This ligament stretches between the C1 tubercles located bilaterally on the medial surface of the C1 lateral masses [19]. It has an *in vitro* strength of 350–1100 N [17, 20, 21] and is a key stabilizer that restricts flexion-extension of the atlantoaxial joint. The alar ligaments also serve as key stabilizers. With an intrinsic failure strength of 200 N on *in vitro* testing, they stretch between the anterolateral surfaces of the superior odontoid process and the medial aspects of the occipital condyles [18]. Their main function is to restrict axial rotation of the craniocervical complex [17] and their disruption results in axial rotatory instability of the craniocervical junction [14]. The alar ligaments also play a lesser role in maintaining tight apposition of the occiput and axis, along with the vertical band of the cruciate ligament and the apical ligament of the dens [8]. The transverse ligament, the atlantoalar ligaments, and atlantodental ligaments are responsible for maintaining apposition of the atlas and odontoid. The apical or suspensory ligament (failure strength ≈ 200 N) [8] stretches from a narrow insertion at the odontoid tip to the basion, lying anterior to the vertical limb of the cruciate ligament and posterior to the alar ligaments [18, 22]. It may have a redundant function to the vertical limb of the cruciate ligament and helps limit flexion-extension of the craniocervical complex [22]. Others have contended it is functionally insignificant though [22].

The anterior atlantooccipital membrane – an extension of the anterior longitudinal ligament (ALL) – and the tectorial membrane – an extension of the posterior longitudinal ligament – additionally contribute to stabilization along the craniocaudal axis [8]. The anterior atlantooccipital membrane (tensile strength ≈230 N) runs from the superior surface of the anterior C1 arch to the anterior foramen magnum, functioning as a tension band that limits extension. The tectorial membrane (tensile strength 76 N) by contrast may help limit flexion [23], though it has been argued that the function is more to prevent the ventral impression of the dura mater [24]. Posterior column ligaments – chiefly the posterior atlantooccipital membrane (tensile strength ≈90 N) and the ligamentum nuchae – work to limit flexion, though their contributions are relatively minor [8]. It has even been argued that the posterior atlantooccipital membrane is contiguous with the deep fascial layer of the rectus capitis posterior minor [23].

Multiple lesser ligaments have also been described that contribute to the stabilization of the craniocervical junction. The anterior atlantodental ligaments run from the anterior base of the dens to the dorsal surface of the anterior C1 arch, immediately inferior to the fovea dentis. These ligaments work synergistically with the transverse atlantal ligament to prevent posterior displacement of the dens relative to the atlas [25]. Additionally, they contribute to stabilization in axial rotation, as they achieve tension prior to the alar ligaments [25]. The articular or capsular ligaments (tensile strength ≈300 N), especially those of the occipitoatlantal joints, restrict motion at the occipitoatlantal and atlantoaxial joints. Specifically, the orientation of the occipitoatlantal capsular ligaments combined with the cup-shaped anatomy of the C1 superior articular surface limits O-C1 motion to flexion-extension only [26]. The looser atlantoaxial capsular ligaments work synergistically with the flat atlantoaxial articular surfaces to enable sliding of the interior articular surfaces of the atlas relative to the superior articular surfaces of C2. This sliding is fundamental to the axial rotation seen at C1–2 [8].

Other ligamentous structures have been described in more recent cadaveric studies, though their contribution to the biomechanics of the craniocervical junction is unclear. The lateral oblique atlantooccipital ligament is a recently described variant traveling between the transverse atlantal process and occipital bone [27]. It may help to serve as a secondary stabilizer of the atlantooccipital joint and restrict movement of the craniocervical junction, but the exact role is unclear. The lateral atlantooccipital ligament (tensile strength 37.5 N) originates from the lateral mass of the atlas, lateral to the joint capsule, and inserts into the jugular process of the occiput. It runs immediately posterior to the rectus capitis lateralis muscle, between the internal jugular vein anteriorly and the vertebral artery (V3) posteriorly, and works to restrict lateral flexion of the atlantooccipital joint [28]. To a lesser degree, it also limits axial rotation of the atlantooccipital joint.

The ligament of Barkow (tensile strength 28 N) works synergistically with the anterior atlantooccipital membrane to help restrain extension at the atlantooccipital joint [29]. It stretches transversely between the occipital condyles, attaching along the anteromedial surface, anterior to the attachment of the alar (check) ligaments. From a surgical standpoint, it may be encountered during a transoral approach and can cue the surgeon to the fact that the dens is immediately deep to the current plane of dissection. By contrast, the transverse occipital ligament (Lauth's ligament) runs posterosuperiorly to the odontoid and alar ligaments, inserting on the medial aspects of the occipital condyle immediately posterior to the alar ligament attachments. It has been postulated to support the alar ligaments in restricting lateral bending, flexion, and axial rotation of the head. The accessory atlantoaxial ligaments (Y-ligament) that lie between the tectorial membrane dorsally and the alar ligaments ventrally similarly help to restrict flexion and axial rotation [30, 31].

## Vertebral Artery and Tumoral Involvement

Arising as the first branch of the subclavian artery (V1 segment), the vertebral arteries ascend through the neck via the transverse foramina of the C2–6 vertebrae (V2 segment) [32, 33]. Accompanying the vertebral arteries in the foramina are vertebral venous plexuses containing 1–3 dominant veins bilaterally [33]. After exiting the foramen of the atlas, the arteries run along the superolateral surface of the posterior C1 arch before bending medially around the lateral mass of the atlas to penetrate the posterior atlantooccipital membrane and run through the sulcus arteriosus [34]. As it exits the sulcus and enters the vertebral canal, the artery penetrates the dura, becoming the V4 segment. The V4 segment travels ventral to the first denticulate ligament [35] – a meningeal extension tethering the spinal cord to the dura laterally that divides the vertebral artery from the dorsally situated spinal accessory nerve. The V4 segments join in the midline to give rise to the basilar artery.

Several anatomic variants to the vertebral artery have been described, the majority of which localize to the V1, V3, or V4 segments; V2 anatomy is relatively constant by comparison [33]. Of interest to pathologies of the craniocervical junction are anomalies in the V3 and V4 segments. Ulm et al. [32]. reported the results of a cadaveric investigation of variants of the V3 segment, in which the V3 segment was subdivided into three sub-segments: (1) the vertical segment between the C2 and C1 foramina, (2) the horizontal part running superomedially along the posterior C1 arch, and (3) the oblique part running from the posterior C1 arch to the dura mater. They found an extradural posterior inferior cerebellar artery (PICA) origin in 3% of specimens, though other series have reported rates up to 23% [33, 36]. Extradural PICA origins should be noted on preoperative films as the iatrogenic injury is uncompensated and results in lateral medullary (Wallenberg's) syndrome. Based upon the study of Ulm et al. [32], the four sites at highest risk for injury to V3 include: (1) the medial edge and (2) the superior border of the V3 horizontal limb along the C1 arch, (3) the medial surface of the vertical limb along the C2 dorsal surface, and (4) the V2/V3 transition along the C2 transverse foramen. In the context of craniocervical approaches to chordoma, the anatomy of the V2/V3 transition point is of particular interest as superior displacement of this transition point – a high-riding vertebral artery – is associated with increased risk of vertebral artery injury during C2 instrumentation. Other anomalies of interest include persistent intersegmental arteries, seen in 4% of cases, and a posterior ponticulus (arcuate foramen), seen in 15% [37].

Because of the potential for angiographic anomalies, preoperative angiography using CT angiography (CTA) [38] or MRI angiography (MRA) [39] is considered a must. Traditional vessel evaluation with a digital subtraction angiogram is not necessary as its diagnostic yield is not substantially different than CTA or MRA. Additionally, the latter two modalities allow for evaluation of the relation of the tumor to the vertebral arteries and more anterolaterally positioned carotid arteries. Knowledge of the tumor-vertebral artery relation along with the presence of sufficient perfusion of the posterior circulation by the bilateral vertebral arteries helps to guide surgical management. Specifically, it informs the surgeon: (1) if vertebral artery sacrifice is necessary to achieve R0 resection, and (2) if vertebral artery sacrifice is feasible based upon the posterior circulation anatomy. Our group [40] recently described an algorithm for vertebral artery management based upon the primary pathology, degree of encasement, and posterior circulation anatomy. For primary lesions such as chordomas, we recommended tumors with ≥180° encasement of the vertebral artery be sacrificed in the absence of posterior circulation anomalies. Those with bilateral involvement or posterior circulation anomalies should undergo vertebral artery skeletonization instead, though this likely precludes R0 resection.

## Surgical Approaches

### Preoperative Planning

As discussed in Chap. 6, preoperative planning for all chordoma patients includes staging, consultation with radiation oncology and neurosurgery or orthopedic oncology (depending upon institutional practice patterns), and anatomic evaluation of the lesion. At bare minimum, staging should include a computed tomography (CT) volume of the chest given the proclivity of chordoma to metastasize first to the lungs. We generally recommend staging with CT of the chest, abdomen, and pelvis, or positron emission tomography to look for metastatic disease.

In cases where staging is negative for metastatic disease, anatomic sequences of the tumor should be acquired to fully evaluate its morphology. We recommend these scans include pre- and post-contrast fat-suppressed T1-weighted magnetic resonance (MRI) sequences and thin-cut (0.75 mm) CT slices through the skull base and occipitocervical junction. Review of the imaging should focus on identifying the borders of the tumor, the presence or absence of epidural invasion, and the joints involved by the tumor. Unlike lesions of the subaxial cervical spine and thoracolumbar spine, lesions of the occipitocervical junction do not conform nicely to the Weinstein-Boriani-Biagini (WBB) system. During surgical staging we focus on whether: (1) the tumor is isolated to the atlantoaxial spine or extends into the subaxial spine, (2) the tumor involves the atlantoaxial or atlantooccipital joints laterally, (3) the tumor envelopes or abuts the vertebral artery/arteries, (4) the tumor extends into the skull base and involves the cranial nerves, and (5) the tumor involves the carotid sheath. Because of this, we routinely also obtain vessel imaging in the form of CT angiography or MRI angiography to evaluate the patency of the bilateral cervical and carotid vessels. Involvement of the dominant vertebral artery may preclude *en bloc* resection if that vessel is involved [40]. Given the complex local anatomy, the construction of a patient-specific three-dimensional model based upon preoperative CT imaging may be useful during preoperative planning [41]. Based upon the tumor morphology, an anterior, posterior, or staged anterior-posterior approach can then be planned. The relative advantages and disadvantages of each are discussed in the sections that follow.

In addition to planning the tumor resection margins, it is also essential to take stock of regional and global radiographic alignment [42]. Cervical deformity is associated with significant pain and disability [43]. It is diagnosed in patients meeting one of the following criteria: C2–7 sagittal Cobb angle ≥10°, C2–7 coronal Cobb angle ≥10°, C2–7 sagittal vertical axis (SVA) ≥4 cm, or chin-brow vertical angle (CBVA) ≥25° (Fig. 7.1) [44]. Appreciation of preoperative alignment is perhaps more important in the treatment of occipitocervical junction lesions than in lesions of the subaxial cervical spine, as nearly three-quarters of cervical lordosis is found in the occiput-C2 interval [45, 46]. Appreciation of global alignment is also essential. Isolated correction of cervical malalignment without consideration of any underlying thoracolumbar deformity may lead to a global sagittal malalignment, which is in turn correlated with greater pain and functional disability [47]. The cervical deformity literature has also suggested that failure to achieve global correction in addition to cervical deformity correction is associated with increased reoperation rates [48]. For this reason, we routinely obtain 36-inch standing films to assess global alignment in addition to cervical alignment.

Due to the great importance of achieving both negative margins and ideal postoperative alignment, preoperative osteotomy planning can greatly facilitate the achievement of surgical goals. The construction of preoperative, patient-specific three-dimensional models may assist with this planning by allowing the surgeon greater appreciation of the local bony anatomy. Several groups have described their use for the treatment of cervical spine tumors [41, 49–52]. The principal drawback of these models is their relatively high price, though it is likely low relative to the cost of surgical implants or revision surgery. A potentially cheaper alternative involves the use of intraoperative navigation based upon preoperative CT volumes [53–57]. Both methods can be used in conjunction with one another, though we have favored navigation-only for most cases. We also favor the use of intraoperative navigation for complex craniocervical lesions as it enables us to correlate intraoperative anatomic findings with preoperative radiographic features. This is particularly beneficial in older patients with significant osteophytes/spondylotic changes and in those with tumors causing significant distortion of the local anatomy.

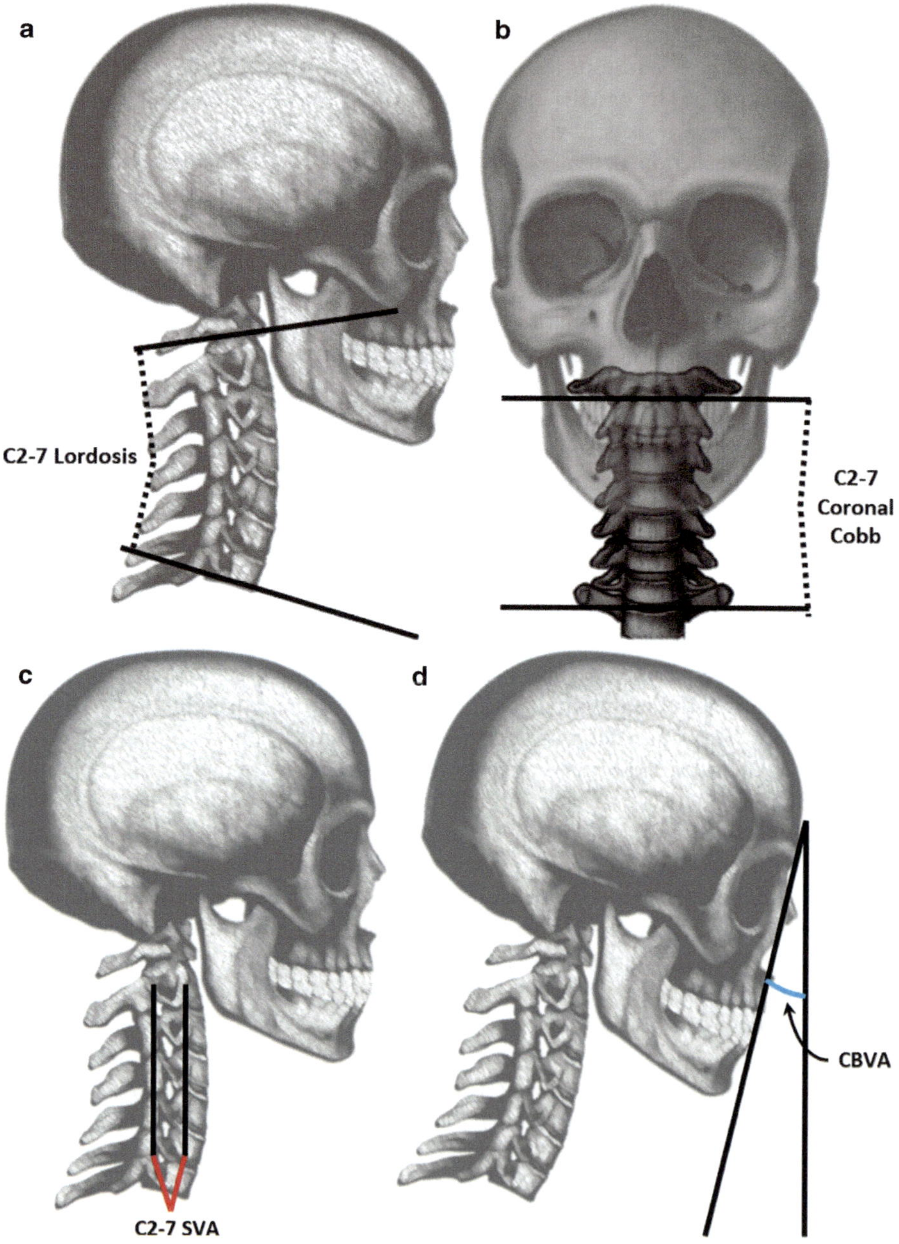

## Posterior Only

The posterior approach is popular as it relies on anatomy that is relatively familiar to surgeons who treat cervical pathologies. It also enables the placement of occipitocervical segmental instrumentation and tumor resection as a single stage. One posterior approach is the extreme-lateral transcondylar approach employed by Shin et al. [5] in their series of primary and metastatic tumors of the occipitocervical junction. A similar approach was also employed by Sen and colleagues in their series of 29 patients treated for chordomas of the craniocervical junction [58].

As occipitocervical junctional lesions can be associated with significant craniocervical instability, patients are intubated supine with in-line stabilization, often using a fiberoptic laryngoscope. Pre-flip motor evoked potentials (MEPs) are acquired and paralytics are held throughout the case to facilitate motor monitoring. The patient is then pinned in a neutral position in a three-pin Mayfield head holder, and the patient is rolled to the prone position on the Jackson table or a standard operating room table equipped with a Wilson frame. We prefer the Jackson table as it enables decompression of the abdomen, lowering central venous pressures, and consequently intraoperative blood loss. The patient's shoulders are then taped down and lateral plain films are acquired to ensure that the postoperative chin-brown angle will leave the patient's face perpendicular to the floor.

A midline incision is carried from the inion inferiorly to the level of the C3 spinous process; additional levels may be exposed depending upon the size of the tumor and the number of levels to be instrumented. Dissection proceeds in the midline avascular plane to the level of the spinous processes. The dissection is then carried laterally to expose the lateral masses of the atlas, axis, and subaxial cervical vertebra(e). Care must be taken when exposing the vertebrae to identify the suboccipital venous plexus, which has the propensity for profuse bleeding and should be coagulated early [34]. It can be found in the posterior suboccipital triangle, bounded superomedially by the rectus capitis posterior major, laterally by the obliquus

**Fig. 7.1** Maintenance of proper cervical alignment is essential to minimize postoperative chronic pain and disability in patients undergoing surgical resection of occipitocervical vertebral column tumors. Though defined in the adult degenerative and spinal deformity literature, the same alignment principles can be applied to the post-resection chordoma patient. Goals should be to have a final C2–7 sagittal Cobb angle <10°, C2–7 coronal Cobb angle <10°, C2–7 sagittal vertical axis (SVA) <4 cm, and a chin-brow vertical angle (CBVA) <25°. C2–7 lordosis or C2–7 sagittal Cobb (**a**) is measured as the angle inscribed by the lines parallel to the C2 and C7 inferior end plates on lateral standing X-rays. C2–7 coronal Cobb (**b**) is similarly the angle inscribed by the intersection of those lines parallel to the inferior C2 and C7 endplates on posterior-anterior standing X-rays. C2–7 SVA (**c**) is defined by the horizontal distance between vertical lines drawn from the C2 centroid (odontoid = C2 plumb line) and the posterior superior endplate of C7. CBVA (**d**) is measured as the angle subtended by a vertical line drawn for the patient's eyebrow and a line connecting the patient's eyebrow to their chin. Chin-brow angle can be measured on photographs or standing radiographs. Iyer et al. [46]. found normative values depend highly on patient age; however, mean values in healthy controls are 21.3 ± 12.1 mm for C2–7 SVA, −1.7 ± 7.8° for CBVA, and −12.2 ± 13.6° for C2–7 lordosis, where a negative angle indicates lordosis capitis superior, and inferiorly by the obliquus capitis inferior. Additionally, within this triangle is the C2 nerve root, which can block visualization of the C1 lateral mass [42, 59]. If sacrificed, it should be ligated proximal to the dorsal root ganglion to prevent postoperative neuropathic pain [59]. As dissection proceeds laterally at the level of the atlantoaxial junction, the surgeon must also be cognizant of the nearby vertebral artery, which courses posteromedially along the superior border of the posterior C1 arch.

As lesions amenable to the posterior approach are predominately on one side of the midline, the approach focuses on gaining access to the affected side of the vertebral column. This starts by removing the C1, C2, and C3 laminae to facilitate access to the vertebral body and prevertebral space [60]. Ligation of the C1 and C2 roots helps to facilitate retraction of the thecal sac and sagittal osteotomy formation. Laterally, the vertebral artery is identified; if it is involved and requires ligation, the facet joints can be drilled away and clips are placed at the distal and proximal ends of the ligated segments. Test occlusion should be performed over 30 minutes with continuously running somatosensory evoked potentials (SSEPs) to look for signs of vertebrobasilar insufficiency. We use thresholds of a 10% increase in SSEP latency or a 50% reduction in SSEP amplitude as signs that vertebral artery ligation will not be tolerated. The thecal sac is mobilized contralateral to the tumor and the ventral epidural space is defined. An ultrasonic bone cutter or high-speed drill is then used to form a parasagittal osteotomy, defining the medial border of the tumor specimen. Transverse osteotomies are also formed proximal and distal to the tumor specimen, freeing it from the healthy bone. Specimen mobilization concludes with soft tissue dissection to define a plane between the prevertebral soft tissues and the tumor. After having mobilized the tumor, the spine is instrumented and the defect reconstructed to provide stability.

The order and location of instrumentation placement is dictated by the tumor location and extent of resection performed. If a significant amount of the vertebral body will be resected, partial instrumentation will be placed first to ensure spine stability during resection. We place the lateral mass and/or pedicle screws at the inferior bound of the construct and install the fixation hardware on the side contralateral to the tumor. The occipital plate is placed and a temporary rod is then placed to maintain spinal stability during tumor resection. If only stabilization is to be pursued, then the contralateral rod is placed and the instrumentation is finalized. Otherwise, the bony work is executed to separate the tumor specimen for the adjacent vertebral column. The tumor is then rotated around the spinal cord and delivered posteriorly. Anterior reconstruction is performed (if necessary), and a second rod is placed. The instrumentation is finalized, graft material is laid down and the wound is closed in layers using a combination of interrupted 0 polyglactin in the fascia, 3-0 polyglactin in the subcutaneous tissue, and a 4-0 subcuticular running poliglecaprone suture. Postoperatively, patients are managed with a cervical collar that is maintained for a minimum of 3 months. When significant vertebral column destabilization occurs (e.g., following C2 corpectomy), additional postoperative treatment with an external orthosis may be required, up to and including placement of a halo device. Plain films are obtained monthly and postoperative CT scans are obtained immediately postoperatively and then at the 3-month, 6-month, and 12-month appointments to look for evidence of hardware failure and to evaluate fusion across the construct.

The biggest limitation of the posterior approach is the limited access to ventrally situated tumors. As previously discussed by the senior author and colleagues [60] the intervening spinal cord poses the greatest restriction in access. Even with ligation of the C1 and C2 nerve roots, exposure is limited from a straight posterior approach and progressively more lateral angles may be required, up to and including resection of the occipital condyle [61]. In the series of Shin et al. [5], the authors had to resect 70% or more of the condyle in 15 of 23 cases undergoing occipitocervical fusion (10 of 15 with chordoma). However, the authors did report extremely high fusion rates, with solid bone fusion in 22 of 23 patients who underwent occipitocervical fusion at a mean long-term follow-up of 66 months.

## Anterior Only

Several options exist for anterior approaches to the craniocervical junction, including the transoral-transpharyngeal approach, the transnasal approach, the transcervical approach, and the transmandibular approach [62]. The transnasal approach is perhaps most familiar to neurosurgeons in the era of modern skull base surgery and is commonly used for resection of clival chordomas [63–65]. It allows for relatively safe, piecemeal resection of clival chordomas with minimal morbidity to the surrounding neurovascular structures. However, the relatively small working window precludes *en bloc* resection via this approach. The transmandibular approach represents the most invasive anterior approach [66], but is capable of offering the greatest surgical exposure. An alternative described by McAfee et al. [67] and later expanded upon by the group at Barrow Neurological Institute [68] is the extraoral or retropharyngeal approach that employs a hockey stick incision along the inferior mandibular margin and anterior border of the sternocleidomastoid muscle. The submandibular approach of Ricciardi and colleagues employs a similar, albeit smaller approach corridor with commensurately less exposure [69]. Transcervical approaches are not commonly used as they generally do not offer enough exposure of the superior tumor pole to facilitate *en bloc* resection. It is generally only an option for tumors to be resected piecemeal. It is similarly impractical or impossible in patients who are obese, have significant cervical kyphosis, or who are barrel chested [70].

A cadaveric study by Baird et al. [71] compared surgical exposure of the lower clivus and craniocervical junction achieved via the endonasal, transoral, and transcervical approach. They found that extended endonasal and transoral approaches offered similar exposure of the craniocervical junction (1305 vs 1406 mm$^2$) with similar working angles (28° vs 30°). However, the extended endonasal approach offered a slightly shorter working distance (94 vs 102 mm). The exposure afforded by the extended endonasal approach stretched from the dorsum sella to the base of the odontoid, whereas the exposure of the transoral extended from the inferior clivus to the superior aspect of the C3 vertebral body. The transcervical exposure offered far less exposure (743 $mm^2$) than the other two approaches and was incapable of accessing pathologies above the level of the basion. In their comparison of the transoral and extraoral approaches, Agrawal and colleagues [68] found the extraoral approach resulted in a significant increase in exposure along the craniocaudal axis. They found the extraoral approach was capable of treating pathologies from the mid-clivus down to the C3/4-disc space. The increase in vertical working length along the dura relative to the transoral approach was 60% (539 vs 336 mm). This was associated with increases in clival and subaxial working area of 62% (874 vs 546 $mm^2$) and 77% (1644 vs 932 $mm^2$), respectively. No high-level clinical evidence exists comparing the complication rates between the different approaches, however in their series of 97 patients treated for craniocervical or upper cervical chordomas, Choi et al. [72] found no difference in the complication rates between the following approaches: transoral approach, transoral approach with soft palate splitting, "open-door" maxillotomy, or the transmandibular approach.

#### Transmandibular

The transmandibular approach represents the most aggressive approach to the craniocervical junction. However, in our experience, it provides the greatest exposure and so may help to facilitate *en bloc* specimen delivery that would be impossible via other approaches. There are three variations to the mandibular approach based upon the site of the osteotomy: (1) the transmandibular-circumglossal-retropharyngeal (TCR), (2) the median labial-mandibular-glossotomy (LMG), and (3) the bilateral-sagittal split mandibular osteotomy (BSSMO) [73]. We favor the TCR approach [66] as it minimizes difficulties associated with reapproximating the mandible.

As with other anterior approaches, patients are placed supine, the neck is draped sterilely and the oral cavity is prepared. Tracheostomy is performed for airway placement to keep the endotracheal tube out of the surgical field. An incision is extended from the mastoid tip inferiorly 2–3 cm along the anterior border of the sternocleidomastoid. The incision is turned medially along the inferior border of the mandible to the mental protuberance at the midline. It is then turned superiorly and extended through the lip. Subplatysmal flaps are elevated and a supra-omohyoid neck dissection is used to identify and protect the lingual and hypoglossal nerve, internal and external carotid, and internal jugular vein. The mandible is exposed along the midline and craniofacial miniplates are placed to ensure reapproximation of the mandible at the end of the operation will lead to perfect apposition. The plates are then removed and a midline mandibulotomy is formed between the two first lower incisors using a reciprocating saw. Some authors advocate for a stair-step mandibulotomy due to concerns regarding postoperative structural stability [66]; however, we generally employ a linear osteotomy for cosmetic purposes.

After dividing the mandible, the dissection proceeds laterally along the floor of the mouth to the glossopharyngeal sulcus. The hemimandible is rotated laterally and the tongue is retracted medially to expose the 10th, 11th, and 12th nerves, the internal carotid artery, and the internal jugular vein. These structures are identified and traced superiorly to the skull base. At the posterior limit of the dissection, the incision splits into superior and inferior limbs. The inferior limb is extended lateral to the Eustachian tube and a retropharyngeal dissection is used to form a plane between the pharynx and longus colli and longus capitis muscles. The Eustachian tube, levator veli palatini, and tensor veli palatini are divided to allow the pharynx to be mobilized from the skull base. The superior limb of the incision extends to the lateral border of the palate. The soft palate is mobilized from its lateral attachment and an ipsilateral hard palate osteotomy may be performed to increase access to the sphenoid sinus. Combined, these allow exposure of the cervical spine and lower clivus. The anterior face of the sphenoid can be drilled away to increase exposure and allow access to the sphenoid sinus and upper clivus.

Osteotomy cuts are then formed on the atlas, axis, and clivus as needed to resect the lesion with negative margins. If the dura is entered, the repair is performed with a combination of subcutaneous fat graft, fascia lata graft, and fibrin glue; collagen-based dural onlay grafts (e.g., DuraGen) can also be employed. After the tumor has been delivered, the superior pharyngeal constrictor is reattached to the skull base and the palatal flap is reapproximated. The soft palate is closed in multiple layers with reabsorbable suture and the pharynx is carefully reapproximated at the posterolateral edges using two layers with absorbable suture. After closing the soft tissue defects of the oropharynx, the hemimandibles are brought back to midline and reapproximated with the previously selected miniplates. Absorbable sutures are then used to close the myocutaneous flaps of the anterior neck and lower face. 5-0 suture is used in the skin and great care should be taken to reapproximate the vermillion border owing to its important role in cosmesis. Postoperative dysphagia is common in patients treated via the transmandibular approach [74] and patients should remain *nil* per os to assist with wound healing. Parenteral feeding may be considered after 2 weeks of healing.

### Transoral Transpharyngeal

The transoral transpharyngeal exposure can be considered an approach intermediate to the transnasal and transmandibular approaches. It provides access to the anterior clivus, atlas, and axis and is reasonable for *en bloc* resection of small skull base lesions [70]. The relevant anatomy in this approach includes the pharyngeal wall – composed of the mucosa and prevertebral fascia – the anterior C1 arch, and prevertebral musculature – the longus capitis and longus colli – that insert onto the ventrolateral aspect of the vertebral bodies [70]. Additionally, within the retropharyngeal space, which is bounded by the 2 layers of the pharyngeal wall, there exist the pharyngeal arteries and veins. At the lateral borders of the pharynx can be found the vertebral arteries, running in the foramina transversaria. One of the biggest drawbacks of the transoral approach is that it necessarily risks inoculating the sterile epidural space with bacterial contaminants from the pharyngeal cavity [70].

For the transoral transpharyngeal approach, the patient is placed supine on the operating table. Intubation can be done via standard endotracheal intubation, with the tube retracted out of view, or via tracheostomy, which is preferable for patients with baseline dysfunction of the glossopharyngeal, hypoglossal, or vagal nerves. Anesthesia is induced and the anterior arch of C1 and body of C2 are identified via palpation. The oral cavity is cleansed with chlorhexidine gluconate oral solution and the patient's face is draped. A self-retaining retractor is placed over the teeth with blades inserted to retract the tongue and buccal mucosa; some advocate for periodic release of compression on the tongue to prevent lingual congestion [75]. At this time the soft palate may be divided in the midline to improve access to the clivus. The palatal flaps are retracted laterally and the posterior pharyngeal mucosa is infiltrated with 1% lidocaine with 1:100,000 epinephrine. A midline incision is made from the lower clivus to the C2/3 junction. The pharyngeal mucosa, pharyngeal constrictors, and anterior prevertebral musculature are elevated and retracted laterally as a single flap, exposing the underlying ALL, C1 anterior arch, and C2 body. Exposure 15–20 mm bilaterally can be obtained from the inferior clivus to the level of the superior C3 body. Further lateral exposure is limited by the presence of the hypoglossal nerve, Eustachian tube, vertebral artery, and vidian nerve. After the specimen is resected, the pharynx is closed in layers, with 3-0 absorbable sutures in the deep muscular and superficial mucosal layers. If the palate was divided, it is re-approximated with absorbable sutures in the nasal mucosa, muscularis, and oral mucosa. If a cerebrospinal fluid (CSF) leak is encountered, primary closure should be attempted; this may be enhanced using fibrin glue, fascia, or bovine pericardium. A lumbar drain should be considered for CSF diversion to facilitate healing and reduce the risk of postoperative meningitis. If additional cephalad exposure is required, endoscopic resection may be considered. An anatomic study by Pillai et al. [76] found that relative to a microscopic approach, an endoscopic approach offers an additional 181 mm$^2$ of posterior pharyngeal exposure and an additional 7 mm of cephalad exposure of the clivus. Commonly, additional cephalad exposure is required [74] and may be achieved through the use of a LeFort I maxillary osteotomy, though this significantly increases the morbidity of the procedure [70]. Options include a unilateral LeFort I osteotomy, bilateral LeFort I osteotomies, and an extended maxillectomy. Of these, the unilateral LeFort I has the lowest associated morbidity and generally provides adequate exposure [70].

The unilateral LeFort I procedure is performed by hydrodissecting the gingival mucosa off the upper alveolar margins with the anesthetic. An incision is then formed under the upper lip from the midline to the maxillary tuberosity; the alveolar tissue is elevated subperiosteally to expose the maxilla. The hardware for craniofacial reconstruction is then planned and placed on the maxilla to ensure proper dental occlusion postoperatively. A unilateral LeFort I and midline parasagittal osteotomy are made through the hard palate and the mobile maxilla is displaced inferolaterally after separation from the pterygoid process and nasal bones. At this point, the pharyngeal dissection proceeds as described above. After the closure of the pharynx, the maxilla is replaced in its native position and the craniofacial plates are placed. The hard palate and sublabial mucosa are closed with absorbable suture and packing is placed in the nares to restore the midline position of the bony septum. Enteral nutrition should be provided to facilitate the healing of the nasal and oral mucosa [70].

### Other Approaches

Other anterior approaches to the craniocervical include the transcervical [77] and endoscopic endonasal approach [78, 79]. While these approaches are reasonable for other pathologies of the craniovertebral junction, the relatively long working distance and narrow operative corridor means that they are not amenable to *en bloc* resection for most lesions. Transnasal approaches are considered a workhorse for clival chordomas, which are generally treated with piecemeal resection [63, 80]. However, the superior survival seen with *en bloc* resection of mobile spine chordomas leads us to recommend the transpharyngeal or transmandibular approaches.

## Anterior-Posterior or Staged

Previous series have reported that staged approaches are the most commonly employed for the treatment of occipitocervical chordoma [81]. Though more morbid by design, staged approaches may help to facilitate R0 resection by employing a second stage to dissect the backside of the tumor and complete the bony cuts. The preference of the senior author when employing a staged approach is lead with a posterior approach to stabilize the spine and release the tumor from the backside. At this time a silastic sheath may also be placed to help identify the tumor and facilitate delivery during the second, anterior approach. The anterior approach is then performed using a transoral or transmandibular approach, depending upon tumor size. At this time the tumor is delivered and vertebral column is reconstructed. Occasionally a third, posterior approach may be required to readjust the positioning of the posterior hardware so as to achieve optimal sagittal and coronal alignment.

## Reconstruction Strategies

The key principle in reconstructing the occipitocervical junction following tumor resection is restoring the functional strength that was lost secondary to: (1) tumor-mediated osseoligamentous destruction and (2) iatrogenic destabilization through soft tissue and bony disruption. In nearly all cases, this will mean restoring strength to both the occipitoatlantal and atlantoaxial joints. Isolated atlantoaxial fixation is unlikely to provide sufficient stabilization of the craniocervical junction. Depending upon the surgical approach adopted, posterior fixation as well as anterior reconstruction will be required.

## Level Selection and Instrumentation Considerations

In selecting levels for instrumentation, the general principal of the senior author is to instrument from the occiput to at least 3 levels below the inferior bound of the tumor resection site (i.e., if the inferior transverse osteotomy cut is made at the C2/3-disc space, instrumentation should include at least C5). This is in contrast to the conventional 2 levels above/2 levels below principle used to reconstruct corpectomy defects in surgery for thoracolumbar metastases. It may be necessary to incorporate additional levels if the tumor is large and involves multiple contiguous vertebrae, or if the inferior bound of the planned construct will place hardware at the cervicothoracic junction. Larger tumors create commensurately large vertebral column defects following reconstruction. This in turn creates a large lever arm and high stress on the relatively weak lateral mass screws included in the subaxial portion of the construct. In the case of a construct ending adjacent to the cervicothoracic junction – lowest instrumented level C7 – extending into the upper thoracic spine (T1, T2, or T3) has been reported to reduce the risk of adjacent segment disease, or distal junctional kyphosis [82]. While this latter point is disputed [82, 83], in our opinion, the higher screw pullout strength of thoracic pedicle screws (600–1000 N) [84, 85] relative to cervical lateral mass screws (300–400 N) [86–88] warrants construct extension across the cervicothoracic junction in the case of long constructs. Additionally, where the fusion construct is extended to the level of the cervicothoracic junction, care should be taken to avoid excessive disruption of the posterior tension band and associated soft tissues. In a cadaveric study, Kretzer et al. [89] demonstrated that disruption of the supraspinous ligament and interspinous ligament at the C7/T1 interface significantly increased the range of motion at the adjacent segment.

For those wishing to conserve levels, but desiring increased construct durability, cervical pedicle screws may be entertained. They have a higher pullout strength than lateral mass screws, [87, 88, 90]; however, they have a much steeper learning curve and a smaller margin for error than lateral mass screws [91]. Cadaveric studies have reported pedicle breaches in 10–65% of screws [87, 92]. These rates are likely to be higher in patients of Southeast Asian [93] and South Asian descent [94], as these patients generally have smaller cervical pedicles, which in many cases are too small to accommodate standard cervical screws. Use of intraoperative navigation may help to reduce the risk of breach occurrence [92].

Isolated occiput to C2 constructs are seldom an option for patients who undergo resection with curative intent. However, for patients who have unresectable lesions or who opt for surgical stabilization without oncologic resection, O-C2 constructs may be reasonable.

When placing the occipital hardware, screws positions should be selected along the midline, the transverse sulcus, and superior nuchal line, as these are the thickest regions of bone [95]. The external occipital protuberance (EOP) is highly variable in its thickness though, ranging from 7.4 to 22.3 mm in healthy, asymptomatic adults [96, 97]. Consequently, its thickness, along with the thickness of the bone at other points along the transverse sulcus and superior nuchal line should be measured preoperatively to determine the ideal fixation points. In general, bone caudal to the transverse sinus is too weak to support occipital instrumentation [42]. Placement of a midline screw might require the EOP to be shaved down to partially recess the plate though, to prevent hardware prominence [42].

Screw-based instrumentation is preferable to older wiring techniques as the wiring constructs have a tendency to stretch and loosen [98], resulting in loss of sagittal correction. The increased mobility of the wired constructs [98] may result in a postoperative cervical kyphotic deformity or dislodgement of an anteriorly placed cage or strut graft. Either unicortical or bicortical screw fixation can be employed with the occipital plate. Bicortical screws have higher pullout strength; however, unicortical placement may be feasible for screws at the occipital protuberance, as cadaveric studies have demonstrated screws in this position have pull-out strength similar to bicortical screws placed elsewhere [99]. Unicortical instrumentation also reduces the risk of incidental durotomy or injury to the underlying dural venous sinuses [42]. Additionally, the bone of the external occipital protuberance is some of the strongest in the body and is consequently unlikely to be the point of construct failure [42]. In cases where an occipital plate cannot be placed, use of an occipital condyle-C1 lateral mass transarticular screw or an occipital condyle-C1 lateral mass construct may be an effective salvage technique [100, 101].

Placing C1 instrumentation can be challenging secondary to difficulty in trying to connect the C1 hardware with the rod joining the occipital plate with C2 and the subaxial spine. Options for C1 fixation include C1 lateral mass screws, C1 pedicle screw, and C1 posterior arch screws. C1 lateral mass screws are the most commonly employed, but biomechanical studies have suggested that C1 pedicle screws may have greater pullout strength [102]. C1 pedicle screws can also be placed with less extensive dissection of the lateral masses [42]. However, the C1 pedicle screw trajectory places the V3 vertebral artery at greater risk than the more inferior C1 lateral mass trajectory [42]. Additionally, where bicortical fixation is pursued, there is an increased risk of internal carotid artery impingement or injury with C1 pedicle screws [3, 42]. This risk is reduced by adopting a 10° medial angulation in the axial plane [103]. Risk of hardware failure is far higher in constructs utilizing C1 posterior arch screws versus lateral mass screws [104] and we do not routinely employ them.

At the level of C2, pars screws, pedicle screws, or translaminar screws can be placed. In a recent meta-analysis of biomechanical studies of atlantoaxial fixation, Du et al. [105] found that existing data are highly heterogeneous. Those data that are available fail to demonstrate a difference between constructs employing C2 pars and C2 pedicle screws; however, constructs incorporating C2 translaminar screws are less rigid than those using C2 pars or pedicle screws. Previous biomechanical studies of occipitoatlantoaxial constructs have suggested that employing C2 pedicle screws or C1/2 transarticular screws offer the greatest stability [106–108]. Despite this, for patients with high-riding vertebral arteries, C2 pars screws may be the preferred option as the narrow C2 pedicles are too small to safely accommodate a screw. In cases with dysmorphic or small pedicles, the use of computer-assisted navigation may help to facilitate screw placement [109].

## Anterior Column Reconstruction

Weight bearing in the cervical spine can be thought of according to the model of Louis [110], where the spine is comprised of a central pillar – the vertebral bodies – and two lateral pillars made up of the lateral masses and zygoapophyseal joints [111]. As the primary weight-bearing portion the spine (approximately 90% in the subaxial cervical spine) [112], the central bony pillar must be reconstructed following resection of any vertebral body tumor. This reconstruction is somewhat unique at the craniocervical junction however. At this junction, the primary load-bearing shifts from the anterolaterally placed occipital condyle-C1 lateral masse junction to the centrally located bony pillar of the axis and subaxial spine. Under normal conditions, the weight of the skull is transferred through the occipital condyles to the C1 lateral masses to the C2 lateral masses. From there, the axis redistributes loading forces into the central bony pillar and lateral masses of the subaxial spine [111]. Following resection of the craniocervical junction for tumor though, weight must now either pass solely through the lateral masses, or it must be passed centrally from the clivus to the subaxial vertebral bodies through a cage or strut graft. The clivus is comprised largely of spongy bone [113] and is non-weight-bearing under normal conditions. Excessive loading on a central anterior construct may therefore lead to failure. Consequently, any anterior construct must necessarily place a larger proportion of the load-sharing on posterior instrumentation than would be necessary in a construct of the subaxial cervical spine or thoracolumbar spine.

Anterior reconstruction has been described using titanium mesh cages with inline fibular structural allograft [41], standalone fibular strut graft [114], titanium mesh cages with morselized allograft [115–117], and expandible titanium cages packed with morselized allograft [118–120]. There is no evidence to support the superiority of one construct over the others; each likely has its merits. The expandible cage has a smaller profile and so may be easier to place. By comparison, the titanium mesh with inline structural graft increases the surface area of the basiocciput-graft interface, potentially reducing von Mises stresses and risk of implant failure. In both cases, the irregular morphology of the clivus and high mobility of the native craniocaudal junction means that the cage should be fixed superiorly to the clivus and inferiorly to the subaxial spine with cancellous screws.

## Graft Material Selection

When selecting graft material, the major considerations are the osteoconductive, osteoinductive, and structural properties of the graft. In general, osteoinductive factors, such as recombinant human bone morphogenetic protein 2 (rhBMP-2), are mitogenic and consequently are contraindicated in patients with active malignancy. To this end, "resected or extant tumor" is a Federal Drug Administration labeled contraindication for the use of rhBMP-2 (PMA P000058). Therefore, we favor osteoconductive materials, such as morselized allograft and demineralized bone matrix, and structural graft materials such as fibular strut graft. As illustrated in the case below, we often favor the use of fibular strut graft as it better approximates the elastic modulus of the clivus [relative to a titanium cage] and may reduce the risk of postoperative pharyngeal dehiscence. In general, we do not place strut grafts along the posterolateral elements though, due to size constraints.

For non-structural graft materials, we prefer morselized allograft, as it is more cost-effective than bioceramics or demineralized bone matrix. Additionally, the non-oncology literature has failed to demonstrate superior fusion outcomes for either of the synthetic alternatives relative to morselized allograft [121]. Similarly, a recent systematic review of different graft materials for patients undergoing instrumented fusion following vertebral column tumor resection found current evidence is insufficient to support the superiority of any single graft material [122].

## Complications and Consequences of Surgery

Surgical management of craniocervical chordomas is associated with high complication rates regardless of approach. For example, in their multi-institutional series, Molina et al. [81] reported a postoperative complication rate of 71%. The major complications of interest include infection, cranial nerve palsy or other new neurological deficit, vertebral artery injury, and hardware breakdown. The relative risk of these different complications is likely to depend upon the surgical approach and size of the resected lesion.

Anterior approaches are often complicated by pharyngeal dehiscence, which can be associated with infection and subsequent bone graft resorption, resulting in deformity and need for surgical revision [123]. CSF leaks and cranial neuropathies are also common, with Colli and Al-Mefty reporting the occurrence of new permanent postoperative neurological deficit in 29% of patients [124]. By comparison, Choi and colleagues reported CSF leaks to occur in only 6% of cases in their series of 97 patients treated for chordomas of the craniocervical junction and upper cervical spine [72]. This is similar to the findings of Hyun et al. [125], who reported the occurrence of a CSF leak in only 1 of 12 patients undergoing anterior or staged anterior-posterior resection of a craniocervical chordoma. A recent review by Shriver et al. [126] including 1238 patients having undergone transoral approaches to the craniocervical junction reported CSF leaks occurred in only 0.8% of cases. These patients underwent odontoidectomy alone and consequently may represent a lower risk surgical population. Nevertheless, pharyngeal dehiscence was noted in 1.7% of cases, meningitis in 1.0%, tracheostomy in 10.8%, velopharyngeal insufficiency in 3.3%, and meningitis in 1.0%. By contrast, Shousha et al. reported a rate of wound infection of 3.6% in their series of 139 patients treated with a transoral approach to pathologies of the craniocervical junction [127]. Yin et al. [128] reported a similar rate of wound infection (3.5%) in their single-site series of 172 patients treated with a transoral approach for complex craniocervical pathologies, including craniocervical tumors. It was noted that five of the six patients experiencing wound infection had undergone placement of anterior hardware, which our personal experience has also suggested to be a risk factor for wound complications. Additionally, postoperative radiation may increase the risk for pharyngeal dehiscence and we routinely recruit the assistance of plastic surgery in pharyngeal closure to decrease the risk of pharyngeal dehiscence and subsequent surgical site infection.

The transmandibular approach has a notably high risk of postoperative complications, with the most common complaints being postoperative sensitivity disturbances, dental, and orthodontic complaints. Choi and colleagues reported complications in four of their nine patients treated with transmandibular approaches to craniocervical chordoma [72]. A similarly high rate was reported by Bertrand et al. [129] in their series of 64 patients having undergone transmandibular approaches for benign or malignant tumors of the head and neck. They found 52% had postoperative sensitivity disturbances (18% on objective testing), 30% had temporomandibular joint pain, 73% had limitations in mandibular joint motion, 10% had cosmetic complaints, and 3% developed periodontal disease. Postoperative dysphagia is also extremely common and patients should be kept *nil* per os to avoid aspiration. In both the series of Choi and Colli, vertebral artery injury was a rare complication, occurring in only 1 of 132 surgeries in the Choi et al. series [72] and 0 of the 63 surgeries in the Colli and Al-Mefty series [124]. It is likely that this risk can be minimized by limiting lateral exposure at the craniocervical junction to 1.5 cm bilaterally [130].

With posterior approaches, chief complications include iatrogenic injury of the horizontal or oblique limbs of the V3 vertebral artery, wound infection, and postoperative hardware failure. While catastrophic, injury to the V3 segment is uncommon and current literature suggests that injury to this vessel is uncommon, occurring in <0.5% of cases [131]. In their series of 29 adult and pediatric patients undergoing staged anterior-posterior surgery for craniocervical chordoma, Shkarubo et al. [132] observed wound dehiscence in 10% of patients. Zuckerman et al. reported a similar rate in their mixed series of patients undergoing posterior surgery for primary or metastatic lesions of the craniocervical junction [133]. Rates of hardware failure appear to be similarly low in small series, though the majority of the literature examining postoperative fusion outcomes for occipitocervical lesions has focused on patients with metastatic disease. In these series, fusion rates range from 92 to 100% [5, 133–137]. A 2010 systematic review of the non-tumor literature reported similar findings, with an average fusion rate of 93% using screw-rod constructs [138].

For constructs instrumenting the occiput to the cervical spine, failure of the construct at C2 in flexion is a common mode of failure [139]. The risk of this complication can be reduced by including additional points of fixation and by including larger diameter rods [140]. In a cadaveric model of posterior occipitocervical (O-C7/T1) fusion, Anderson and colleagues [140] demonstrated that progressively larger rods were associated with notable increases in construct stiffness. Risk of rod failure can be further reduced by reducing rod notching (e.g., due to overly aggressive bending) [139, 141] or by employing a hinged rod [142, 143]. Some authors have argued that if non-hinged rods are used, they should never be bent in more than one direction or bent back [if the initial bend is too extreme] as this may lead to failure in the early postoperative period [42].

Additionally, Cheng et al. [144] reported that implant density in long occipitocervical fusions may significantly impact the rigidity of the construct. Using an O-T1 cadaveric spine, the authors compared the range of motion in flexion-extension, axial rotation, and lateral bending using three-point fixation at the occiput, C4, and T1 or total fixation (i.e., fixation at every level from occiput to T1). They found that the lower density, three-point fixation construct had a significantly higher range of motion in axial rotation and lateral bending. Similar issues may present themselves in the context of occipitocervical tumors that require resection of the central bony pillar at multiple levels, which precludes fixation at those levels. In such cases, unilateral fixation at the osteotomized levels should be pursued to help limit lateral bending and axial rotation.

## Example Case

A 61-year-old female presented to an outside facility with complaints of progressive, midline neck pain. Imaging was obtained that demonstrated a T2-hyperintense, T1-hypointense, heterogeneously enhancing mass involving the right lateral masses of the C2 and C3 vertebral bodies with prevertebral and epidural extension (Fig. 7.2). CT-guided biopsy of the lesion was positive for brachyury, consistent with a diagnosis of chordoma. The patient was neurologically non-focal on exam; however, given her good overall health and the lesion's epidural extension, it was recommended that she undergo *en bloc* resection with curative intent. A two-staged posterior-anterior procedure was planned, including a transmandibular anterior stage. Neoadjuvant radiation was not recommended given that the transmandibular approach already placed her at high risk for infection. The procedure is illustrated in Fig. 7.3.

The first stage comprised a midline occipito-cervico-thoracic approach with instrumentation placed from the occiput to the level of T2. C1–4 laminectomies were performed and parasagittal three-column osteotomies were performed at C1–4 to define the medial border of the surgical specimen. Care was taken to remain extracapsular and a silastic sheath was placed for the anterior stage. Outrigger rods were placed given the substantial instability that was expected following anterior column resection. A tracheostomy was placed and the anterior stage was performed the next day using a transmandibular circumglossal approach and right-sided radical neck dissection. The superior and inferior borders of the specimen were defined by an inferior clivectomy and C4/5 diskectomy, respectively. The sample was removed *en bloc* with negative margins on microscopic examination. A vascularized fibular strut autograft was placed in the resultant anterior column defect and anastomosed to the external carotid artery and facial vein. The graft was secured using a kick plate affixed to the C5 vertebra and a lag screw placed through the graft and into the clivus. The wound closure was performed by plastic surgery. The patient was successfully discharged but unfortunately required a revision of her posterior wound shortly after discharge, with the extension of her posterior fusion construct to T4. She has not required subsequent surgical intervention though and is now 12 months out with no evidence of tumor recurrence. She remains at her neurological baseline and has successfully had her trachea decannulated.

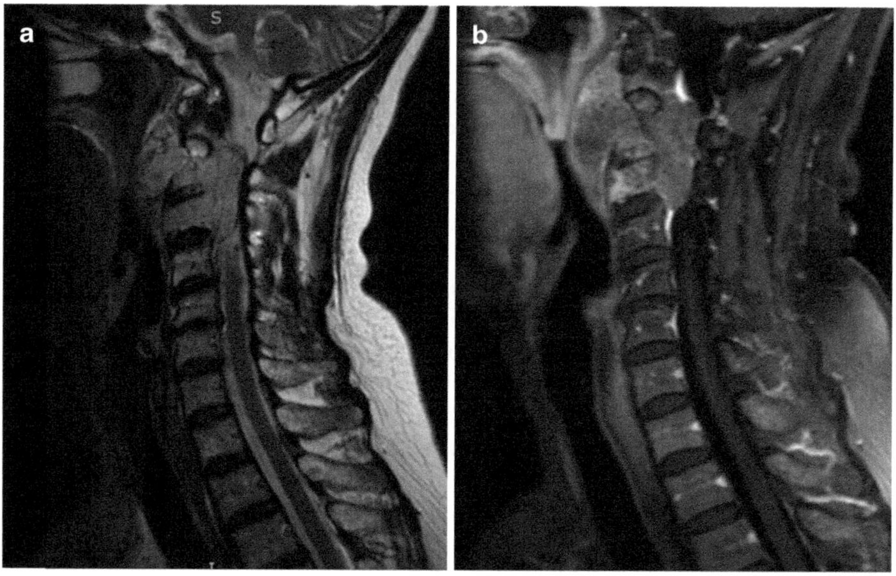


**Fig. 7.2** Preoperative imaging of a craniocervical chordoma. Sagittal MRI demonstrated a lesion involving the C2 and C3 bodies that was mildly hyperintense to bone on T2-weighted imaging (**a**) and demonstrated mild, heterogeneous enhancement on T1-weighted imaging (**b**). Axial sections through the C2 body (**c**), C2/3-disc space (**d**), and C3 body (**e**, **f**) show an eccentric mass arising from the right side of the C2–3 vertebrae, enveloping the right vertebral artery and expanding into the right prevertebral space. Additionally, the tumor invades through the C2/3 foramen and into the epidural space, displacing and deforming the cervical spinal cord. Bone-windowed sagittal (**g**) and axial (**h**) multi-detector CT images demonstrate near-complete erosion of the C3 body and erosion of the posteroinferior aspect of the axis. Three-dimensional CT reconstructions (**i**–**o**) demonstrated encasement of the right vertebral artery and lateral displacement of the right internal carotid artery and right internal jugular vein. (**i**–**m**) illustrate coronal reconstructions and (**n**–**o**) illustrate sagittal reconstructions

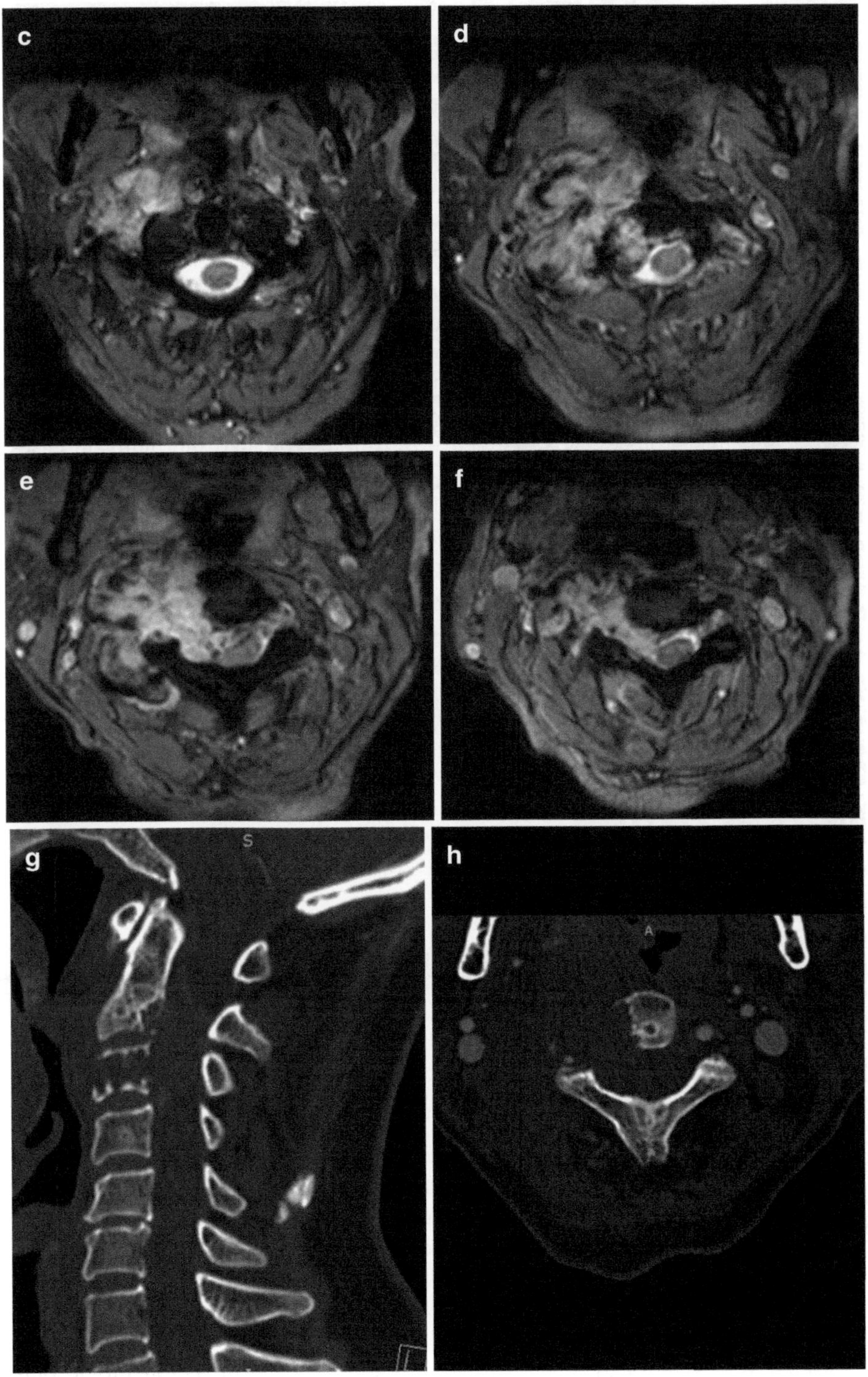


**Fig. 7.2** (continued)

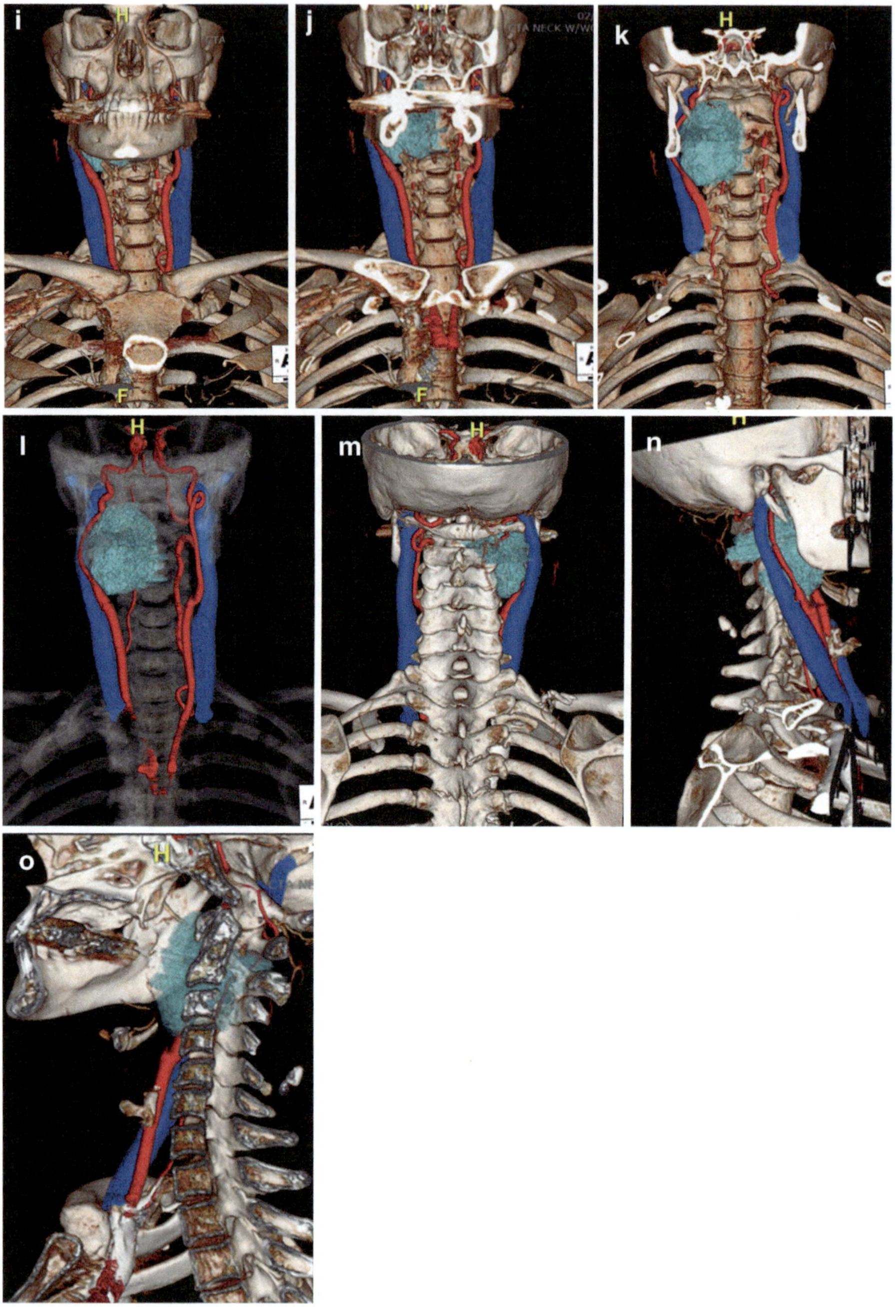


**Fig. 7.2** (continued)

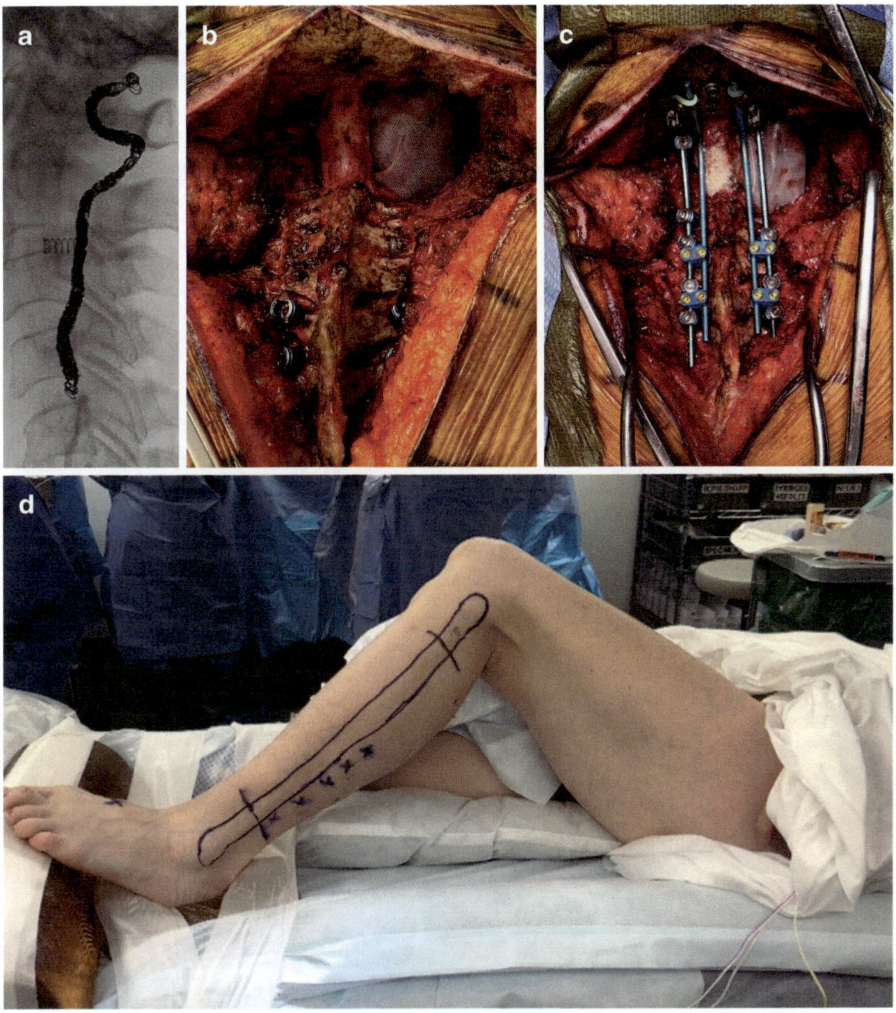

**Fig. 7.3** After demonstrating bilateral vertebral artery sufficiency, the patient underwent right vertebral artery sacrifice with endovascular coils placed by interventional radiology (**a**). The first stage employed a posterior approach (**b**, **c**) with a C1–4 laminectomy to decompress the spinal cord and expose the tumor. A silastic sheath was placed (**c**) to protect the spinal cord during the subsequent anterior stage. Instrumentation was placed from the occiput to T2 with accessory rods for additional stabilization (**c**). The second, anterior stage, was then executed using a transmandibular approach. The left leg was prepared (**d**) for harvesting of a vascularized fibular strut graft (**e**). The mandible was pre-plated (**f**) to ensure accurate reapproximation after resection of the tumor. A large soft tissue exposure was then performed, extending along the midline from the inferior lip to the mental protuberance. It was extended laterally along the inferior right mandibular border to the level of the mastoid tip (**g**). Multiple narrow malleable retractor blades were placed to expose the anterior aspect of the tumor (**h**), with vessel loops being used to tag essential neurovascular structures. The anterior osteotomy cuts were completed and the tumor delivered (**i**), allowing visualization of the posterior instrumentation (**j**). After placing the fibular strut graft, a kick-plate was secured to the superior aspect of the C5 body to prevent dislodgement of the strut graft (**k**). Superiorly the strut graft was affixed to the clivus using a lag screw (**l**). The wound was then reapproximated and the patient was taken to the neurocritical care unit

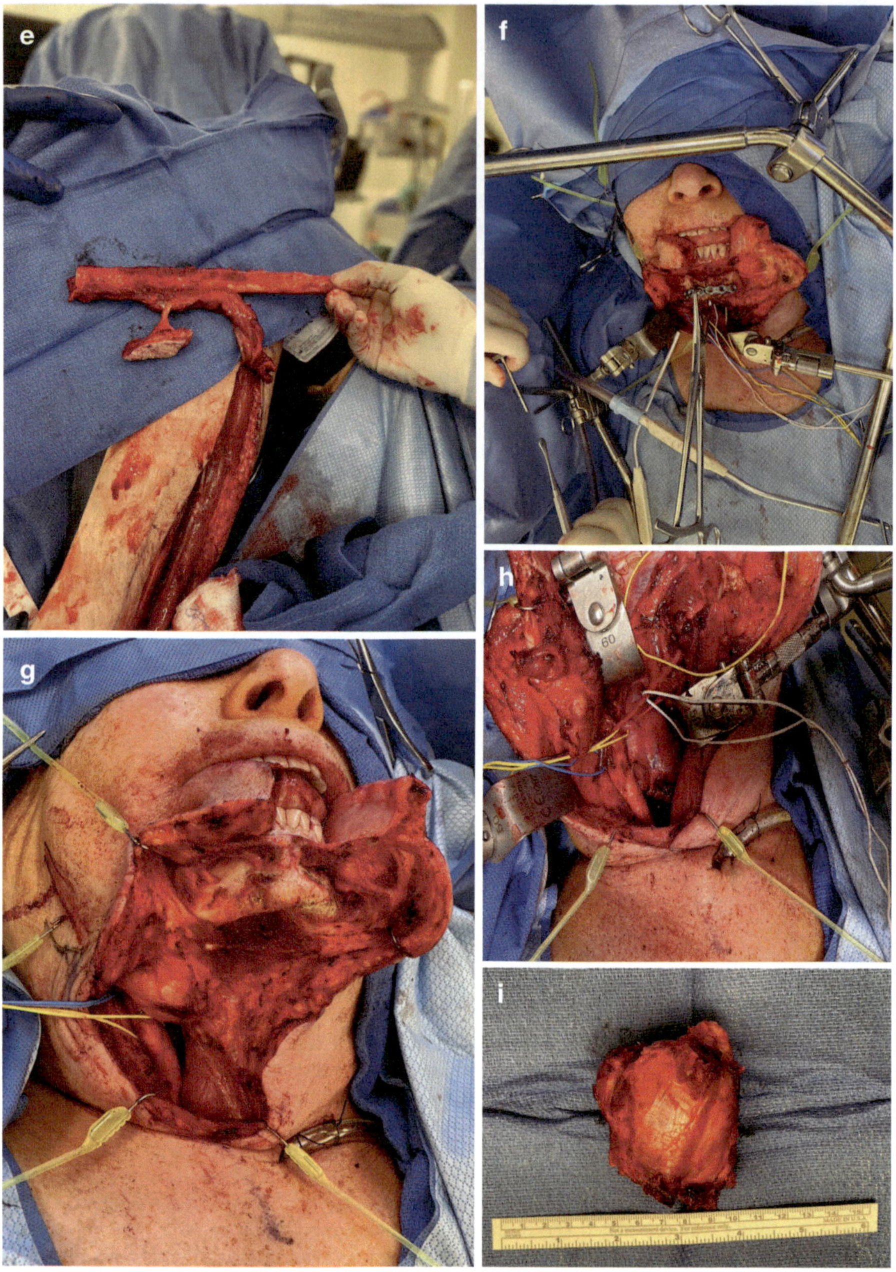


**Fig. 7.3** (continued)

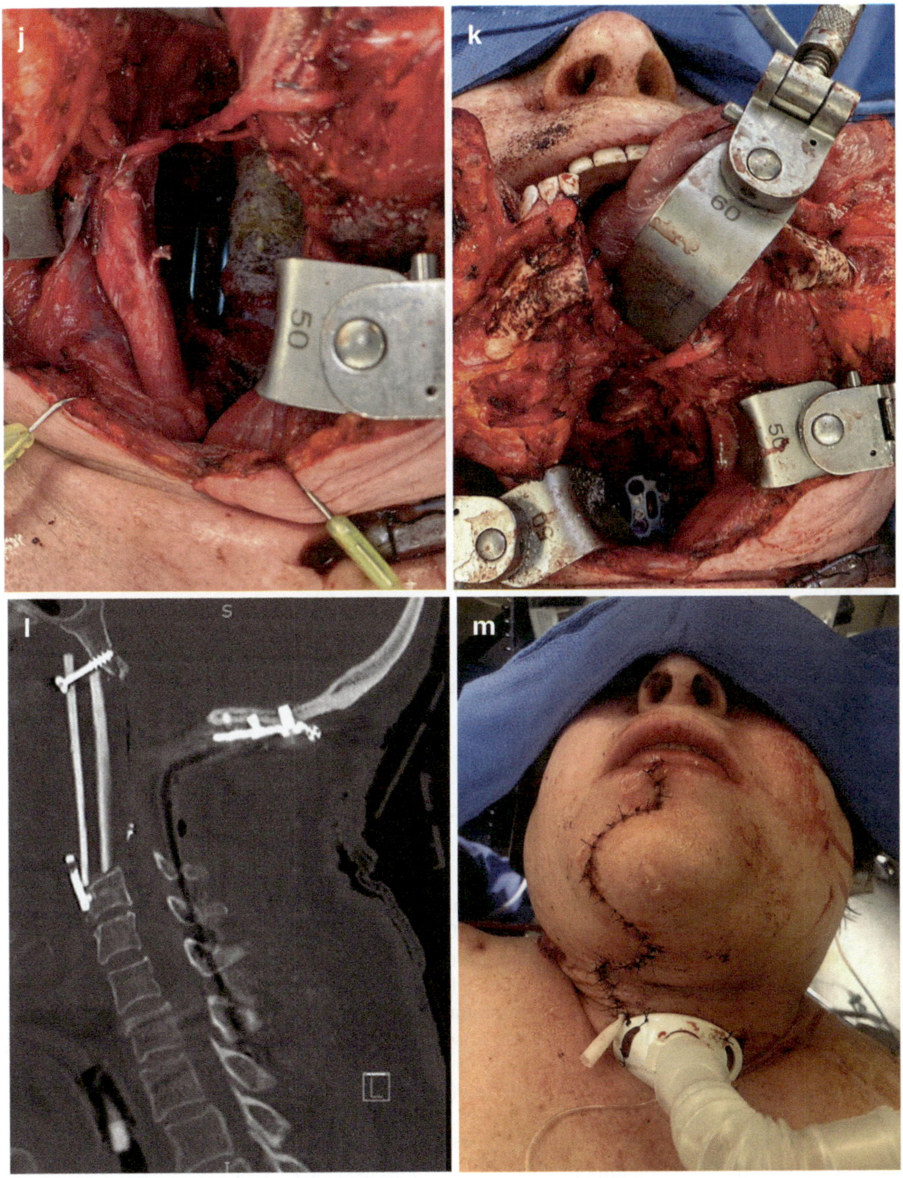


**Fig. 7.3** (continued)

## Conclusion

The craniocervical junction is a biomechanically complex segment of the mobile spine that can become involved primarily by chordomas of the atlantoaxial complex or secondarily by chordomas of the clivus or subaxial spine that extend along the craniocaudal axis. R0 resection with negative margins likely provides survival benefit and can be pursued via an anterior-only, posterior-only, or combined anterior-posterior approach, as dictated by the tumor morphology. The high mobility and complex anatomy of the craniocervical junction make *en bloc* resection with negative margins difficult. Additionally, *en bloc* resection is highly destabilizing and in the overwhelming majority of cases, reconstruction and instrumented fusion is required. We feel that the optimal reconstruction relies on a combination of anterior column support and posterior segmental instrumentation, though the current evidence is insufficient to support any singular approach. Intervention requires a multidisciplinary team and extensive preoperative planning; however, effective planning can lead to optimal patient outcomes.

**Disclosures** Daniel M. Sciubba Consultant for Baxter, DePuy-Synthes, Medtronic, Stryker.

**IRB Approval** IRB approval was not required for the present chapter. All images included have had patient identifiers removed.

## References

1. Fischer B, Steiner H. Über ein malignes Chordom der Schädel Rückgratshöhle. Beiträge zur Pathol Anat und zer Allg Pathol. 1907;40:109–19.
2. Wu KK, Mitchell DC, Guise ER. Chordoma of the atlas. J Bone Joint Surg Am. 1979;61:140–1.
3. Currier BL, Todd LT, Maus TP, Fisher DR, Yaszemski MJ. Anatomic relationship of the internal carotid artery to the C1 vertebra: a case report of cervical reconstruction for chordoma and pilot study to assess the risk of screw fixation of the atlas. Spine (Phila Pa 1976). 2003;28:E461–7.
4. Yang S, Gao Y. Clinical results of the transoral operation for lesions of the craniovertebral junction and its abnormalities. Surg Neurol. 1999;51:16–20.
5. Shin H, Barrenechea IJ, Lesser J, Sen C, Perin NI. Occipitocervical fusion after resection of craniovertebral junction tumors. J Neurosurg Spine. 2006;4:137–44.
6. Gokaslan ZL, Zadnik PL, Sciubba DM, et al. Mobile spine chordoma: results of 166 patients from the AOSpine Knowledge Forum Tumor database. J Neurosurg Spine. 2016;24:644–51.
7. Offiah CE, Day E. The craniocervical junction: embryology, anatomy, biomechanics and imaging in blunt trauma. Insights Imaging. 2017;8:29–47.
8. Crawford N, Hurlbert R. Anatomy and biomechanics of the craniocervical junction. Semin Neurosurg. 2002;13:101–10.
9. Dvorak J, Antinnes JA, Panjabi M, Loustalot D, Bonomo M. Age and gender related normal motion of the cervical spine. Spine (Phila Pa 1976). 1992;17:S393–8.

10. Panjabi M, Dvorak J, Duranceau J, Yamamoto I, Gerber M, Rauschning W, Bueff HU. Three-dimensional movements of the upper cervical spine. Spine (Phila Pa 1976). 1988;13:726–30.
11. Benzel EC. Biomechanics of spine stabilization. 2015; https://doi.org/10.1055/b-003-106374.
12. Ishii T, Mukai Y, Hosono N, Sakaura H, Nakajima Y, Sato Y, Sugamoto K, Yoshikawa H. Kinematics of the upper cervical spine in rotation. Spine (Phila Pa 1976). 2004;29:E139–44.
13. Penning L, Wilmink JT. Rotation of the cervical spine. Spine (Phila Pa 1976). 1987;12:732–8.
14. Dvorak J, Hayek J, Zehnder R. CT – functional diagnostics of the rotatory instability of the upper cervical spine. Spine (Phila Pa 1976). 1987;12:726–31.
15. Vishteh AG, Crawford NR, Melton MS, Spetzler RF, Sonntag VKH, Dickman CA. Stability of the craniovertebral junction after unilateral occipital condyle resection: a biomechanical study. J Neurosurg Spine. 1999;90:91–8.
16. Radcliff KE, Hussain MM, Moldavsky M, Klocke N, Vaccaro AR, Albert TJ, Khalil S, Bucklen B. In vitro biomechanics of the craniocervical junction—a sequential sectioning of its stabilizing structures. Spine J. 2015;15:1618–28.
17. Dvorak J, Schneider E, Saldinger P, Rahn B. Biomechanics of the craniocervical region: the alar and transverse ligaments. J Orthop Res. 1988;6:452–61.
18. Panjabi MM, Oxland TR, Parks EH. Quantitative anatomy of cervical spine ligaments. Part I. Upper cervical spine. J Spinal Disord. 1991;4:270–6.
19. Mueller K, MacConnell A, Berkowitz F, Voyadzis J-M. Morphological classification of the tubercle of insertion of the transverse atlantal ligament: a computer tomography–based anatomical study of 200 subjects. Neuroradiol J. 2019;32:426–30.
20. Fielding JW, van Cochran GB, Lawsing JF, Hohl M. Tears of the transverse ligament of the atlas. A clinical and biomechanical study. J Bone Joint Surg Am. 1974;56:1683–91.
21. Spence KF, Decker S, Sell KW. Bursting atlantal fracture associated with rupture of the transverse ligament. J Bone Joint Surg Am Vol. 1970;52:543–9.
22. Tubbs RS, Grabb P, Spooner A, Wilson W, Oakes WJ. The apical ligament: anatomy and functional significance. J Neurosurg Spine. 2000;92:197–200.
23. Tubbs RS, Hallock JD, Radcliff V, Naftel RP, Mortazavi M, Shoja MM, Loukas M, Cohen-Gadol AA. Ligaments of the craniocervical junction. J Neurosurg Spine. 2011;14:697–709.
24. Tubbs RS, Kelly DR, Humphrey ER, Chua GD, Shoja MM, Salter EG, Acakpo-Satchivi L, Wellons JC, Blount JP, Oakes WJ. The tectorial membrane: anatomical, biomechanical, and histological analysis. Clin Anat. 2007;20:382–6.
25. Tubbs RS, Mortazavi MM, Louis RG, Loukas M, Shoja MM, Chern JJ, Benninger B, Cohen-Gadol AA. The anterior atlantodental ligament: its anatomy and potential functional significance. World Neurosurg. 2012;77:775–7.
26. Phuntsok R, Ellis BJ, Herron MR, Provost CW, Dailey AT, Brockmeyer DL. The occipitoatlantal capsular ligaments are the primary stabilizers of the occipitoatlantal joint in the craniocervical junction: a finite element analysis. J Neurosurg Spine. 2019;30:593–601.
27. Kikuta S, Iwanaga J, Oskouian RJ, Tubbs RS. A new variant ligament of the atlantooccipital joint: the lateral oblique atlantooccipital ligament. Eur Spine J. 2019;28:1188–91.
28. Tubbs RS, Stetler W, Shoja MM, et al. The lateral atlantooccipital ligament. Surg Radiol Anat. 2007;29:219–23.
29. Tubbs RS, Dixon J, Loukas M, Shoja MM, Cohen-Gadol AA. Ligament of Barkow of the craniocervical junction: its anatomy and potential clinical and functional significance. J Neurosurg Spine. 2010;12:619–22.
30. Bodon G, Kiraly K, Tunyogi-Csapo M, Hirt B, Wilke H-J, Harms J, Patonay L. Introducing the craniocervical Y-ligament. Surg Radiol Anat. 2019;41:197–202.
31. Tubbs RS, Salter EG, Oakes WJ. The accessory atlantoaxial ligament. Neurosurgery. 2004;55:400–4.
32. Ulm AJ, Quiroga M, Russo A, Russo VM, Graziano F, Velasquez A, Albanese E. Normal anatomical variations of the V3 segment of the vertebral artery: surgical implications. J Neurosurg Spine. 2010;13:451–60.

33. Heary RF, Albert TJ, Ludwig SC, Vaccaro AR, Wolansky LJ, Leddy TP, Schmidt RR. Surgical anatomy of the vertebral arteries. Spine (Phila Pa 1976). 1996;21:2074–80.
34. Joaquim AF, Ghizoni E, Rubino PA, Anderle DV, Tedeschi H, Rhoton AL, de Oliveira E. Lateral mass screw fixation of the atlas: surgical technique and anatomy. World Neurosurg. 2010;74:359–62.
35. Tubbs RS, Mortazavi MM, Loukas M, Shoja MM, Cohen-Gadol AA. The intracranial denticulate ligament: anatomical study with neurosurgical significance. J Neurosurg. 2011;114:454–7.
36. Isaji T, Yasuda M, Kawaguchi R, Aoyama M, Niwa A, Nakura T, Matsuo N, Takayasu M. Posterior inferior cerebellar artery with an extradural origin from the V3 segment: higher incidence on the nondominant vertebral artery. J Neurosurg Spine. 2018;28:154–9.
37. Hong JT, Lee SW, Son BC, Sung JH, Yang SH, Kim IS, Park CK. Analysis of anatomical variations of bone and vascular structures around the posterior atlantal arch using three-dimensional computed tomography angiography. J Neurosurg Spine. 2008;8:230–6.
38. Skutta B, Fürst G, Eilers J, Ferbert A, Kuhn FP. Intracranial stenoocclusive disease: double-detector helical CT angiography versus digital subtraction angiography. Am J Neuroradiol. 1999;20:791–9.
39. Dagirmanjian A, Ross JS, Obuchowski N, Lewin JS, Tkach JA, Ruggieri PM, Masaryk TJ. High resolution, magnetization transfer saturation, variable flip angle, time-of-flight MRA in the detection of intracranial vascular stenoses. J Comput Assist Tomogr. 1995;19:700–6.
40. Westbroek EM, Pennington Z, Ehresman J, Ahmed AK, Gailloud P, Sciubba DM. Vertebral artery sacrifice versus Skeletonization in the setting of cervical spine tumor resection: case series. World Neurosurg. 2020;139:e601–7.
41. Ahmed AK, Pennington Z, Molina CA, Xia Y, Goodwin CR, Sciubba DM. Multidisciplinary surgical planning for en bloc resection of malignant primary cervical spine tumors involving 3D-printed models and neoadjuvant therapies: report of 2 cases. J Neurosurg Spine. 2019;30:424–31.
42. Joaquim AF, Osorio JA, Riew KD. Occipitocervical fixation: general considerations and surgical technique. Glob Spine J. 2020;10:647–56.
43. Soroceanu A, Smith JS, Lau D, et al. Establishing the minimum clinically important difference in Neck Disability Index and modified Japanese Orthopaedic Association scores for adult cervical deformity. J Neurosurg Spine. 2020;33:441–5.
44. Tan LA, Riew KD, Traynelis VC. Cervical spine deformity—part 1: biomechanics, radiographic parameters, and classification. Neurosurgery. 2017;81:197–203.
45. Ames CP, Blondel B, Scheer JK, et al. Cervical radiographical alignment: comprehensive assessment techniques and potential importance in cervical myelopathy. Spine (Phila Pa 1976). 2013;38:S149–60.
46. Iyer S, Lenke LG, Nemani VM, Fu M, Shifflett GD, Albert TJ, Sides BA, Metz LN, Cunningham ME, Kim HJ. Variations in occipitocervical and cervicothoracic alignment parameters based on age. Spine (Phila Pa 1976). 2016;41:1837–44.
47. Glassman SD, Bridwell K, Dimar JR, Horton W, Berven S, Schwab F. The impact of positive sagittal balance in adult spinal deformity. Spine (Phila Pa 1976). 2005;30:2024–9.
48. Kudo Y, Toyone T, Endo K, et al. Impact of spinopelvic sagittal alignment on the surgical outcomes of dropped head syndrome: a multi-center study. BMC Musculoskelet Disord. 2020;21:382.
49. Salazar D, Huff TJ, Cramer J, Wong L, Linke G, Zuniga J. Use of a three-dimensional printed anatomical model for tumor management in a pediatric patient. SAGE Open Med Case Rep. 2020;8:2050313X2092760.
50. Li Y, Zheng G, Liu T, Liang Y, Huang J, Liu X, Huang J, Cheng Z, Lu S, Huang L. Surgical resection of solitary bone plasmacytoma of atlas and reconstruction with 3-dimensional–printed titanium patient-specific implant. World Neurosurg. 2020;139:322–9.
51. Xiao J-RR, Huang WD, Yang X-HH, Yan W-JJ, Song D-WW, Wei HF, Liu T-LL WZP, Yang C. En bloc resection of primary malignant bone tumor in the cervical spine based on 3-dimensional printing technology. Orthop Surg. 2016;8:171–8.

52. Yamazaki M, Akazawa T, Okawa A, Koda M. Usefulness of three-dimensional full-scale modeling of surgery for a giant cell tumor of the cervical spine. Spinal Cord. 2007;45:250–3.
53. Detchou DK, Dimentberg R, Vaughan KA, Kolster R, Braslow BM, Malhotra NR. Navigated ultrasonic osteotomy to aid in en bloc chordoma resection via spondylectomy. World Neurosurg. 2020;143:319–24.
54. Vedantam A, Vigneswaran K, Rao G, Walsh GL, Rhines LD, Tatsui CE. Use of navigated ultrasonic bone cutting tool for en bloc resection of thoracic chondrosarcoma: technical report. Oper Neurosurg. 2020;19(5):551–6. https://doi.org/10.1093/ons/opaa239.
55. Petrov D, Spadola M, Berger C, Glauser G, Mahmoud AF, O'Malley B, Malhotra NR. Novel approach using ultrasonic bone curettage and transoral robotic surgery for en bloc resection of cervical spine chordoma: case report. J Neurosurg Spine. 2019;30:788–93.
56. Konakondla S, Albers JA, Li X, Barber SM, Nakhla J, Houghton CE, Telfeian AE, Oyelese AA, Fridley JS, Gokaslan ZL. Maximizing sacral chordoma resection by precise 3-dimensional tumor modeling in the operating room using intraoperative computed tomography registration with preoperative magnetic resonance imaging fusion and intraoperative neuronavigation: a case series. World Neurosurg. 2019;125:e1125–31.
57. Zoccali C, Walter CM, Favale L, Di Francesco A, Rossi B. A computer-assisted navigation technique to perform bone tumor resection without dedicated software. Comput Assist Surg. 2016;21:166–71.
58. Sen C, Shrivastava R, Anwar S, Triana A. Lateral transcondylar approach for tumors at the anterior aspect of the craniovertebral junction. Neurosurgery. 2010;66:A104–12.
59. Elliott RE, Kang MM, Smith ML, Frempong-Boadu A. C2 nerve root sectioning in posterior atlantoaxial instrumented fusions: a structured review of literature. World Neurosurg. 2012;78:697–708.
60. McLoughlin GS, Sciubba DM, Suk I, Bydon A, Witham T, Wolinsky J-P, Gokaslan ZL. Resection of a retropharyngeal craniovertebral junction chordoma through a posterior cervical approach. J Spinal Disord Tech. 2010;23:359–65.
61. Alzhrani G, Gozal YM, Eli I, Sivakumar W, Raheja A, Brockmeyer DL, Couldwell WT. Extreme lateral transodontoid approach to the ventral craniocervical junction: cadaveric dissection and case illustrations. J Neurosurg. 2019;131:920–30.
62. Singh H, Harrop J, Schiffmacher P, Rosen M, Evans J. Ventral surgical approaches to craniovertebral junction chordomas. Neurosurgery. 2010;66:A96–A103.
63. Wang Q, Wang Y, Wang J, Wang Y. Clinical classification of clival chordomas for transnasal approaches. Neurosurg Rev. 2020;43:1201–10.
64. Cavallo LM, Mazzatenta D, D'Avella E, et al. The management of clival chordomas: an Italian multicentric study. J Neurosurg. 2020:1–10.
65. Zoli M, Milanese L, Bonfatti R, et al. Clival chordomas: considerations after 16 years of endoscopic endonasal surgery. J Neurosurg. 2018;128:329–38.
66. DeMonte F, Diaz E, Callender D, Suk I. Transmandibular, circumglossal, retropharyngeal approach for chordomas of the clivus and upper cervical spine. Neurosurg Focus. 2001;10:1–5.
67. McAfee PC, Bohlman HH, Riley LH, Robinson RA, Southwick WO, Nachlas NE. The anterior retropharyngeal approach to the upper part of the cervical spine. J Bone Joint Surg Am. 1987;69:1371–83.
68. Agrawal A, Cavalcanti DD, Garcia-Gonzalez U, Chang SW, Crawford NR, Sonntag VKH, Spetzler RF, Preul MC. Comparison of extraoral and transoral approaches to the craniocervical junction: morphometric and quantitative analysis. World Neurosurg. 2010;74:178–88.
69. Ricciardi L, Sturiale CL, Izzo A, et al. Submandibular approach for single-stage craniovertebral junction ventral decompression and stabilization: a preliminary cadaveric study of technical feasibility. World Neurosurg. 2019;127:206–12.
70. Hsu W, Wolinsky J-P, Gokaslan ZL, Sciubba DM. Transoral approaches to the cervical spine. Neurosurgery. 2010;66:A119–25.
71. Baird CJ, Conway JE, Sciubba DM, Prevedello DM, Quiñones-Hinojosa A, Kassam AB. Radiographic and anatomic basis of endoscopic anterior craniocervical decompres-

sion: a comparison of endonasal, transoral, and transcervical approaches. Oper Neurosurg. 2009;65:ons158–64.
72. Choi D, Melcher R, Harms J, Crockard A. Outcome of 132 operations in 97 patients with chordomas of the craniocervical junction and upper cervical spine. Neurosurgery. 2010;66:59–65.
73. Feiz-Erfan I, Lettieri SC, Spetzler RF, Porter RW, Beals SP, Joganic EF, DeMonte F. Transmandibular approaches to the skull base. In: Badie B, editor. Neurosurgical operative. Atlas neuro-oncology. 2nd ed. New York: Georg Thieme Verlag; 2011. p. 301–7.
74. Choi D, Gleeson M. Surgery for chordomas of the craniocervical junction: lessons learned. Skull Base. 2010;20:041–5.
75. Hsu W, Sciubba DM, Daniel Sasson A, Khavkin Y, Wolinsky J-P, Gailloud P, Gokaslan ZL, Murphy K. Intraoperative localization of thoracic spine level with preoperative percutaneous placement of intravertebral polymethylmethacrylate. J Spinal Disord Tech. 2008;21:72–5.
76. Pillai P, Baig MN, Karas CS, Ammirati M. Endoscopic image-guided transoral approach to the craniovertebral junction: an anatomic study comparing surgical exposure and surgical freedom obtained with the endoscope and the operating microscope. Oper Neurosurg. 2009;64:ons437–44.
77. McGirt MJ, Attenello FJ, Sciubba DM, Gokaslan ZL, Wolinsky J-P. Endoscopic transcervical odontoidectomy for pediatric basilar invagination and cranial settling. J Neurosurg Pediatr. 2008;1:337–42.
78. Liu JK, Patel J, Goldstein IM, Eloy JA. Endoscopic endonasal transclival transodontoid approach for ventral decompression of the craniovertebral junction: operative technique and nuances. Neurosurg Focus. 2015;38:E17.
79. Dlouhy BJ, Dahdaleh NS, Menezes AH. Evolution of transoral approaches, endoscopic endonasal approaches, and reduction strategies for treatment of craniovertebral junction pathology: a treatment algorithm update. Neurosurg Focus. 2015;38:E8.
80. Fernandes Cabral DT, Zenonos GA, Fernandez-Miranda JC, Wang EW, Gardner PA. Iatrogenic seeding of skull base chordoma following endoscopic endonasal surgery. J Neurosurg. 2018;129:947–53.
81. Molina CA, Ames CP, Chou D, Rhines LD, Hsieh PC, Zadnik PL, Wolinsky J-P, Gokaslan ZL, Sciubba DM. Outcomes following attempted en bloc resection of cervical chordomas in the C-1 and C-2 region versus the subaxial region: a multiinstitutional experience. J Neurosurg Spine. 2014;21:348–56.
82. Ibaseta A, Rahman R, Andrade NS, et al. Crossing the cervicothoracic junction in cervical arthrodesis results in lower rates of adjacent segment disease without affecting operative risks or patient-reported outcomes. Clin Spine Surg. 2019;32:377–81.
83. Huang KT, Harary M, Abd-El-Barr MM, Chi JH. Crossing the cervicothoracic junction in posterior cervical decompression and fusion: a cohort analysis. World Neurosurg. 2019;131:e514–20.
84. Yüksel KZ, Adams MS, Chamberlain RH, Potocnjak M, Chan Park S, Sonntag VKH, Crawford NR. Pullout resistance of thoracic extrapedicular screws used as a salvage procedure. Spine J. 2007;7:286–91.
85. White KK, Oka R, Mahar AT, Lowry A, Garfin SR. Pullout strength of thoracic pedicle screw instrumentation. Spine (Phila Pa 1976). 2006;31:E355–8.
86. Koo KH, Yoon ST, Kim SB, Hutton WC. The effect of hubbing on the pull-out strength of lateral mass screws in the cervical spine. J Spinal Disord Tech. 2015;28:E45–8.
87. Jones EL, Heller JG, Silcox DH, Hutton WC. Cervical pedicle screws versus lateral mass screws: anatomic feasibility and biomechanical comparison. Spine (Phila Pa 1976). 1997;22:977–82.
88. Ito Z, Higashino K, Kato S, Kim SS, Wong E, Yoshioka K, Hutton WC. Pedicle screws can be 4 times stronger than lateral mass screws for insertion in the midcervical spine: a biomechanical study on strength of fixation. J Spinal Disord Tech. 2014;27:80–5.
89. Kretzer RM, Hu N, Umekoji H, Sciubba DM, Jallo GI, McAfee PC, Tortolani PJ, Cunningham BW. The effect of spinal instrumentation on kinematics at the cervicothoracic junction:

emphasis on soft-tissue response in an in vitro human cadaveric model. J Neurosurg Spine. 2010;13:435–42.
90. Johnston TL, Karaikovic EE, Lautenschlager EP, Marcu D. Cervical pedicle screws vs. lateral mass screws: uniplanar fatigue analysis and residual pullout strengths. Spine J. 2006;6:667–72.
91. Oh S-H, Min W-K. Analysis of cervical pedicle with reconstructed computed tomography imaging in Korean population. J Spinal Disord Tech. 2014;27:E99–E103.
92. Ludwig SC, Kramer DL, Balderston RA, Vaccaro AR, Foley KF, Albert TJ. Placement of pedicle screws in the human cadaveric cervical spine: comparative accuracy of three techniques. Spine (Phila Pa 1976). 2000;25:1655–67.
93. Yusof MI, Ming LK, Abdullah MS, Yusof AH. Computerized tomographic measurement of the cervical pedicles diameter in a Malaysian population and the feasibility for transpedicular fixation. Spine (Phila Pa 1976). 2006;31:E221–4.
94. Patwardhan A, Srivastava S, Nemade P, Bhosale S, Srivastava S. Computed tomography-based morphometric analysis of cervical pedicles in Indian population: a pilot study to assess feasibility of transpedicular screw fixation. J Postgrad Med. 2012;58:119.
95. Roberts DA, Doherty BJ, Heggeness MH. Quantitative anatomy of the occiput and the biomechanics of occipital screw fixation. Spine (Phila Pa 1976). 1998;23:1100–7.
96. Batista UC, Joaquim AF, Fernandes YB, Mathias RN, Ghizoni E, Tedeschi H. Computed tomography evaluation of the normal craniocervical junction craniometry in 100 asymptomatic patients. Neurosurg Focus. 2015;38:E5.
97. Zarghooni K, Boese CK, Siewe J, Röllinghoff M, Eysel P, Scheyerer MJ. Occipital bone thickness: implications on occipital-cervical fusion. A cadaveric study. Acta Orthop Traumatol Turc. 2016;50:606–9.
98. Hurlbert RJ, Crawford NR, Choi WG, Dickman CA. A biomechanical evaluation of occipitocervical instrumentation: screw compared with wire fixation. J Neurosurg Spine. 1999;90:84–90.
99. Haher TR, Yeung AW, Caruso SA, Merola AA, Shin T, Zipnick RI, Gorup JM, Bono C. Occipital screw pullout strength. Spine (Phila Pa 1976). 1999;24:5–9.
100. Takigawa T, Simon P, Orías AAE, Hong JT, Ito Y, Inoue N, An HS. Biomechanical comparison of occiput-C1–C2 fixation techniques. Spine (Phila Pa 1976). 2012;37:E696–701.
101. Uribe JS, Ramos E, Youssef AS, Levine N, Turner AWL, Johnson WM, Vale FL. Craniocervical fixation with occipital condyle screws. Spine (Phila Pa 1976). 2010;35:931–8.
102. Ma X-Y, Yin Q-S, Wu Z-H, Xia H, Liu J-F, Xiang M, Zhao W-D, Zhong S-Z. C1 pedicle screws versus C1 lateral mass screws. Spine (Phila Pa 1976). 2009;34:371–7.
103. Murakami S, Mizutani J, Fukuoka M, Kato K, Sekiya I, Okamoto H, Abumi K, Otsuka T. Relationship between screw trajectory of C1 lateral mass screw and internal carotid artery. Spine (Phila Pa 1976). 2008;33:2581–5.
104. Zarro CM, Ludwig SC, Hsieh AH, Seal CN, Gelb DE. Biomechanical comparison of the pull-out strengths of C1 lateral mass screws and C1 posterior arch screws. Spine J. 2013;13:1892–6.
105. Du JY, Aichmair A, Kueper J, Wright T, Lebl DR. Biomechanical analysis of screw constructs for atlantoaxial fixation in cadavers: a systematic review and meta-analysis. J Neurosurg Spine. 2015;22:151–61.
106. Oda I, Abumi K, Sell LC, Haggerty CJ, Cunningham BW, McAfee PC. Biomechanical evaluation of five different occipito-atlanto-axial fixation techniques. Spine (Phila Pa 1976). 1999;24:2377.
107. Nassos JT, Ghanayem AJ, Sasso RC, Tzermiadianos MN, Voronov LI, Havey RM, Rinella AS, Carandang G, Patwardhan AG. Biomechanical evaluation of segmental occipitoatlanto-axial stabilization techniques. Spine (Phila Pa 1976). 2009;34:2740–4.
108. Finn MA, Fassett DR, Mccall TD, Clark R, Dailey AT, Brodke DS. The cervical end of an occipitocervical fusion: a biomechanical evaluation of 3 constructs. J Neurosurg Spine. 2008;9:296–300.
109. Hur J-W, Kim J-S, Ryu K-S, Shin M-H. Accuracy and safety in screw placement in the high cervical spine. Clin Spine Surg. 2019;32:E193–9.

110. Louis R. Spinal stability as defined by the three-column spine concept. Anat Clin. 1985;7:33–42.
111. Pal GP, Routal RV. A study of weight transmission through the cervical and upper thoracic regions of the vertebral column in man. J Anat. 1986;148:245–61.
112. Goel VK, Clausen JD. Prediction of load sharing among spinal components of a C5–C6 motion segment using the finite element approach. Spine (Phila Pa 1976). 1998;23:684–91.
113. Hofmann E, Prescher A. The clivus: anatomy, normal variants and imaging pathology. Clin Neuroradiol. 2012;22:123–39.
114. Bailey CS, Fisher CG, Boyd MC, Dvorak MFS. En bloc marginal excision of a multilevel cervical chordoma. J Neurosurg Spine. 2006;4:409–14.
115. Alberto O-PL, Ernesto C-AE, Nicasio A-M, Luis G-AJ, Martín G-G, Juan B-C. Operative technique for en bloc resection of upper cervical chordomas: extended transoral transmandibular approach and multilevel reconstruction. Asian Spine J. 2014;8:820–6.
116. Jeszenszky D, Fülöp Fekete T, Harms J, Fekete TF, Melcher R, Harms J. C2 prosthesis: anterior upper cervical fixation device to reconstruct the second cervical vertebra. Eur Spine J. 2007;16:1695–700.
117. Yang J, Yang X-H, He S-H, Jiao J, Jia Q, Hu J-B, Xiao J-R. A novel reconstruction using a combined anterior and posterior approach after axis tumor spondylectomy. Clin Spine Surg. 2020;33:E299–306.
118. Wewel JT, Nunna RS, Tan LA, Kasliwal MK, O'Toole JE. Novel reconstruction of the anterior craniocervical junction using an expandable cage with integrated fixation after total C2 spondylectomy for chordoma. J Clin Neurosci. 2016;30:157–60.
119. Eco LC, Brayton A, Whitehead WE, Jea A. Reconstruction of the anterior craniocervical junction using an expandable cage after resection of a C1 chordoma in a 5-year-old child: case report. J Neurosurg Pediatr. 2019;24:62–5.
120. Ozpinar A, Liu JJ, Whitney NL, Tempel ZJ, Choi PA, Andersen PE, Coppa ND, Hamilton DK. Anterior spinal reconstruction to the clivus using an expandable cage after C2 chordoma resection via a labiomandibular glossotomy approach: a technical report. World Neurosurg. 2016;90:372–9.
121. Kadam A, Millhouse PW, Kepler CK, Radcliff KE, Fehlings MG, Janssen ME, Sasso RC, Benedict JJ, Vaccaro AR. Bone substitutes and expanders in spine surgery: a review of their fusion efficacies. Int J Spine Surg. 2016;10:33.
122. Elder BD, Ishida W, Goodwin CR, Bydon A, Gokaslan ZL, Sciubba DM, Wolinsky J-P, Witham TF. Bone graft options for spinal fusion following resection of spinal column tumors: systematic review and meta-analysis. Neurosurg Focus. 2017;42:E16.
123. Wei F, Liu Z, Liu X, Jiang L, Dang G, Passias PG, Yu M, Wu F, Dang L. An approach to primary tumors of the upper cervical spine with spondylectomy using a combined approach. Spine (Phila Pa 1976). 2018;43:81–8.
124. Colli BO, Al-Mefty O. Chordomas of the skull base: follow-up review and prognostic factors. Neurosurg Focus. 2001;10:1–11.
125. Hyun S-J, Kim J-W, Kim K-J, Jahng T-A, Roh SW, Ra Y-S, Kim H-J, Rhim S-C. Long-term results following surgical resection of chordomas in the craniocervical junction and the upper cervical spine: review of 12 consecutive cases. Oper Neurosurg. 2018;14:112–20.
126. Shriver MF, Kshettry VR, Sindwani R, Woodard T, Benzel EC, Recinos PF. Transoral and transnasal odontoidectomy complications: a systematic review and meta-analysis. Clin Neurol Neurosurg. 2016;148:121–9.
127. Shousha M, Mosafer A, Boehm H. Infection rate after transoral approach for the upper cervical spine. Spine (Phila Pa 1976). 2014;39:1578–83.
128. Yin Q, Xia H, Wu Z, Ma X, Ai F, Zhang K, Wang J, Zhang T, Bai Z, Wang Z. Surgical site infections following the transoral approach. Clin Spine Surg. 2016;29:E502–8.
129. Bertrand J, Luc B, Philippe M, Philippe P. Anterior mandibular osteotomy for tumor extirpation: a critical evaluation. Head Neck. 2000;22:323–7.

130. Güvençer M, Men S, Naderi S, Kiray A, Tetik S. The V2 segment of the vertebral artery in anterior and anterolateral cervical spinal surgery: a cadaver angiographic study. Clin Neurol Neurosurg. 2006;108:440–5.
131. Elliott RE, Tanweer O, Frempong-Boadu A, Smith ML. Impact of starting point and C2 nerve status on the safety and accuracy of C1 lateral mass screws. J Spinal Disord Tech. 2015;28:171–85.
132. Shkarubo AN, Andreev DN, Konovalov NA, Zelenkov PV, Lubnin AJ, Chernov IV, Koval KV. Surgical treatment of skull base tumors, extending to craniovertebral junction. World Neurosurg. 2017;99:47–58.
133. Zuckerman SL, Kreines F, Powers A, Iorgulescu JB, Elder JB, Bilsky MH, Laufer I. Stabilization of tumor-associated craniovertebral junction instability: indications, operative variables, and outcomes. Neurosurgery. 2017;81:251–8.
134. Abumi K, Takada T, Shono Y, Kaneda K, Fujiya M. Posterior occipitocervical reconstruction using cervical pedicle screws and plate–rod systems. Spine (Phila Pa 1976). 1999;24:1425–34.
135. Luksanapruksa P, Buchowski JM, Wright NM, Valone FH, Peters C, Bumpass DB. Outcomes and effectiveness of posterior occipitocervical fusion for suboccipital spinal metastases. J Neurosurg Spine. 2017;26:554–9.
136. Fourney DR, York JE, Cohen ZR, Suki D, Rhines LD, Gokaslan ZL. Management of atlantoaxial metastases with posterior occipitocervical stabilization. J Neurosurg Spine. 2003;98:165–70.
137. George B, Archilli M, Cornelius JF. Bone tumors at the cranio-cervical junction. Surgical management and results from a series of 41 cases. Acta Neurochir. 2006;148:741–9.
138. Winegar CD, Lawrence JP, Friel BC, Fernandez C, Hong J, Maltenfort M, Anderson PA, Vaccaro AR. A systematic review of occipital cervical fusion: techniques and outcomes. J Neurosurg Spine. 2010;13:5–16.
139. Steinmetz MP, Mroz TE, Benzel EC. Craniovertebral junction. Neurosurgery. 2010;66:A7–A12.
140. Anderson PA, Oza AL, Puschak TJ, Sasso R. Biomechanics of occipitocervical fixation. Spine (Phila Pa 1976). 2006;31:755–61.
141. Lindsey C, Deviren V, Xu Z, Yeh R-F, Puttlitz CM. The effects of rod contouring on spinal construct fatigue strength. Spine (Phila Pa 1976). 2006;31:1680–7.
142. Abode-Iyamah K, Dlouhy B, Lopez A, Menezes A, Hitchon P, Dahdaleh N. Comparison of hinged and contoured rods for occipitocervical arthrodesis in adults: a clinical study. J Craniovertebr Junction Spine. 2016;7:171.
143. Iyer RR, Elder BD, Garzon-Muvdi T, Sacks JM, Suk I, Wolinsky J-P. Use of an articulating hinge to facilitate cervicothoracic deformity correction during vertebral column resection. Oper Neurosurg. 2018;15:278–84.
144. Cheng BC, Hafez MA, Cunningham B, Serhan H, Welch WC. Biomechanical evaluation of occipitocervicothoracic fusion: impact of partial or sequential fixation. Spine J. 2008;8:821–6.

# Surgical Management of Chordoma of the Cervical Spine

# 8

Oliver G. S. Ayling and Nicolas Dea

## Abbreviations

| | |
|---|---|
| C | Cervical |
| CT | Computed tomography |
| MR | Magnetic resonance |
| T | Thoracic |
| WBB | Weinstein-Boriani-Biagini |

## Introduction

The cervical spine is a relatively uncommon location for primary chordoma. As with chordomas of other spinal regions, *en bloc* resection with negative margins is considered the standard of care owing to the superior odds of achieving long-term overall and progression-free survival [1–4]. However, achieving such resection is often difficult owing to the intimate association of the subaxial cervical vertebrae with multiple vital neurovascular structures, notably the vertebral arteries and the nerve roots feeding the brachial plexus. Additionally, resection of lesions at the cervicothoracic junction places instability at a stress riser within the mobile spine, which demands complex reconstruction to provide adequate biomechanical support. Here, we review the principles and techniques employed for the management of chordomas of the subaxial cervical spine.

O. G. S. Ayling · N. Dea (✉)
Combined Neurosurgical and Orthopedic Spine Program, Vancouver General Hospital, University of British Columbia, Vancouver, BC, Canada
e-mail: nicolas.dea@vch.ca



D. M. Sciubba, J. H. Schwab (eds.), *Chordoma of the Spine*,
https://doi.org/10.1007/978-3-030-76201-8_8

## Anatomy of the Cervical Spine

The anatomy of the cervical spine and neck has many critically important structures all of which can lead to morbidity for the patient via intentional sacrifice as part of the surgical plan or inadvertent injury. These unique challenges lead to specific technical intricacies that are not encountered in the thoracic, lumbar, and sacral regions [5]. Extra-spinal anatomy includes the esophagus, trachea, paraspinal musculature, carotid arteries, as well as cranial nerve branches of the vagus nerve, glossopharyngeal nerve, hypoglossal, nerve, recurrent laryngeal nerve, accessory nerve, and sympathetic chain. As well, the lesser-known cervical plexus, comprised of C1–C4 nerve roots and located deep to the sternocleidomastoid, must be avoided in order to maintain sensation to the posterior neck and scalp, and motor function to the strap muscles and diaphragm. Additionally, there are cervical nerve roots bilaterally at each level that exit above their corresponding pedicles, except for C8, which exits below the C7 vertebral body. Particular attention must be paid to the nerve roots and whether they will be removed during the surgery as the associated motor and sensory deficits will impact patient function and quality of life. The vertebral artery is intimately involved with the cervical spine as it enters the foramen transversarium, typically at the C6 level but in ~10% of patients may enter at C7. The vertebral artery then travels up to C1 where it begins to course posteriorly along the posterior arch of C1 prior to piercing the dura intracranially and merging to form the basilar artery. It is vital to obtain preoperative vascular imaging with computed tomography (CT) or magnetic resonance (MR) angiography followed by conventional catheter angiograms. Careful study of the preoperative vascular imaging allows one to determine the dominant vertebral artery, the extent of tumor involvement with the vertebral arteries, and whether there is sufficient collateral flow from the contralateral vertebral artery. Utilization of preoperative catheter angiograms allows for assessment of collateral flow during occlusion tests, embolization of the involved arteries, and provides exquisite anatomical details unafforded by CT and MR imaging. In particular, it must be noted if the anterior spinal artery has a unilateral vertebral artery origin or if a vertebral artery ends as a posterior inferior cerebellar artery where the sacrifice of that vertebral artery would lead to spinal cord or cerebellar infarction.

There are seven cervical vertebral bodies with their corresponding intervertebral disk spaces. As discussed in Chap. 7, the atlas (C1) and axis (C2) support the head on the spine and provide ~50% of the rotation of the cervical spine. Involvement of tumor at C1–C2 will often necessitate an occipital-cervical fusion of the patient's spine, significantly impacting their mobility. Furthermore, the angle of the mandible obscures access to the atlas and axis making their surgical access inherently more challenging. In most patients, access to the C3–C7 vertebral segments is straightforward from either an anterior or posterior approach but lower cervical-thoracic segments can be obscured by the sternum and chest wall anteriorly. *En bloc* surgery in the cervical spine leads to significant instability and the reconstruction must attempt to achieve a solid fixation while maintaining as much biomechanical function of cervical spine as possible. Moreover, as the surgical intent is often cure, methods to ensure solid bony union are desirable, especially in a hostile environment like the cervico-thoracic junction or in patients who will have high-dose postoperative radiation [6].

## Surgical Approaches

Stefano Boriani, a pioneer of *en bloc* surgical resections for spinal tumors, eloquently highlighted a fundamental principle delivered by Bertil Stener, who is credited with innovating spine oncology care with his early *en bloc* surgeries, "it does not exist a single surgical technique able to perform *en bloc* resection of all bone tumors in the spine, but the surgical technique should be planned according to the tumor extension, the spine location, the histology, the margins to be achieved" [7, 8]. It then follows from this that the fundamental underpinning of cervical surgery for resection of chordomas should adhere to oncological principles, chiefly Enneking appropriate resections, when this can be achieved with acceptable morbidity to the patient. To aid in the planning of *en bloc* surgical resections of primary spinal tumors, the Weinstein-Boriani-Biagini (WBB) surgical system was proposed in 1997 [9]. This system was created to expand on the Enneking system [10] and address some of the shortcomings of applying a system for the appendicular skeleton to the spine.

### The Role of Biopsy, Surgical Staging, and Surgical Planning

A fundamental tenet of surgery for primary spinal tumors, such as chordomas, is the inclusion of the biopsy route with a margin of healthy tissue in the resection specimen. Once a biopsy has been planned and performed, leading to a diagnosis, then surgical staging via the WBB system is undertaken to determine the extension of the tumor. The oncologic spine surgeon should be involved in the planning of the biopsy, to facilitate resection of its tract during the definitive surgery. Transoral biopsy and other biopsy tracts that violate multiple fascial layers should be avoided. The vertebra is divided into 12 wedge-shaped regions in the transverse plane, akin to a clock-face, that radiates around the spinal cord. On top of this, five concentric zones from outside to inside are used to describe the extent of osseous and dural involvement [9]. Utilization of the WBB system leads to three fundamental approaches for *en bloc* resections of spinal tumors: a vertebrectomy when only one pedicle is involved, a sagittal resection when anterior and posterior elements are involved, and resection of the posterior arch for tumors involving only the posterior elements. This system allows for surgical planning to maintain oncological resections with the goal of reducing local recurrence and increasing survival rates. In total, there are up to ten different surgical strategies outlined by the WBB system for primary spinal tumors [8].

## Combined Approaches for Cervical Chordomas

In general, wide or marginal *en bloc* excisions of cervical chordomas require multi-staged procedures with a multidisciplinary team including spine surgeons, plastic surgeons, and otolaryngologists [11, 12]. In the largest case series of *en bloc* resections for cervical chordomas by Molina et al. [13], only 3 of 16 patients underwent a one-sided surgical approach. For the vast majority of subaxial cervical chordoma resections, the first stage is performed via a posterior approach. There are many goals to the posterior approach. Beginning with a posterior approach allows placement of instrumentation for stabilization, performing releasing osteotomies, facetectomies, and laminectomies, as well as ligation of involved nerve roots and vertebral artery. Spinal navigation is used to facilitate screw insertion but more importantly to guide osteotomy cuts and tumor delineation. For positioning, the head is fixated in the Mayfield skull clamp to maintain neutral spine alignment. Posteriorly, lateral mass screws and connecting rods are typically used for stabilization with consideration of occipital fixation for higher tumors. If the vertebral artery needs to be sacrificed, we would typically have it embolized preoperatively to decrease the risks of bleeding intraoperatively. Preoperative angiography is crucial in these cases to better delineate the anatomy and to assess if the vertebral artery can be safely sacrificed, as mentioned above. In patients where there is doubt about the safety of vessel occlusion, a balloon occlusion test can be done in conjunction with a wake-up test to make sure the patient is stable neurologically. Once embolized with coils, the artery is easier to identify and to dissect during the surgery. The vertebral artery can then be cut during the posterior approach. The C1–C4 nerve roots can often be taken with minimal functional impairment to the patient, in contrast to the substantial morbidity of taking C5–T1 nerve roots. Nevertheless, hemi-diaphragmatic paralysis can be seen with unilateral upper cervical nerve root sacrifice. In our experience, however, this has not resulted in serious clinical consequences. Posterior tumor dissection and development of a clear plane between the tumor pseudocapsule and dural interface can also be achieved posteriorly. The posterior longitudinal ligament is also cut at the level of the disk spaces and the discectomy is often also initiated from the back to facilitate the second stage of the surgery. We would also typically try to do as much tumor dissection during the posterior approach as more work during the first stage will significantly facilitate the second stage. This includes posterolateral tumor dissection as anterior as possible. Nerve roots that are to be saved will be dissected and marked with vessel loops to facilitate their identification during the anterior part. Depending on the surgical plan, the final rods can be placed during the initial stage, but it may be necessary to finalize the construct after the anterior approach if the tumor is in the way or if the spine needs to be mobile to facilitate anterior exposure. After completion of the posterior portion of the case, the incision is closed and the second stage of the operation occurs, typically the next day. The assistance of plastic surgery colleagues is invaluable to ensure proper soft tissue coverage and decrease wound complications in patients with previous surgery, radiation therapy, or when the incision involves the cervicothoracic junction [14].

The anterior portion of the operation involves anterior dissection of the tumor, any remaining osteotomy cuts, and *en bloc* delivery of the specimen followed by any required anterior reconstruction. The second operative stage may, in some cases, require lateral positioning of the patient in order to have simultaneous anterior and posterior access [12] but is more commonly performed in a typical supine position. During anterior approaches, particularly for higher cervical cases, otolaryngology surgeons may be of valuable assistance in the exposure and preservation of the larynx, esophagus, carotid artery, and cranial nerve branches. In these circumstances, a large anterior incision extending from the mastoid along the anterior border of the sternocleidomastoid is performed, allowing wide exposure to safely access the tumor as well as to deliver it in *en bloc* fashion. Some have performed resections of cervical chordomas from this anterior approach alone but led to intralesional and or subtotal resections in all patients as it is a significant challenge to effectively remove any tumor posterior to the pedicle or spinal cord [5]. Critical structures to be preserved are identified, discectomies and osteotomies are completed, and the tumor is delivered. Anterior reconstruction is tailored to the resection performed. For symmetrical reconstructions expandable cages and anterior plating are used [11] while asymmetrical reconstructions can be achieved with iliac or fibular grafts and secured in place with screws [18]. As mentioned previously, a solid bony union should be the goal. Due to the highly unstable nature of *en bloc* resections of chordomas in the cervical spine, external bracing may be considered to facilitate fusion and prevent hardware complications or pseudarthrosis.

Surgery for resection of chordomas at C1–C2 and the craniocervical junction is technically more demanding than the subaxial spine and associated with a higher rate of complications [13]. Despite this, *en bloc* resections following oncological principles, rather than intralesional operations, are possible to achieve. In order to assist with this goal, the utilization of transoral or transmandibular approaches may be necessary in conjunction with otolaryngology surgeons [15]. Surgery of chordomas at the craniocervical junction is discussed in further detail in Chap. 7.

## Complications

Complications during and after surgery for cervical chordomas are common [16]. The importance of a multidisciplinary team in an experienced quaternary center cannot be overstated. Even in very experienced hands, these cases are very challenging and rigorous planning is mandatory [17]. Although the overall reported number of case series in this patient population is relatively small they all have complications related to the operations [16]. Broadly, complications occur due to the associated inherent morbidity of the surgical approach with dysphagia [12, 13, 18], nerve palsies leading to weakness of the limbs or diaphragm [11, 13, 18], hardware complications with pseudoarthrosis or instrument failures [11, 13, 18], and medical complications with wound infections, pneumonia, and shock [11, 13, 18]. Dysphagia is the most common adverse event after cervical *en bloc* tumor resections because of the extensive circumferential approaches, retraction, and often sacrifice of neural structure and muscles involved in swallowing, with up to ≈30% reported in the literature [19]. As dysphagia postoperatively is so common it has been our practice to consider early PEG tube insertion to ensure proper nutritional intake early postoperatively. Similarly, a tracheostomy may also be used upfront if prolonged intubation is anticipated as respiratory adverse events are as common as dysphagia in this patient population [19]. Expected neurological deficits should be thoroughly discussed with the patients ahead of time. To aid in recovery after such extensive operations, rehabilitation may be necessary for patients with significant deficits, and nerve or tendon transfer can be considered as well. Molina et al. [13] compared attempted *en bloc* resections of cervical chordomas at C1–2 to those at C3–C7 and demonstrated a significantly higher rate of complications (71% vs. 22%) and lower rates of marginal resections (29% vs. 78%), highlighting the immense technical challenge of surgery at the C1–2 levels.

## Quality of Life

Oncologic resection of cervical chordomas is a significant undertaking that can lead to substantial morbidity. The patient should be central in the shared decision-making process as some of this morbidity may be unacceptable to individual patients. More important than crude complication rates are the quality-of-life changes secondary to these massive surgeries. We know however that in long-term survivors, quality of life scores return to normative data and that recurrence is the most important factor negatively impacting the quality of life in these patients [17, 20]. As such, aggressive surgeries to decrease local recurrence is justified from a quality-of-life standpoint. However, the significant morbidity of surgery for cervical chordomas has pushed some groups to reconsider oncologic resections for these cases [21]. In an international survey of major cancer centers, up to 30% of respondents preferred intralesional resection and relied more heavily on adjuvant treatment rather than attempting *en bloc* resections for tumors that would result in high morbidity, such as high cervical chordomas. As discussed in Chap. 14, some promising outcomes are available to support these intralesional resections followed by high-dose radiation therapy, but long-term outcome data are lacking before such a management strategy can be suggested [22]. Despite this, in patients who refuse maximally aggressive surgical resection or in medically unstable patients, such an approach may be the best one. Many advances have been made in the radiation oncology world including stereotactic body radiation therapy, intensity-modulated photons radiation therapy, and heavy particles radiation therapy like protons and carbon ion. These will be discussed in more details in Chap. 15 of this book.

## Case

A 66-year-old man presented with worsening neck pain and dysphagia but was otherwise neurologically intact. MRI and CT scan of the cervical spine demonstrated a large mass centered at C3 and extending from C2 to C4 with associated pathological fracture of the C3 vertebral body (Fig. 8.1a, b). A CT-guided biopsy confirmed the diagnosis of chordoma. Given the involvement of the vertebral artery, coil embolization was performed preoperatively (Fig. 8.1c).

A two-stage surgery over two days was planned with the goal of an *en bloc* resection. The first stage consisted of an occipital to T2 posterior instrumented fusion. Screws were placed at C1, C2, C6, T1, T2, and an occipital plate. After the posterior instrumentation was placed, laminectomies at C2–C5 were completed. The lateral masses at C3 and C4 on the right and C4 and C5 on the left were then removed. The pedicles of C4 and C5 were then cut to ensure anterior-posterior connection. The vertebral artery was then divided just distal to where it was embolized. At this point, with a corridor to the tumor, the tumor was progressively dissected anteriorly to the carotid sheath. Then, C2 was osteotomized to the vertebral foramen and connected to the C2/3-disk space, this allowed the vertebral artery to then be mobilized out of the way. In order to continue the anterior dissection of the tumor around the pseudocapsule the left C3 and C4 nerve roots were taken at the dural take off and again distal to the tumor (Fig. 8.2a). In total this allowed an open corridor to dissect tumor off of the dura. Next, discectomies were performed at C2/3 and C4/5. A Penrose drain was then placed anteriorly to the thecal sac and cottonoid patties placed bilaterally to mark the boundaries to be identified during the anterior approach. Prior to closure temporary right-side rod from C1–T2 was placed to provide some stabilization but still allow for the extension of the neck to facilitate the second-stage anterior approach. The patient was kept intubated and sedated overnight.

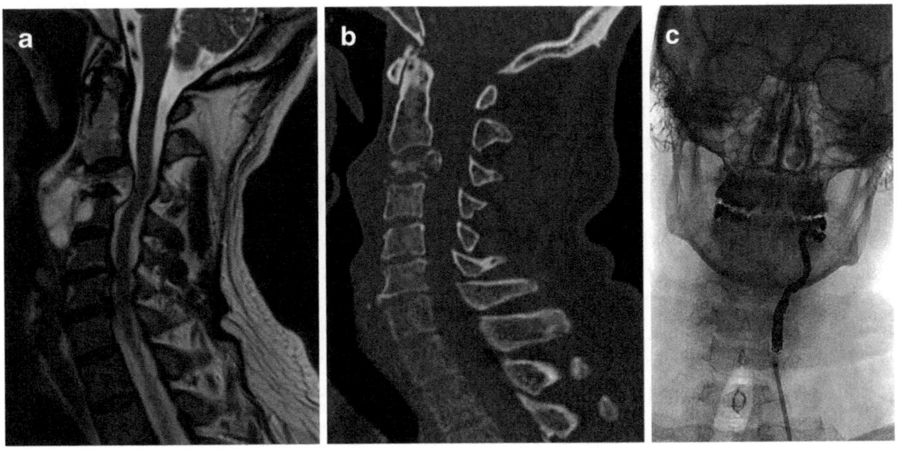


**Fig. 8.1** Preoperative imaging. (**a**) Sagittal T2-weighted MRI image of C3 lesion. (**b**) Sagittal CT image of C3 lesion. (**c**) Preoperative embolization of left vertebral artery

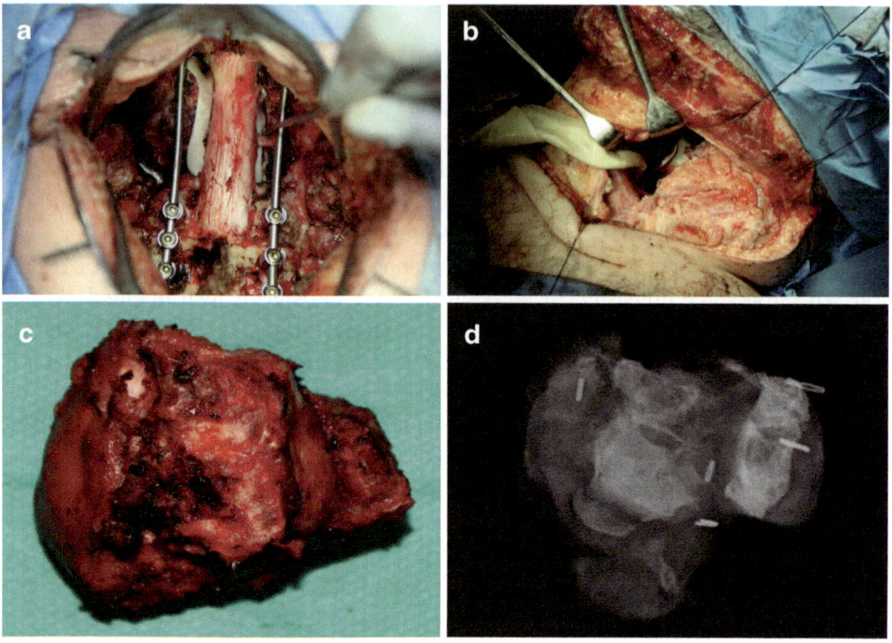


**Fig. 8.2** Intraoperative images of the cervical chordoma *en bloc* resection. (**a**) Posterior approach highlighting the posterior dissection plane of the tumor and resection of left C3 and C4 nerve roots. (**b**) Anterior approach via incision extending from mastoid to mastoid for tumor dissection and anterior delivery. (**c**) Image of specimen after *en bloc* resection. (**d**) X-ray of the *en bloc* specimen

The second stage of the operation was performed via an anterior approach in conjunction with the otolaryngology team (Fig. 8.2b). A large anterior incision from the left to the right mastoid tip bilaterally was performed with the raising of platysmal flaps. The sternocleidomastoid was skeletonized and the marginal mandibular, hypoglossal, superior laryngeal, recurrent laryngeal, accessory, and vagus nerves were identified. The cervical fascia and prevertebral fascia were dissected to expose the anterior cervical spine from the base of the skull down to C6. Once the anterior dissection was complete it was possible to identify the Penrose drain and cottonoid patties placed during the prior posterior approach. Discectomies were completed at C2/3 and C4/5, paying careful attention to remain outside of tumor capsule. The posterior longitudinal ligament was then completely freed between C2–C5 and then final cuts were made anterior to posterior in order to connect the osteotomies made the prior day. At this point, the tumor was free and was then delivered by progressively mobilizing it out. Iliac crest graft was harvested, measured, and cut to size to fill the C3–4 defect from the *en bloc* resection, from C2–C5. An anterior plate from C2–C6 was then fixated in place. The anterior neck incision was closed and then the patient was placed prone on the operative table. The posterior incision was re-opened and the temporary rod was removed. Appropriately sized rods were contoured into shape and placed from the occiput to T2 bilaterally and then the wound

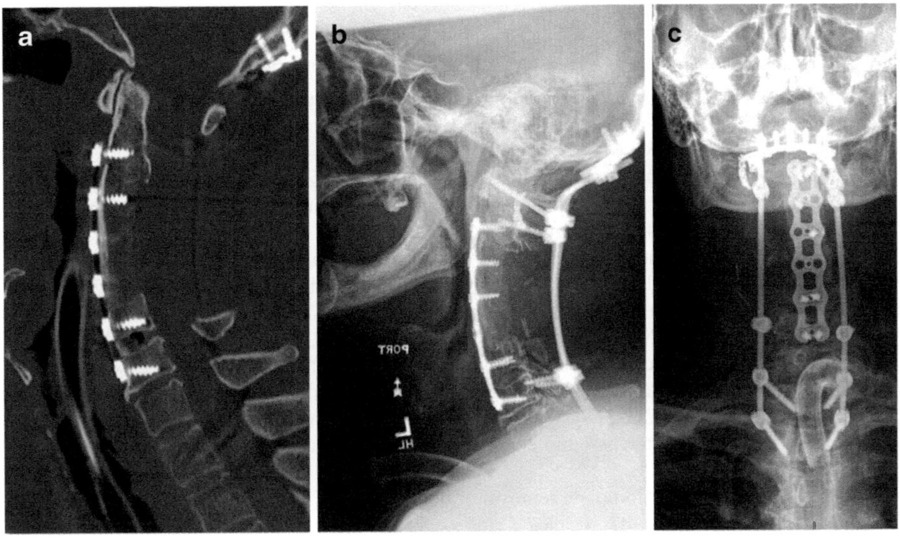


**Fig. 8.3** Postoperative imaging. (**a**) Postoperative sagittal CT scan. Postoperative lateral (**b**) and AP X-rays (**c**) showing anterior and posterior instrumented reconstruction

was closed. The patient was kept intubated and then taken to the intensive care unit for ongoing postoperative care. Postoperatively a tracheostomy was placed for supportive care during treatment of pneumonia. The surgical specimen was consistent was a chordoma, all surgical margins were negative for tumor (Fig. 8.2c, d). Postoperative imaging demonstrated the anterior-posterior reconstruction with appropriate cervical lordosis (Fig. 8.3).

## Conclusion

Cervical chordomas are rare and present an immense challenge for management. The best available evidence indicates that the preferred treatment of cervical chordomas is an aggressive surgical approach with *en bloc* surgical resection in order to achieve negative surgical margins. This strategy offers the lowest recurrence rate, and higher quality of life in long-term survivors. *En bloc* resections for cervical chordomas are performed in multidisciplinary fashion, often in multi-staged posterior-anterior approaches requiring meticulous planning to minimize morbidity and achieve negative margins. Morbidity is substantial and as such other strategies to decrease the surgical footprint and decrease surgical morbidity while still maintaining a low recurrence rate are being explored but long-term data are still lacking.

**IRB Approval** IRB approval was not required for the present work.

## References


1. Gokaslan ZL, Zadnik PL, Sciubba DM, et al. Mobile spine chordoma: results of 166 patients from the AOSpine Knowledge Forum Tumor database. J Neurosurg Spine. 2016;24:644–51.
2. Bongers MER, Dea N, Ames CP, Schwab JH. Surgical strategies for chordoma. Neurosurg Clin N Am. 2020;31:251–61.
3. Fisher CG, Saravanja DD, Dvorak MF, et al. Surgical management of primary bone tumors of the spine: validation of an approach to enhance cure and reduce local recurrence. Spine (Phila Pa 1976). 2011;36:830–6.
4. Charest-Morin R, Fisher CG, Sahgal A, Boriani S, Gokaslan ZL, Lazary A, Reynolds J, Bettegowda C, Rhines LD, Dea N. Primary bone tumor of the spine—an evolving field: what a general spine surgeon should know. Glob Spine J. 2019;9:108S–16S.
5. Barrenechea IJ, Perin NI, Triana A, Lesser J, Costantino P, Sen C. Surgical management of chordomas of the cervical spine. J Neurosurg Spine. 2007;6:398–406.
6. Glennie RA, Rampersaud YR, Boriani S, Reynolds JJ, Williams R, Gokaslan ZL, Schmidt MH, Varga PP, Fisher CG. A systematic review with consensus expert opinion of best reconstructive techniques after osseous en bloc spinal column tumor resection. Spine (Phila Pa 1976). 2016;41:S205–11.
7. Stener B, Johnsen OE. Complete removal of three vertebrae for giant-cell tumor. J Bone Joint Surg Br. 1971;53-B:278–87.
8. Boriani S. En bloc resection in the spine: a procedure of surgical oncology. J Spine Surg. 2018;4:668–76.
9. Boriani S, Weinstein JN, Biagini R. Primary bone tumors of the spine: terminology and surgical staging. Spine (Phila Pa 1976). 1997;22:1036–44.
10. Enneking WF, Spanier SS, Goodman MA. A system for the surgical staging of musculoskeletal sarcoma. Clin Orthop Relat Res. 1980;153:106–20.
11. Hsieh PC, Gallia GL, Sciubba DM, Bydon A, Marco RAW, Rhines L, Wolinsky J-P, Gokaslan ZL. En bloc excisions of chordomas in the cervical spine: review of five consecutive cases with more than 4-year follow-up. Spine (Phila Pa 1976). 2011;36:E1581–7.
12. Bailey CS, Fisher CG, Boyd MC, Dvorak MFS. En bloc marginal excision of a multilevel cervical chordoma: case report. J Neurosurg Spine. 2006;4:409–14.
13. Molina CA, Ames CP, Chou D, Rhines LD, Hsieh PC, Zadnik PL, Wolinsky J-P, Gokaslan ZL, Sciubba DM. Outcomes following attempted en bloc resection of cervical chordomas in the C-1 and C-2 region versus the subaxial region: a multiinstitutional experience. J Neurosurg Spine. 2014;21:348–56.
14. Altaf F, Weber M, Dea N, Boriani S, Ames C, Williams R, Verlaan J-J, Laufer I, Fisher CG. Evidence-based review and survey of expert opinion of reconstruction of metastatic spine tumors. Spine (Phila Pa 1976). 2016;41:S254–61.
15. Choi D, Melcher R, Harms J, Crockard A. Outcome of 132 operations in 97 patients with chordomas of the craniocervical junction and upper cervical spine. Neurosurgery. 2010;66:59–65.
16. Charest-Morin R, Flexman AM, Srinivas S, et al. Perioperative adverse events following surgery for primary bone tumors of the spine and en bloc resection for metastases. J Neurosurg Spine. 2020;32:98–105.
17. Dea N, Charest-Morin R, Sciubba DM, Bird JE, Disch AC, Mesfin A, Lazáry Á, Fisher CG, Ames C. Optimizing the adverse event and HRQOL profiles in the management of primary spine tumors. Spine (Phila Pa 1976). 2016;41:S212–7.
18. Cloyd JM, Chou D, Deviren V, Ames CP. En bloc resection of primary tumors of the cervical spine: report of two cases and systematic review of the literature. Spine J. 2009;9:928–35.
19. Pham M, Awad M. Outcomes following surgical management of cervical chordoma: a review of published case reports and case series. Asian J Neurosurg. 2017;12:389–97.
20. Charest-Morin R, Dea N, Fisher CG. Health-related quality of life after spine surgery for primary bone tumour. Curr Treat Options in Oncol. 2016;17:9.

21. Dea N, Fisher CG, Reynolds JJ, et al. Current treatment strategy for newly diagnosed chordoma of the mobile spine and sacrum: results of an international survey. J Neurosurg Spine. 2019;30:119–25.
22. Lockney DT, Shub T, Hopkins B, et al. Spinal stereotactic body radiotherapy following intralesional curettage with separation surgery for initial or salvage chordoma treatment. Neurosurg Focus. 2017;42:E4.

# Surgical Management of Chordoma in the Thoracic Spine

9

Daniel G. Tobert, John H. Shin, and Joseph H. Schwab

## Abbreviations

| | |
|---|---|
| ASA | Anterior spinal artery |
| EBR | En bloc resection |
| ICU | Intensive care unit |
| MAP | Mean arterial pressure |
| MRI | Magnetic resonance image |

## Introduction

This chapter discusses the relevant surgical anatomy to consider when approaching a chordoma of the thoracic spine. The challenges associated with tumors in this region are unique in some ways and shared in others. One of the unique features of thoracic spine chordomas is that some of the tumors, like distal sacral tumors, can be managed from a posterior-only approach. However combinatorial posterior and anterior approaches are still common and often safer. The purpose of this chapter is to discuss relevant anatomy that must be considered with either approach. A case example is shown to help further illustrate the anatomy and to prompt the reader to consider various factors when approaching these tumors surgically.

D. G. Tobert · J. H. Schwab (✉)
Department of Orthopaedic Surgery, Massachusetts General Hospital, Harvard Medical School, Boston, MA, USA
e-mail: jhschwab@mgh.harvard.edu

J. H. Shin
Department of Neurologic Surgery, Massachusetts General Hospital, Harvard Medical School, Boston, MA, USA



D. M. Sciubba, J. H. Schwab (eds.), *Chordoma of the Spine*,
https://doi.org/10.1007/978-3-030-76201-8_9

## Thoracic Spine Vascular Anatomy

The aorta holds a dominant position in the vascular anatomy of the thorax. The position relative to the spine and tumor must be considered closely. Thoracic chordomas can compress the thoracic aorta but it is rare in the primary setting for invasion into the adventitia. In general, one can develop a plane between the chordoma and the aorta. The segmental vessels coming off the aorta at each level must be appreciated and appropriately managed to prevent uncontrolled bleeding. The arch of the aorta has several important large branches including the brachiocephalic trunk on the far right, the common carotid artery and then the subclavian artery on the left. These vessels can be a variable during an anterior approach toward upper thoracic chordomas. They are typically not an issue posteriorly. While the arteries are clearly important, they are somewhat more resistant to injury due to their robust muscular layers. The most frequent injuries that occur to these large arteries are related to the avulsion of the smaller segmental vessels. If this occurs, it is usually during the removal of the tumor. A chordoma that abuts these large vessels should be looked upon with suspicion, especially in revision settings if someone has had high-dose radiation therapy. While a plane is typically developed even in this setting, there are circumstances where a chordoma can invade into the lining of the large arterial vessels. In these cases, one must decide whether or not to remove the vessel and replace it with the help of cardiothoracic surgery or to accept a close or positive margin. In the revision setting, we often plan for large vessel reconstruction to increase the change of obtaining negative margins, but this is necessary in only a subset of cases.

The azygos system is a venous drainage system that is often underappreciated. This is potentially due to its smaller caliber relative to the neighboring aortocaval system. However, it is the azygos system that is more likely to be associated with bleeding than the arterial system. The azygos system typically contains a larger azygous vein on the right side of the spine and a smaller hemi-azygos vein on the left side. These veins are the continuation of ascending lumbar veins as well as subcostal veins. The azygos system begins at the caudal end of the thoracic spine (T12). As the azygos system proceeds caudally it collects segmental, subcostal vessel contributions. Toward the arch of the aorta, the azygos cranes over the right main bronchus posteriorly and eventually anastomoses with the superior vena cava. The origin and the course of the azygos system and the presence of its associated accessory hemi-azygos vein are quite variable. Close inspection of the preoperative imaging can help to delineate the caliber and number of these vessels in each case. They must be carefully considered preoperatively and contended with intraoperatively to avoid large volume and potentially catastrophic blood loss. The azygos vessels are easily avulsed during resection or passage of instruments in the thoracic spine.

## Spinal Cord Blood Supply

The thoracic region spinal cord blood supply is derived primarily from the aorta and in some cases from the subclavian vessels. The anterior spinal artery (ASA) is the main blood supply to the ventral thoracic cord parenchyma. The aorta supplies the anterior spinal artery through radiculo-medullary branches. There are fewer radiculo-medullary arteries in the thoracic spine (one to four is typical) and less collateralization of the blood supply in the thoracic spine. In addition, the distance between these arteries is greater in the thoracic spine. Furthermore, there is little communication between the central and peripheral regions of the thoracic spinal cord. The dominant radiculo-medullary artery in the thoracic spine is termed the artery of Adamkiewicz. It arises from the aorta and enters the spinal cord from the left in most cases between T9 and T-12. The artery of Adamkiewicz gives off a hairpin shaped, descending branch, and a smaller branch that ascends. The ASA in the thoracic spine is in continuity throughout the spinal cord in this region but the caliber of the ASA fluctuates depending upon the region of the cord. Areas supplied by a vessel of diminutive caliber are more at risk for vascular insult [1].

Iatrogenic vascular injury to the thoracic spinal cord was closely studied during the advent and subsequent evolution of thoraco-abdominal aortic aneurysm (TAAA) repair. TAAA was at one point associated with spinal cord ischemia in up to 32% of cases [2, 3]. This finding initially led some vascular surgeons to reconstruct the segmental spinal arteries to their graft to help prevent the risk of cord ischemia. Subsequent research in this area has improved our understanding of spinal cord blood supply. For instance, loss of the artery of Adamkiewicz by itself is not associated with cord ischemia in all cases. Cord ischemia is multifactorial and also partly based on patient factors such as renal and vascular disease as well as perioperative hemodynamic fluctuations [2]. Several studies have noted the importance of maintaining an elevated mean arterial pressure to perfuse the spinal cord. Additionally, the insertion of intrathecal drains to control the intrathecal pressure and facilitate a gradient between the mean arterial pressure (MAP) became commonplace in TAAA. Several studies noted that cord ischemia often occurred in a delayed fashion up to several days after an operation [3]. Cord ischemia was found to be associated with drops in MAP and increases in intrathecal pressure, which further illustrates the importance of maintaining this pressure gradient.

The number of segmental vessels that are occluded or ligated during tumor resection is an important determinant for spinal cord perfusion. One study in the thoracic surgery literature investigated cases in which four or more segmental vessels were occluded by a vascular stent. They included eight cases, and in six of the eight cases, the dominant radiculo-medullary vessel was occluded. The authors noted intraoperatively that two of the eight patients had changes in their motor evoked potentials. However, both of these cases responded to increasing the MAP. This small series of patients did not report any occurrence of postoperative paraplegia [4].

As described in Chap. 13, the role of the artery of Adamkiewicz has been investigated in the setting of en bloc resection (EBR) in the thoracic spine. In a case series of 15 patients, the authors removed the artery of Adamkiewicz as well as the cephalad and caudal adjacent segmental vessels bilaterally [5]. No cases demonstrated postoperative neurologic changes in this series. This clinical study corresponds with an animal study using a canine model performed by the same authors. The anatomy is notably different in canines as the dominant radiculo-medullary vessel typically occurs at L5. The authors reported a change in spinal cord blood flow after removing the dominant radiculo-medullary vessel along with the adjacent two vessels. However, none of the canine subjects demonstrated neurologic compromise afterward [6, 7]. Yet, despite this evidence, it should not be a foregone conclusion that removing the dominant radiculo-medullary vessel along with the adjacent two segmental vessels is safe. As mentioned in Chap. 13, the authors report anecdotal experience of postoperative neurologic deficits attributable to ischemia. In the author's experience, patients with spinal cord compression or deformation of the spinal cord with preoperative neurologic deficits are at higher risk and the spinal cord is not in a stable physiologic state in this setting. Furthermore, a patient with preexisting renal and/or vascular disease may be more at risk for developing cord ischemia. The non-zero risk of an ischemic event with resection and catastrophic clinical sequelae warrants a thorough discussion with the patient preoperatively. Close monitoring of the MAP is an important component and is recommended in the perioperative setting. In our institution, we utilize the intensive care unit (ICU) in between staged procedures and for 48–72 hours postoperatively to ensure the MAP remains adequate. In certain cases where the risk of cord ischemia is felt to be high, an intrathecal drain is placed in order to more fully control the pressure gradient. It is important to consider preoperative angiography in patients where spondylectomy is considered, particularly at the cord level. The results of angiography can help inform intraoperative and postoperative management. In addition, the results of angiography can help guide preoperative risk discussions with patients and families.

## Segmental Nerve Roots

Each of the paired segmental nerve roots of the thoracic spine exits the spinal canal under the pedicle of their vertebral body with the same numbering. As such, the first thoracic segmental nerve root leaves the spine under the pedicle of the T1 vertebral body. The C8 segmental nerve root leaves the spine between C7 and T1. These nerve roots must be carefully managed in the case of upper thoracic chordoma. They are both functional nerve roots and can lead to significant hand dysfunction if damaged or sacrificed. This must be discussed with the patient in advance. Both C8 and T1 contribute to multiple motor endpoints in the upper limb. However, the most profound changes seen after removing these segmental nerve roots are in hand function where the loss of intrinsic and finger flexion can be profound and debilitating. It is important to recognize that inadvertent and irreparable damage to nerve roots is possible even in the absence of frank injury. Extensive dissection of the nerve roots can devascularize and lead to similar dysfunction seen in overt ligation. The use of radiation therapy can potentiate the dysfunction through pain and upper extremity swelling. The remaining thoracic nerve roots from T2 through T12 also contain important motor function. However, removing these segmental nerve roots leads to less disability than observed at C8 and T1. Resection of the remaining segmental nerve roots leads to numbness in their distribution, but it can also lead to dysesthetic pain. In addition, the work of breathing may change depending on how many segmental nerve roots are removed and the degree of intercostal muscle dysfunction. Resection of nerve roots in the lower thoracic spine may lead to changes in the flank musculature and lead to the appearance of a hernia. Dyesthesia related to nerve root resection can create challenges with acute postoperative pain and progress to chronic pain. The patient is aware of this potential outcome in advance of surgery. The segmental nerve roots also serve as the conduit for the segmental arterial and venous supply to the spinal cord as described in the previous section.

## Relevant Osseous Anatomy

Each of the 12 thoracic vertebrae typically has an associated rib. The rib articulates with the transverse process as well as the vertebral body. If EBR is considered, it is usually necessary to remove a portion of singular or multiple ribs. From a posterior approach, one can identify large segments of the ribs if the trapezius and latissimus musculature is gently elevated from the dorsal aspect of the ribs. It is important to consider these muscular structures when one is dissecting far lateral on the ribs because they may be necessary for flap coverage in the future. Depending upon the exposure that is necessary and the position of the tumor, it is often possible to leave a portion of the proximal aspect of the rib in place. Leaving the articulation of the rib with the vertebral body and the transverse process in its original position can simplify the approach. Transection of the rib lateral to the transverse process followed by a second transection further lateral allows removal of the rib and access to the thoracic spine from a posterior approach.

The ribs can be an important source of non-vascularized autogenous graft. However, one can also use a vascularized rib for reconstructive purposes. During the approach to the spine, one must keep this in mind if a vascular reconstruction is needed. Posterior vascular reconstruction using a rib is possible and it has the advantage of not requiring anastomosis since the rib is left attached to its segmental vessel. The ribs chosen for these purposes are typically cephalad or caudal to the primary levels of the tumor since the segmental vessels are typically removed from the ribs to access the tumor. Further discussion of this will occur later in this chapter during the case example.

The osseous anatomy of the vertebral bodies from T1 through T12 is better covered in a general spine textbook. The preoperative plan should involve scrutiny of imaging for any morphometric deviation in the patient's anatomy. This includes the shape and dimensions of the pedicles as well as the size of the vertebral bodies. Evaluating bone density and considering preoperative radiation therapy is important and has implications for reconstruction efforts. It is not uncommon to have a poor bone structure in patients who are being treated for cancer and this is particularly true if a patient has undergone radiation therapy. If bone quality is of concern, then one might consider alternative forms of instrumentation such as laminar hooks. This is also a consideration if the pedicle anatomy is such that a standard pedicle screw will not be possible.

## Case Example

The following case example is meant to illustrate some of the difficulties posed by an upper thoracic tumor. A 66-year-old woman had a cough for several months and presented to her primary care doctor, which prompted further imaging. Figure 9.1 demonstrates a chest radiograph revealing a widened mediastinum, which then led to a magnetic resonance image (MRI). Figure 9.2 demonstrates a T2-sequence hyperintense mass on MRI at the level of the third thoracic vertebrae. Note this corresponds to the level of the aortic arch. A subsequent biopsy confirmed chordoma as the pathology. Figure 9.2 also demonstrates that the esophagus is being compressed by the mass, which is depicted by a white arrow in the figure. Anterolateral to the esophagus is the aortic arch. Compression of the esophagus complicates the patient's management in two ways. First, if one were to consider radiation therapy alone for

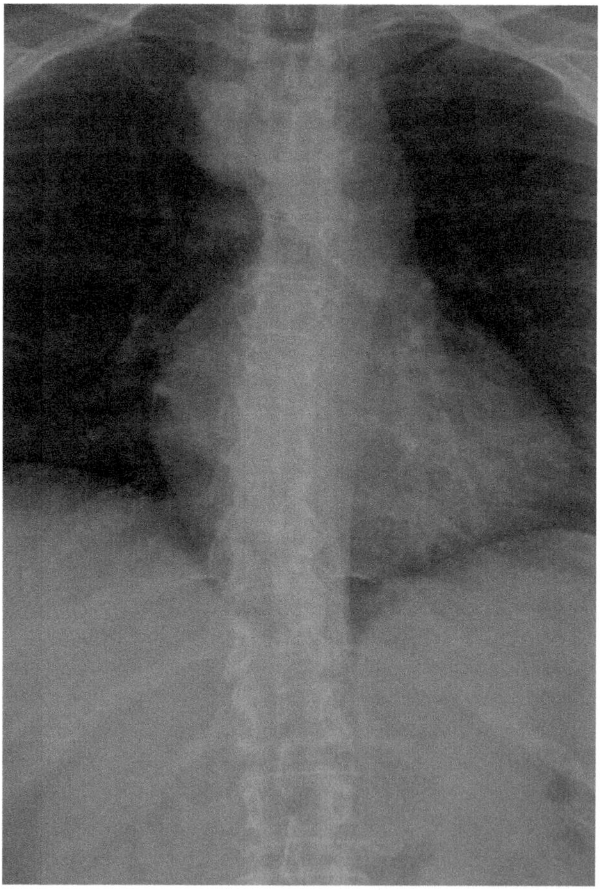

**Fig. 9.1** Posterior anterior chest radiograph revealing widened mediastinum concerning for malignancy

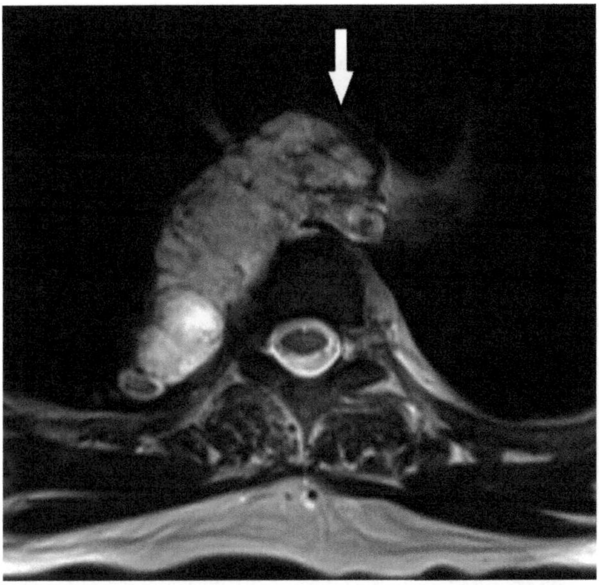

**Fig. 9.2** This axial T2-weighted image of the third thoracic vertebrae revealing a lobular mass. The mass is compressing the esophagus which is delineated by the white inverted vertical arrow

treatment of this mass, which some patients may opt for, this would have a low probability of success. The position of the esophagus would mandate a lower dose of radiation to this region. A suboptimal dose of radiation, which would spare esophageal injury, would not be able to control the tumor. For that reason, surgery with or without radiation therapy is a better option in this situation. Although the appearance on imaging may give the impression that the tumor is growing into the esophagus, it is more likely that the esophagus is being compressed rather than invaded. Figure 9.3 reveals that the mass involves portions of three vertebrae (T2–T4) and contacts a total of five vertebrae (T1–T5). This observation lays the foundation for the spondylectomy. In this case, our plan was to transect through the vertebral body above and below the main 3 impacted vertebrae. This patient has a robust azygos vein reversing along the right side of the vertebral bodies. Figure 9.4 demonstrates the large caliber azygos vein as well as many of the segmentals coming off of the azygos and traveling along the lateral border of the vertebral bodies. It is important to characterize the venous structures in the planned operative field as these will need to be managed during the approach. Preoperative angiography revealed that the dominant radiculo-medullary artery enters the spinal cord along the left side through the T9 segmental nerve root (Fig. 9.5).

Stage one of the operation involved a posterior approach with instrumentation as well as the development of a plane circumferentially around the vertebrae above and below the level of the tumors [8, 9]. Figure 9.6 reveals the blunt dissection that is performed in order to develop a plain dorsal to the great vessels of the thoracic spine and ventral to the vertebral body. In the thoracic spine, several ribs must be removed

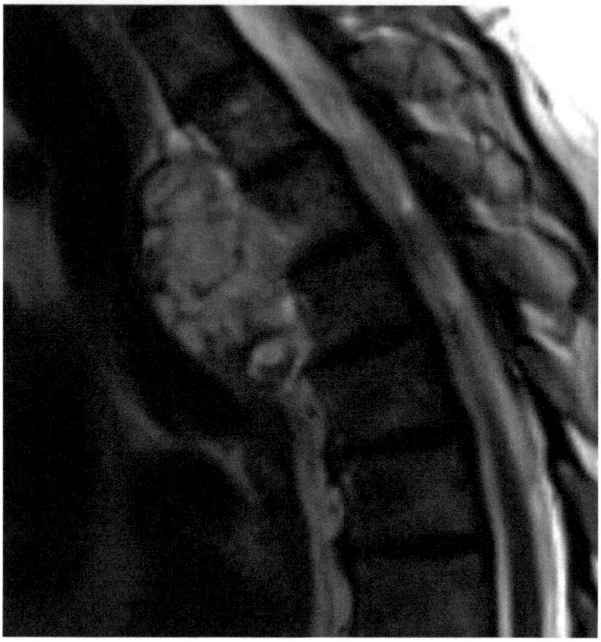

**Fig. 9.3** This sagittal T2-weighted image reveals the lobular mass again. It involves three main vertebrae but the cephalad and caudal aspects of adjacent vertebrae are also impacted. This must be considered during the surgical planning

to develop these planes. The amount of rib removed is determined based on the size of the tumor and the space needed to adequately and safely access the tumor. Typically, 5–7 centimeters lateral to the costotransverse joint is enough rib removal to allow access. When dissecting around the dorsal convexity of the ribs, one eventually begins to visualize the mid-portion of the rib both caudally and in the cephalad direction. At these levels, one can see Sharpey's fibers where the intercostal musculature inserts into the ribs. The intercostal muscle and the associated Sharpey's fibers can be removed sharply. Once these areas have been carefully released gentle blunt dissection can occur typically in the extra plural compartment. Gentle release of the adventitial tissue deep to the rib can be done bluntly. Once the rib has been mobilized it can be transected and removed. The rib is an important structure and can be used for structural grafting or morselized for autograft. During the process of removing the ribs, the segmental subcostal neurovascular bundle is also isolated. Depending upon the planned reconstruction, these intercostal vessels can be used for vascularized rib graft. However, in most cases, the segmental nerve artery and vein are removed to allow access to the thoracic cavity for spondylectomy. Once the ribs have been removed at the level of the tumor and typically one level above and below on both sides, then one can begin to bluntly elevate the pleural tissue off the lateral border of the vertebrae. With a gentle retraction of the lung tissue, the segmental vessels coming off the azygos system and the aorta can be identified. These

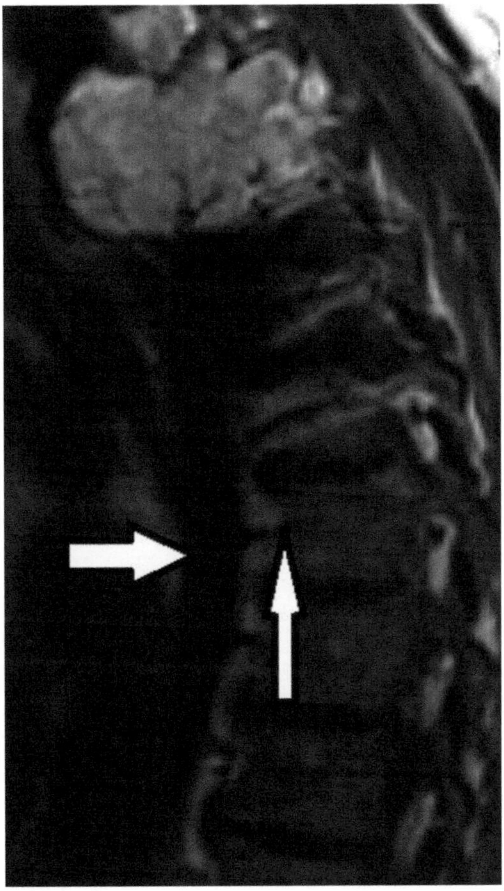

**Fig. 9.4** This sagittal T2-weighted image reveals the azygos vein (horizontal arrow) as it ascends the right side of the anterolateral thoracic spine. The vertical arrow reveals the segmental vessels coming from the azygos. An appreciation of the segmental vessels is crucial when one is planning en bloc spondylectomy

segmental vessels can be ligated and gently elevated away from the vertebral body. This allows for blunt dissection ventral to the vertebral body and dorsal to the great vessels. It is important to fully develop the plane between the vessels and the vertebral body.

Once the blunt dissection has been carried out the vertebrae can be osteotomized above and below the tumor. At our center, we often utilize threadwire saws to complete the osteotomy. We generally pass these during the posterior portion of the surgery and then utilize their cutting function during the anterior portion of the surgery, which was performed in this case. Figures 9.7 and 9.8 reveal how the Penrose drains are initially passed through the plane created by blunt dissection. The purpose of passing the Penrose drain is to eventually pass the threadwire saws through the Penrose drain. In this way, the Penrose drain acts as a conduit. After the Penrose drain has served its purpose it is removed, leaving the threadwire saws in place (Fig. 9.9). After the threadwire saws have been passed dorsal to the great vessels and ventral to the spinal cord we secure them in the field with clamps. We then performed removal of the posterior vertebral elements. The posterior elements are

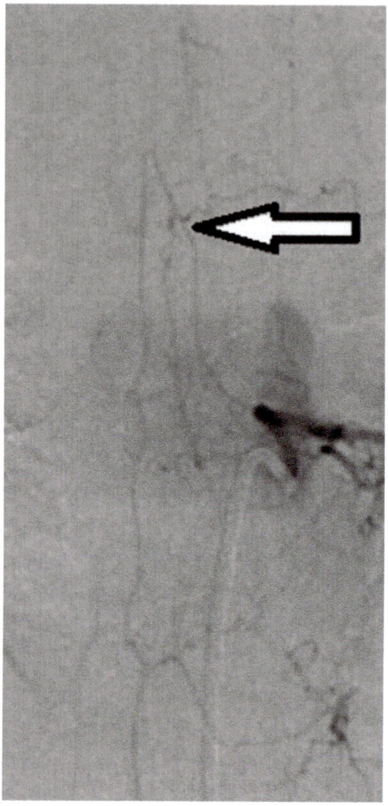

**Fig. 9.5** Preoperative angiogram demonstrating the hairpin loop formed by the dominant radiculo-medullary artery at T9

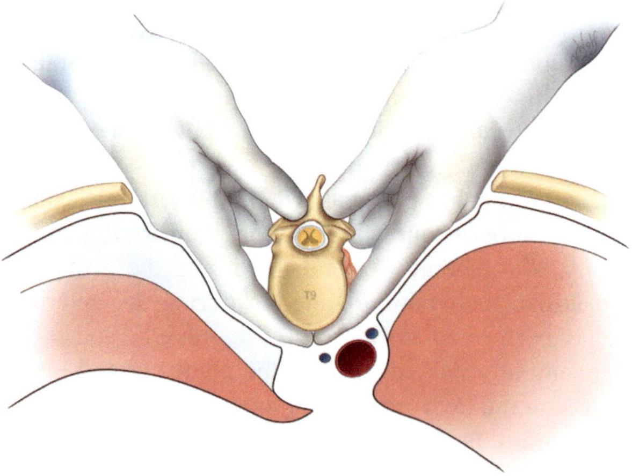

**Fig. 9.6** This diagram demonstrates the blunt dissection associated with stage one. The dissection occurs dorsal to the great vessels of the thorax and ventral to the vertebral body. This was initially described for passage of the threadwire saws by Tomita et al.

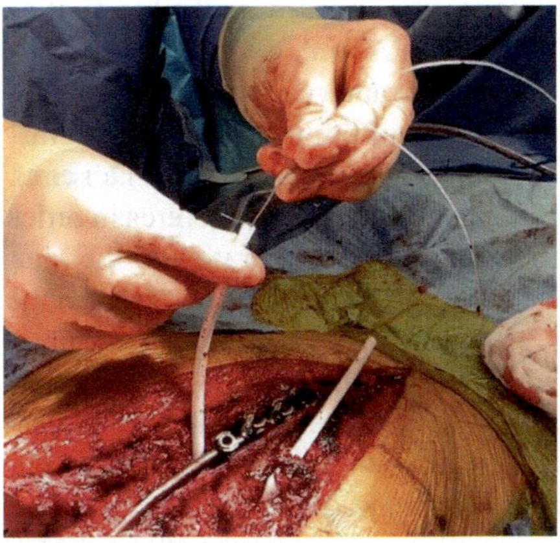

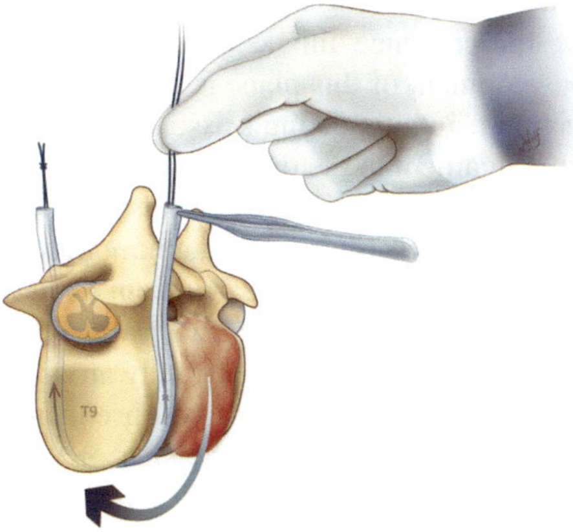


**Figs. 9.7 and 9.8** An intraoperative photograph as well as an artistic rendition with the Penrose drain in place. The Penrose drain is placed in the plane and bluntly dissected as demonstrated in Fig. 9.6. In this figure, the threadwire saws are passed through the Penrose drain, which is serving as a conduit

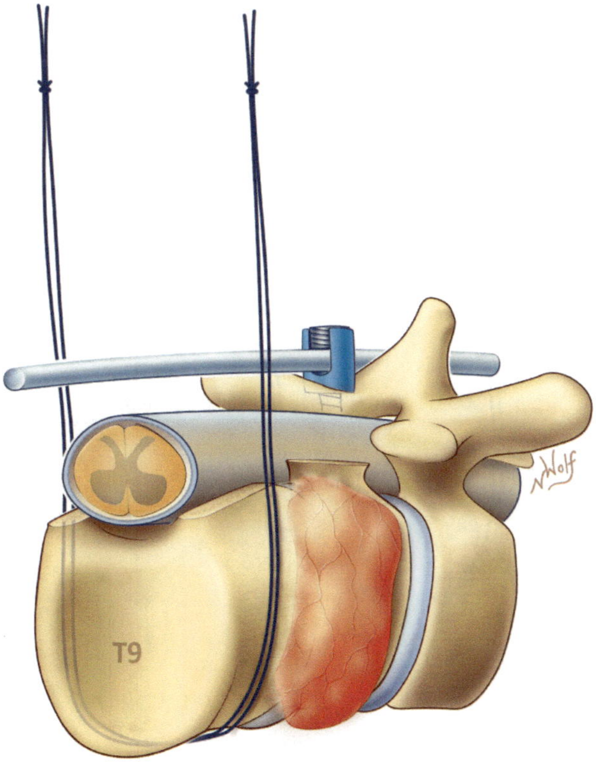


**Fig. 9.9** This figure demonstrates the position of the threadwire saw after the Penrose drain has been removed. Notice there are two threadwire saws. This is done because the threadwire saws can break if they are caught on a screw or on particularly hard bone and the second wire is kept in reserve

removed (including the pedicles) where it is safe to do so based on the location of the tumor. Once this is done, we develop a plane ventral to the spinal cord. Development of this plane is done with bipolar electrocautery as well as sharp dissection using dissecting scissors to cut any attachments from the posterior longitudinal ligament to the dura. This is done throughout the ventral surface of the spinal cord at the level of the tumor. It is very important to detach these structures in order to facilitate the removal of the tumor away from the spinal cord in stage two. Once this dissection has been carried out one can safely pass the threadwire saws ventral to the spinal cord as seen in Figs. 9.10 and 9.11. Once the threadwire saws have been safely past circumferentially around the vertebrae they are coiled and sutured together with silk sutures and subsequently sutured to a posterior rod. This is typically done to the rod on the side of the planned anterior approach (usually left) (Fig. 9.12). After the posterior incision is closed and stage one completed, the patient is transferred to the ICU. This level of care allows maintenance of mean arterial pressures and frequent neurologic checks. In addition, we often obtain a CT to help elucidate the final position of the threadwire saws. It is useful to see their position and also their relative trajectory. It is possible to inadvertently pass one of the threadwire saws ventral to a component of the azygos venous system. It is important to recognize this to avoid transection of the vessel during the anterior approach.

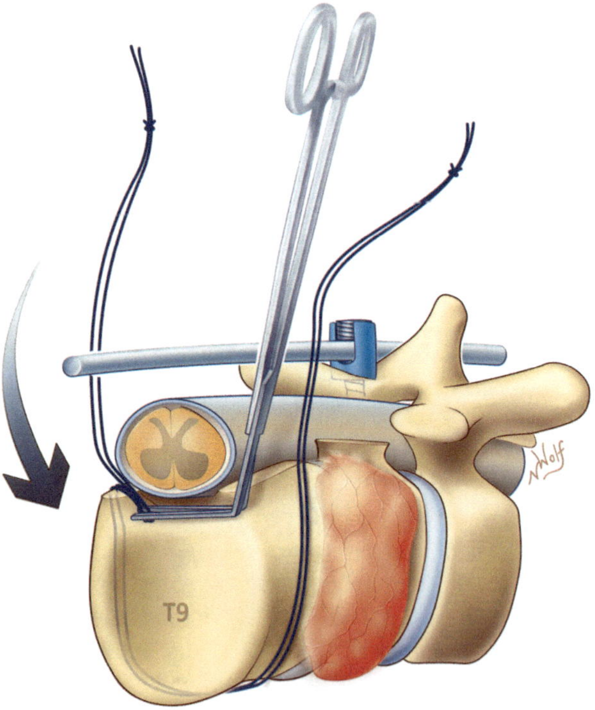


**Fig. 9.10** The threadwire saw is being passed ventral to the spinal cord

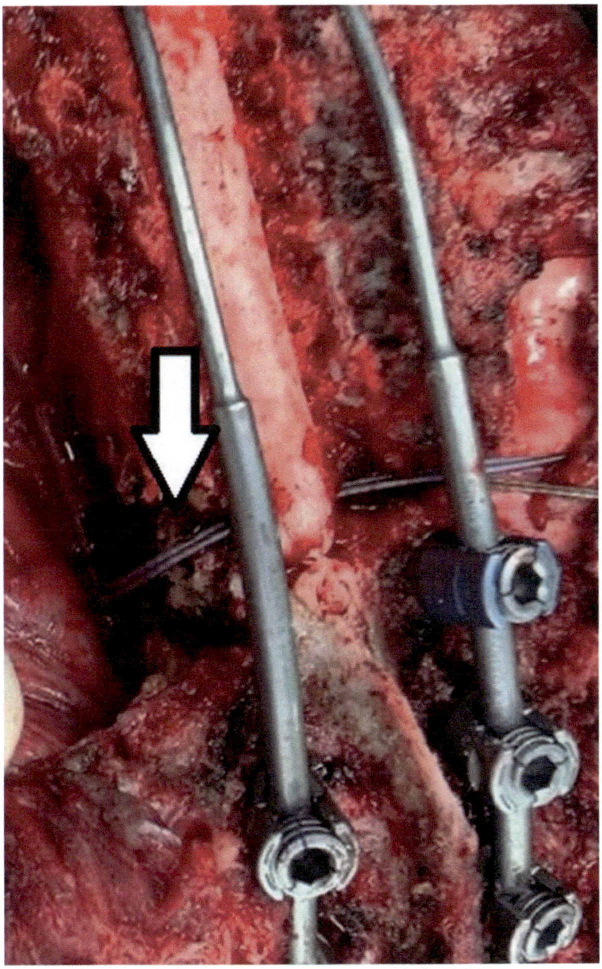

**Fig. 9.11** This intraoperative photograph demonstrates the threadwire saw in position prior to the end of stage one. The arrow demonstrates the threadwire saw, which is wrapped around the vertebral body in a 360° manner ventral to the spinal cord

In this example, the patient's tumor is difficult to access from an anterior approach. While it may have been possible to remove this tumor completely from a posterior approach, we felt that the compression of the esophagus as well as the proximity to segmental vessels off of the arch of the aorta and azygos system made it relatively unsafe to remove this all posteriorly. Therefore, we planned an anterior approach with the help of a thoracic surgeon who performed a sternotomy (Figs. 9.13 and 9.14). Isolation and deflation of the left lung field by the anesthesiologist aided the exposure. We were able to identify and ligate further segmental vessels and develop a plane between the esophagus and the tumor. This allowed us to identify

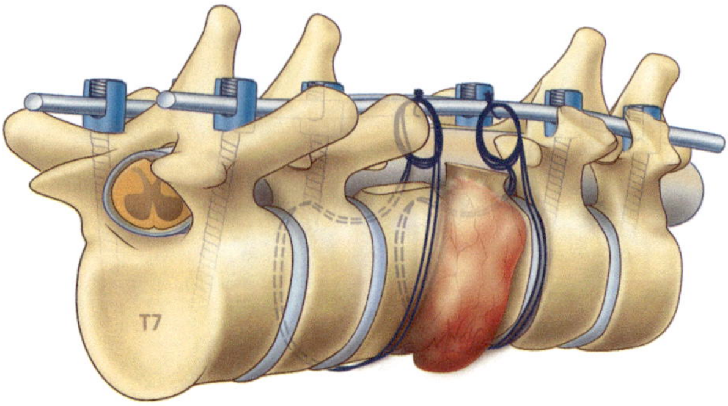


**Fig. 9.12** This diagram demonstrates the threadwire saws after they have been coiled and sutured to the posterior rod in preparation for closure of the wound so that in stage two they can be released and used as a saw

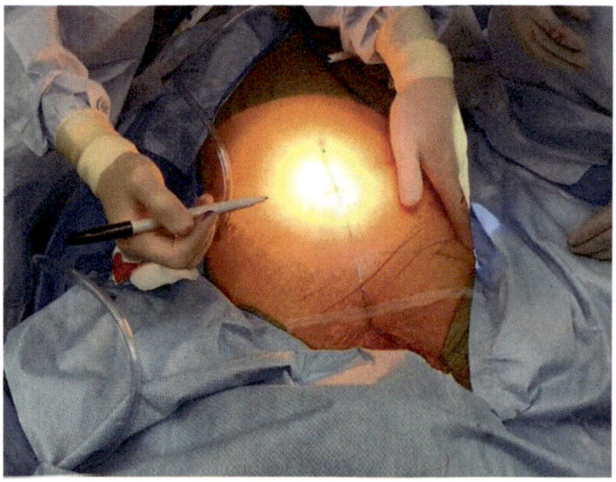

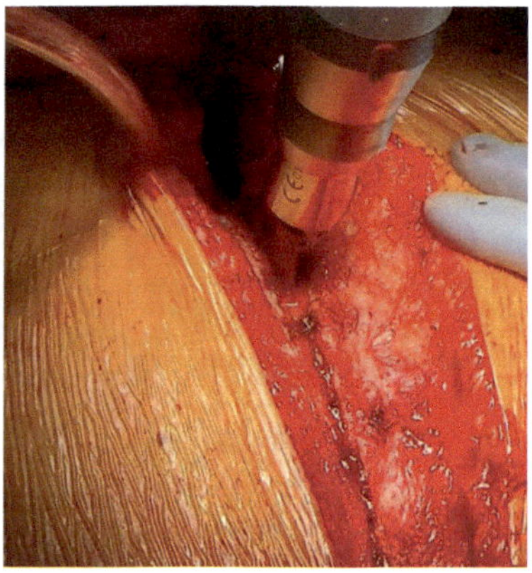

**Figs. 9.13 and 9.14** These intraoperative photographs reveal the planned sternotomy incision as well as the sternotomy being performed

the threadwire saws which had been sutured to the posterior rods. We released the saws by cutting the silk sutures which held them in position. The saws were then placed into their saw handles and a gentle back in forth action with the hands was used to cut through the vertebral bodies (Fig. 9.15). Great care was taken to retract the deflated lung as well as to protect the heart which was directly in the field (Fig. 9.16). Once the vertebrae are cut, the specimen should be relatively mobile. However, there are often soft tissue attachments that were not completely appreciated during the posterior approach. Sharp dissection of these attachments allows delivery of the specimen. Often, there are attachments between the posterior longitudinal ligament and the spinal cord which need to be transected. This can be done by gently rotating the specimen while protecting the spinal cord. Figure 9.17 reveals the specimen immediately after it was removed from the field (Fig. 9.17). Figure 9.18 shows an anterior viewpoint of the specimen. One can see the spinal cord in the

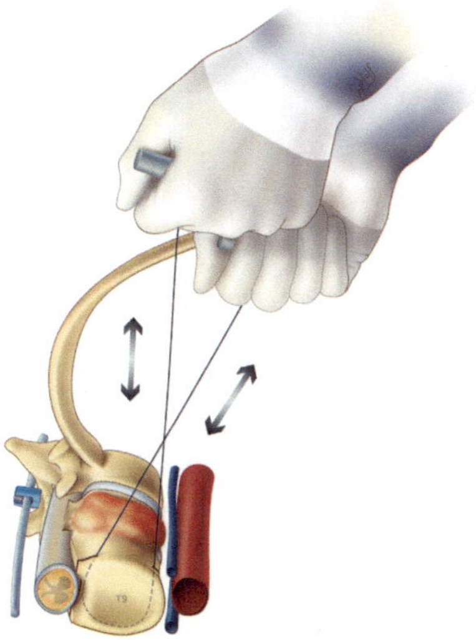

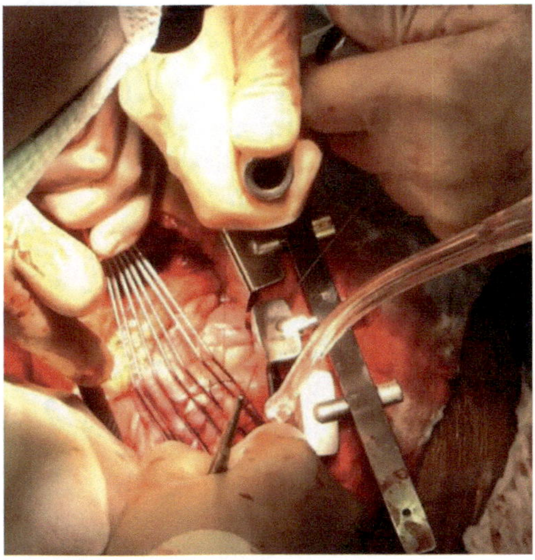

**Figs. 9.15 and 9.16** This figure demonstrates the threadwire saw being used to section the vertebral body. The intraoperative photograph also demonstrates the threadwire saw in action with the lungs being gently retracted

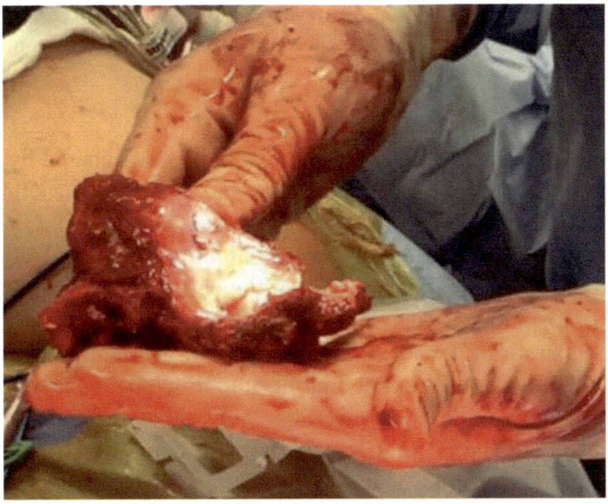

**Fig. 9.17** This is an intraoperative photograph of the specimen immediately after excision

upper left portion of the image. The heart is designated with the five-pointed star and the deflated lung is designated by the hexagon. Reconstruction of the defect can be carried out in multiple ways. We prefer vascularized bone grafts as described in Chap. 13. Figure 9.19 reveals further complexity associated with an upper thoracic tumor as this shows the vascularized fibular graft delivered into the operative field.

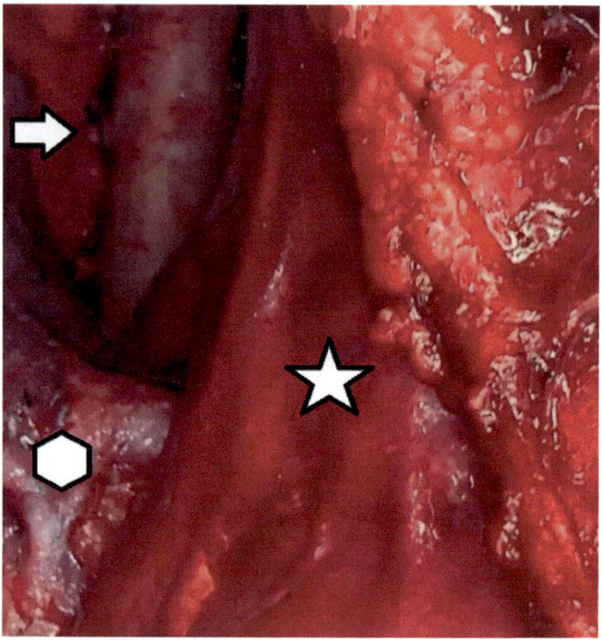

**Fig. 9.18** This intraoperative photograph reveals the relevant anatomy from an anterior perspective once the specimen has been removed. The arrow delineates the spinal cord where one can see the segmental nerve roots have been ligated with zero silk sutures. The five-pointed star is on the heart. The hexagon is on the deflated lung

One can also see the brachiocephalic artery, which is designated by an arrow and complicated both the extirpation of the tumor and also reconstruction (Fig. 9.19). Figures 9.20 and 9.21 reveal a radiograph of the gross specimen. Gross and microscopic examination of the specimen with our pathologist revealed negative margins (Figs. 9.20 and 9.21). After reconstruction of the defect using a vascularized fibular graft, the anastomosis was carried out using a segmental vessel from the azygos and aortic arch. Postoperative CT scan and standing x-rays are demonstrated in Figs. 9.22 and 9.23. Postoperatively, the patient continues to do well 2 years out from her surgery at the time of this writing. However, one notes several findings from a sagittal balance point of view. She is compensating a positive sagittal balance with pelvic retroversion and hyperlordosis of the lumbar spine. This positive sagittal balance was likely iatrogenic from the reconstruction and not fully appreciated at the time of surgery. Positive sagittal balance has been linked to poor quality of life after en bloc spondylectomy [10].

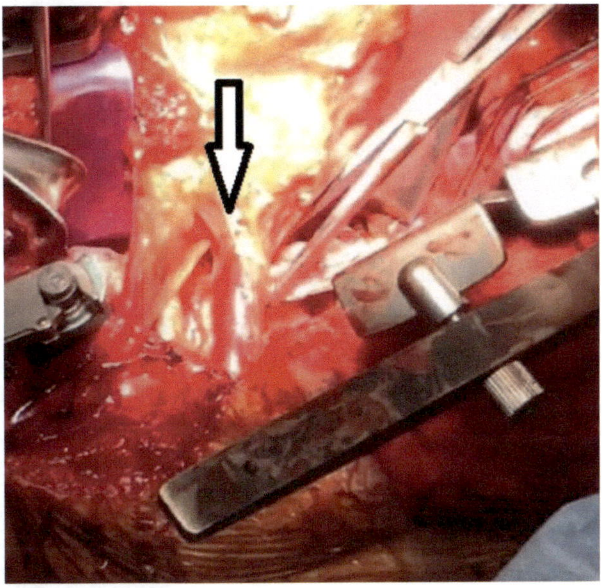

**Fig. 9.19** This intraoperative photograph reveals the vascularized fibular graft being delivered into the field. The vascularized fibular graft is being held by a Coaker clamp. The inverted arrow is demonstrating the brachiocephalic artery

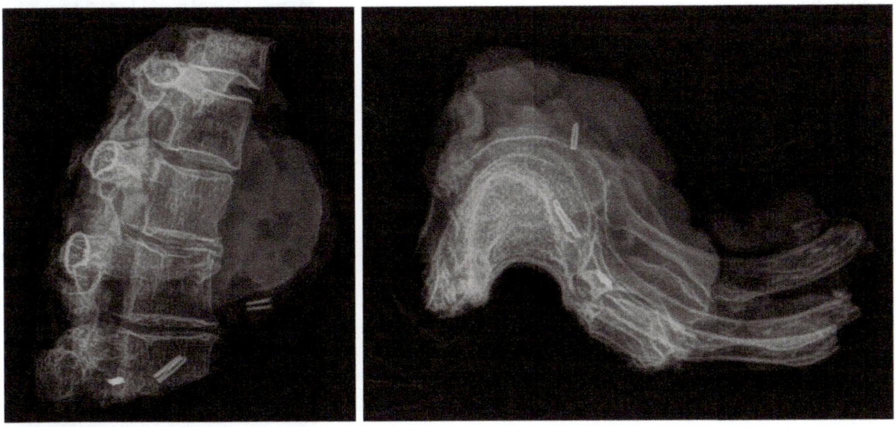

**Figs. 9.20 and 9.21** These intraoperative radiographs reveal the specimen from a lateral view and an axial view

**Fig. 9.22** Postoperative CT scan demonstrating the position of the vascularized fibular graft

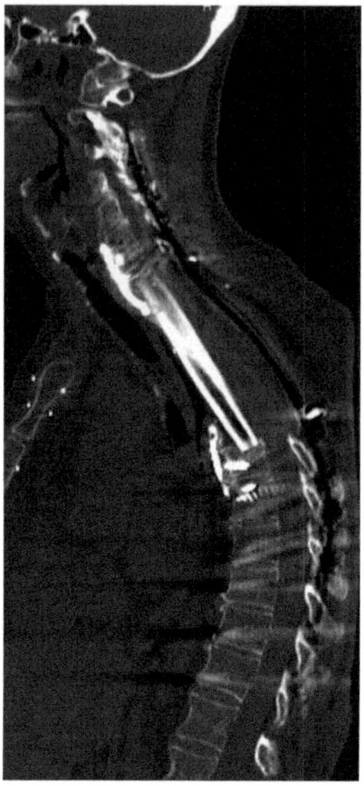

**Fig. 9.23** Standing postoperative full length spinal radiograph

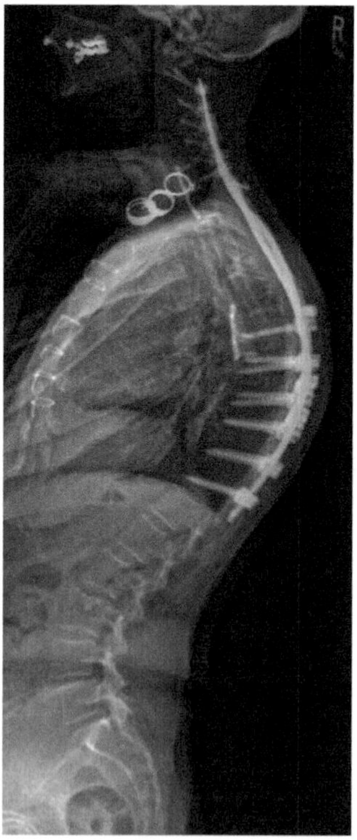

## References


1. Colman MW, Hornicek FJ, Schwab JH. Spinal cord blood supply and its surgical implications. J Am Acad Orthop Surg. 2015;23:581–91.
2. Crawford ES, et al. Thoracoabdominal aortic aneurysms: preoperative and intraoperative factors determining immediate and long-term results of operations in 605 patients. J Vasc Surg. 1986;3:389–404.
3. Svensson LG, Crawford ES, Hess KR, Coselli JS, Safi HJ. Experience with 1509 patients undergoing thoracoabdominal aortic operations. J Vasc Surg. 1993;17:357–68; discussion 368–70.
4. Schurink GW, et al. Assessment of spinal cord circulation and function in endovascular treatment of thoracic aortic aneurysms. Ann Thorac Surg. 2007;83:S877–81; discussion S890–2.
5. Murakami H, et al. Does interruption of the artery of Adamkiewicz during total en bloc spondylectomy affect neurologic function? Spine (Phila Pa 1976). 2010;35:E1187–92.
6. Fujimaki Y, Kawahara N, Tomita K, Murakami H, Ueda Y. How many ligations of bilateral segmental arteries cause ischemic spinal cord dysfunction? An experimental study using a dog model. Spine (Phila Pa 1976). 2006;31:E781–9.
7. Kato S, et al. Effects on spinal cord blood flow and neurologic function secondary to interruption of bilateral segmental arteries which supply the artery of Adamkiewicz: an experimental study using a dog model. Spine (Phila Pa 1976). 2008;33:1533–41.
8. Tomita K, Kawahara N, Murakami H, Demura S. Total en bloc spondylectomy for spinal tumors: improvement of the technique and its associated basic background. J Orthop Sci. 2006;11:3–12.
9. Shah AA, et al. Modified en bloc spondylectomy for tumors of the thoracic and lumbar spine: surgical technique and outcomes. J Bone Joint Surg Am. 2017;99:1476–84.
10. Massier JRA, et al. Sagittal spinal parameters after en bloc resection of mobile spine tumors. Spine J. 2019;19:1606–12.

# Surgical Management of Chordoma of the Lumbar Spine

# 10

Sutipat Pairojboriboon, Amanda Sacino, and Sheng-Fu Larry Lo

## Abbreviations

| | |
|---|---|
| ALL | Anterior longitudinal ligament |
| ASIS | Anterior superior iliac spine |
| BMI | Body mass index |
| EA | Enneking appropriate |
| EI | Enneking inappropriate |
| IMRT | Intensity-modulated radiotherapy |
| LECA | Lateral extracavitary approach |
| PLL | Posterior longitudinal ligament |
| PSIS | Posterior superior iliac spine |
| RT | Radiation therapy |
| S2AI | S2-alar-iliac |
| TES | Total en bloc spondylectomy |
| TMC | Titanium mesh cage |
| VBR | Vertebral body replacement |

S. Pairojboriboon
Department of Neurosurgery, Johns Hopkins University School of Medicine, Baltimore, MD, USA

Department of Orthopaedic Surgery, Phramongkutklao Hospital and College of Medicine, Bangkok, Thailand

A. Sacino
Department of Neurosurgery, Johns Hopkins University School of Medicine, Baltimore, MD, USA

S.-F. L. Lo (✉)
Department of Neurosurgery, Johns Hopkins University School of Medicine, Baltimore, MD, USA

Department of Neurosurgery, Zucker School of Medicine at Hofstra/Northwell, Hempstead, NY, USA
e-mail: larrylo@northwell.edu



D. M. Sciubba, J. H. Schwab (eds.), *Chordoma of the Spine*,
https://doi.org/10.1007/978-3-030-76201-8_10

## Introduction

Surgical management for chordoma of the lumbar spine is challenging due to the fact that they arise in the vertebral body and grow to compress the spinal cord and nerves or into paraspinal soft tissues. The idea of surgical margins was pioneered by Enneking, which correlates with the local recurrence rate and the length of disease-free survival [1]. Wide (en bloc) margins can be categorized as Enneking appropriate (EA) while the intralesional margins are Enneking inappropriate (EI) [2]. According to a systematic review and multicenter cohort study from Boriani et al., en bloc chordoma resection leads to a decrease in local recurrence, longer disease-free survival, and a reduction of death rates [3].

## Anatomy of the Lumbar Spine

The lumbar spine consists of five vertebrae which are distinguished by their larger size compared with the cervical and thoracic spine. The lumbar pedicle diameter width is narrowest at L2 (~6 mm) and widest at L5 (~15 mm) [4]. The zygapophyseal or facet joints are trochoid joints, as the inferior articular processes glide in the hollow grooves of the superior articular processes. The orientation of the joint lines in the craniocaudal direction help to maintain lumbar lordosis [4]. Due to lumbar lordosis, the sagittal orientation of the L1 pedicle is about 5 degrees and L5 is almost parallel to the endplate. In the transverse plane, L1 convergence is approximately 10 degrees then it progressively increases to almost 30 degrees at L5 [5]. The lumbar vertebral bodies are connected by intervertebral fibrocartilaginous disks, anterior longitudinal ligament (ALL), and posterior longitudinal ligament (PLL). The lumbar spinal canal shape changes from ovoid at its upper part to trefoil in the lower part [6]. The average minimum anteroposterior diameter of the lumbar spinal canal is 15 mm [7].

The muscles overlying the posterior lumbar spine are composed of superficial and deep layers. The superficial layer consists of the latissimus dorsi and thoracolumbar fascia. The deep layer consists of erector spinae, multifidus, and rotator muscles [8]. On the lateral side, the transverse processes at L1-L5 are the origin of the deep part of psoas major muscles, while the superficial part originates from the lateral surfaces of the T12-L4 intervertebral disks [9]. The lumbar plexus, consisting of the L1-L4 ventral rami, emerges between the psoas major muscles and the lumbar transverse process. The genitofemoral nerve lies anterior to the psoas muscle. The ureter runs between the psoas muscle and peritoneum [8]. The anterior surface of upper lumbar vertebrae are attachment sites of the diaphragmatic crura (L1-3 on the right and L1-2 on the left) [10]. The aorta and vena cava run anterior to the lumbar spine then bifurcate into the common iliac vessels at the L4 vertebral body or L4-L5 intervertebral disk [11].

## Surgical Approaches

Although total en bloc spondylectomy (TES) for lumbar chordoma has the best clinical outcome, it is not always feasible to achieve a negative (EA) margin with large extra-compartmental tumors. Local recurrence rates are 50–100% in cases of subtotal or EI resection compared to 0–53% with en bloc resection with negative margins or EA resection [12, 13]. Strategies combining adjuvant high-dose radiation therapy (RT) after subtotal excision were superior to subtotal resection alone in terms of local control rates [13]. Generally, the optimal dose of conventional RT to acquire local control is excess of 60 Gy, [14] but this dose can cause collateral damage to normal soft tissues. Intensity-modulated radiotherapy (IMRT) is able to solve this problem by delivering precise radiation to the tumors, thus achieving a higher dose to the target while minimizing the dose to surrounding healthy tissue [15]. According to an international survey from the AOSpine Knowledge Forum Tumor, there is treatment variability among some of the world's most experienced cancer centers ranging from en bloc resection alone to intralesional resection followed by postoperative RT (Fig. 10.1) [16]. Interestingly, the experienced groups who had treated more than 10 cases of chordoma per year preferred a more aggressive approach than the less-experienced groups.

Injury to the artery of Adamkiewicz, which supplies the lower one-third of the thoracolumbar spinal cord, is one of the major concerns during TES. Its location originates from the left side in 68–73% of cases and at the level of the ninth intercostal to the second lumbar artery in 85% of cases [17, 18]. A planned sacrifice of the artery of Adamkiewicz is sometimes unavoidable for upper lumbar TES. Nonetheless, Murakami et al. studied changes in neurologic function after

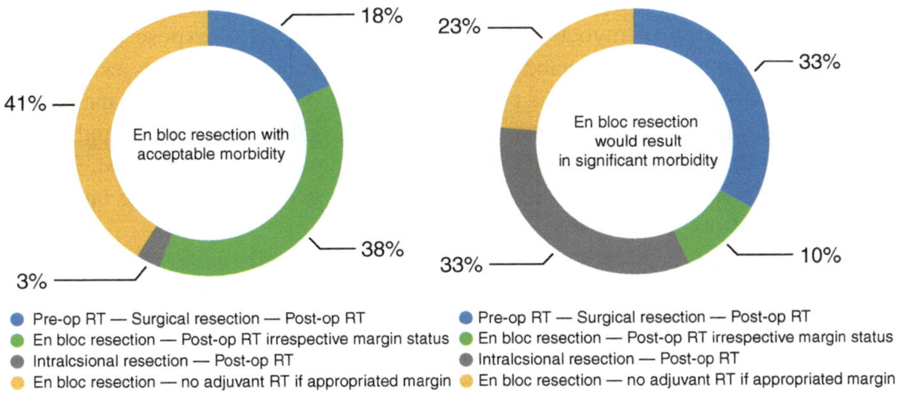


**Fig. 10.1** International survey of the strategic treatment of newly diagnosed chordoma of the lumbar spine and sacrum; en bloc resection with acceptable morbidity (left) and en bloc resection with significant morbidity (right) [16]

interruption of the Adamkiewicz artery during TES in a series of 15 cases. They concluded that three pairs of segmental arteries, including the Adamkiewicz artery, could be sacrificed without neurologic deterioration sequelae [17, 19].

The lumbar spine is a challenging region for performing TES due to many anatomic reasons: the presence of the great vessels in front of the vertebrae, the necessity to preserve the lumbar plexus, and the close relationship to abdominal organs and psoas muscles. In general, en bloc resection of the lumbar spine usually requires two-staged (posterior-anterior, posterior-anterolateral) approaches because of anatomic limitations of the lumbar spine and pelvis [20]. Nonetheless, the posterior-only TES of the fifth lumbar vertebrae is a viable option for surgical treatment depending on the patients' anatomy and tumor size and location [21]. Posterior-only TES of the first lumbar vertebrae is also an option due to the acceptable neurological sequalae from sacrifice of the first lumbar nerve root that is necessary to deliver the tumor posteriorly. We will defer specific discussion of a posterior-only TES for the first lumbar vertebrae with L1 nerve root sacrifice given that the surgical principles are similar to a thoracic posterior-only TES with thoracic nerve root sacrifice and will be covered in a separate chapter.

## Posterior-Anterior Approach

The lateral extracavitary approach (LECA) provides dorsal and ventrolateral access to the thoracolumbar spine from T3 to S1, allowing for ventral resection and posterior instrumentation in one setting. Although this approach can provide ventral access, it still does not compare to an anterior approach which provides a clear visualization of adjacent ventral intracavitary structures (e.g., aorta and vena cava). The patient is positioned prone. The thoracolumbar fascia is incised in a T-shape or a separate erector spinae flap that can be rotated medially and laterally is elevated. The lateral retraction of myocutaneous flap was conducted to expose the erector spinae muscles, which are retracted medially. Next the transverse processes, lamina, and pedicles can be removed. This corridor allows the surgeon access to the neural foramina, the dissecting plane between the anterolateral vertebral body and psoas muscles, and the superior and inferior disk spaces at the vertebrectomy site. During surgery, the patient can be rotated away from the surgeon by tilting the operating table to facilitate exposure across the midline [22, 23].

The anterior approach (transperitoneal or retroperitoneal) enables better margin dissection in cases where the tumor is complicated by adhesions and scar tissue with close proximity to great vessels and allows delivery of the tumor without lumbar nerve root sacrifice in selected cases. Additionally, the anterior approach allows for better control of segmental vessels. In general, collaboration with a general or vascular surgeon is recommended. Pfannenstiel, horizontal, or vertical incisions may all be appropriate; however, a vertical incision may allow for superior exposure if needed. After entering the posterior peritoneum, the aorta, vena cava, and sacral promontory should be identified. Then the disk spaces and vertebral bodies should be identified by using a Kittner swab to perform blunt dissection. The use of electrocautery should be avoided due to the risk of hypogastric plexus injury leading to retrograde ejaculation [24]. The fluoroscope or plain radiographs may be used to confirm the correct spinal level. Essentially, the iliolumbar vein and middle sacral artery should be ligated prior to mobilization of the aorta, vena cava, and iliac vessels [25].

## Posterior-Anterolateral Approach

This modified TES technique, which is described by Shah et al. [26], consists of two stages. The first stage is the posterior approach. After soft tissue exposure of the osseous elements of the spine, dissection is conducted anteriorly between the vertebral body and the great vessels in order to develop a circumferential tunnel which is enlarged enough to pass a half-circle clamp configuration. A Penrose drain is passed via this clamp through the tunnel created between the great vessels and vertebral body followed by passing thread-wire saws (Mani Diamond Tomita-Saw) into the sheath. Intraoperative XR should be used to confirm the appropriate position. The removal of the posterior osseus elements and posterior instrumentation are then performed. The end of each saw is passed through the plane between the thecal sac and PLL in order to lasso around the vertebral body and anchor to the posterior instrumentation.

The patient is then positioned in the lateral position in order to perform the flank incision. The anterolateral approach was performed to identify the saw and release the anchor from the posterior instrumentation. The saw is then used to perform cephalad and caudal osteotomies until the tumor is gently mobilized. The remaining parts are dissected then the specimen is removed en bloc [26].

## Posterior-Only Approach

In order to preserve the lumbar nerve roots, a posterior-only TES is only performed at the L5 vertebral level. Yang et al. [21] reported this technique with reconstruction using an iliac graft. The gluteus maximus, gluteus medius, iliacus, and quadratus lumborum muscles were partially detached from the iliac wing. The osteotomies are made horizontally at L5-S1, followed by a vertical cut at the midpoint between anterior superior iliac spine (ASIS) and posterior superior iliac spine (PSIS). The bone excised from the osteotomies is to be used as the iliac graft. After dissection of the tumor is complete, it is rotated en bloc out toward the cavity created by the osteotomies. The L4 and L5 nerve roots are retracted away. For the reconstruction, the iliac graft was fixed back into place [21].

## Reconstruction Principle

TES is a destabilizing procedure; however, combined anterior-posterior stabilizations comprising two or more adjacent segments of posterior fixation and vertebral body replacement (VBR) allows for sufficient stability [27].

### Anterior Reconstruction

A titanium mesh cage (TMC) provides anterior column stability and restores lumbar column height. The sharp teeth on the cage prevent graft dislodgement from its bite into the vertebral endplate on impaction [28]. However, expandable cages have a 17% risk of significant subsidence and the possibility of adjacent vertebral fractures [29]. The TMC may be packed with morselized allogenic bone graft. The fusion rate using a TMC with bone graft is 76.7%. The significant predictive factors for instrumentation failure are perioperative radiotherapy, the cage in the oblique position, and a body mass index (BMI) >28 kg/m$^2$ [30]. A fibula graft is another construct option, which is composed of either non-vascularized or vascularized bone grafts with anterior plating. Additional disadvantages of fibular allografts are immunological rejection, the rare possibility of disease transmission, and longer times to achieve fusion [29]. Even though the vascularized fibular autografts are stronger and have a better osseous union rate of 80–90% than non-vascularized grafts, they require an end-to-side microanastomosis to recipient vessels (e.g., lumbar segmentals, the iliac vessels, the inferior mesenteric vessels, or the aorta) [31].

### Posterior Reconstruction

Generally, the posterior instrumentation should span at least two levels above and below the area of the spondylectomy, and usually involve lumbosacral as well as sacropelvic fixation. The long arthrodesis without fusion over the lumbosacral junction can lead to pseudarthrosis rates up to 41% [32]. According to one biomechanical study, S1 screws should be supplemented with two iliac screws in cases of instrumented fusion extending above L3 [33]. The incorporation of the ilium into the spinal construct provides greater stability and fusion rates across the lumbosacral junction. Currently, the most widely used techniques are iliac and S2-alar-iliac (S2AI) screws, which achieve pelvic anchorage and improve the fusion rate greater than 90% [34, 35]. Rod fracture is also a frequent complication. A 6.35-mm rod may be a good option to increase stability in these cases [36].

## Outcomes

Clarke et al. reported a case of a three-level TES from L3 to L5. The total estimated blood loss and total operative time were 6200 mL and 29 h. The patient recovered well from surgery and there was no local recurrence nor instrumentation failure at the 8-month follow-up [37]. Sciubba and colleagues reported outcomes on 23 cases of TES of the lumbar spine. The median total estimated blood loss and total operative time were 3200 mL and 18.5 h. The local recurrence and 5-yr survival was 8.7% and 84.4% [38]. Kawahara et al. reported 10 cases of TES of the lower lumbar spine. The mean operative time and blood loss were 15.45 h and 5120 mL. There was no local recurrence at 52-month follow-up [39]. Yang et al. reported the outcomes of posterior-only TES on L5 tumors. The average blood loss and operative time were 2514 mL and 6 hr. (Table 10.1) [21].

**Table 10.1** Comparison of total en bloc spondylectomy (TES) studies of lumbar spine

| | No. of cases | Total estimated blood loss (mL) | Total operative time (h.) | Negative margin | Contaminated margin | Instru-mentation failure during f/u | Local recurrence |
|---|---|---|---|---|---|---|---|
| Sciubba et al. [38] | 23 | 3200 | 18.5 | 17 (73.9%) | 6 (26.1%) | 9 (39.1%) | 2 (8.7%) |
| Kawahara et al. [39] | 10 | 5370 | 17.9 | 2 (20%) | 8 (80%) | 2 (20%) | 0 |
| Yang et al. [21] | 7 | 2514 | 6 | NA | NA | 0 | 0 |

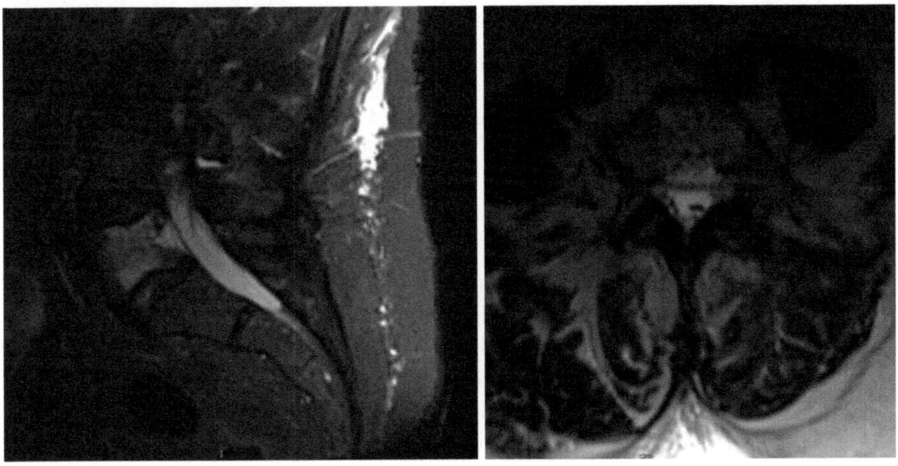

**Fig. 10.2** Sagittal and axial MRI demonstrating a T2 hyperintense lesion within the L5 vertebral body with erosion through the posterior cortex and trace extension into the ventral epidural space

## Illustrative Case

A 53-year-old female with BMI 32.12 kg/m$^2$ presented with chronic lower back pain over the past 5 years. MRI showed an abnormal signal intensity at the L5 vertebral body with ventral epidural extension (Fig. 10.2). The results of a core needle biopsy revealed histology consistent with chordoma. She was referred to Neurosurgery for surgical treatment options. Her case was presented at a multidisciplinary spine tumor board, which agreed that the best treatment plan was preoperative neoadjuvant RT followed by TES at L5.

### Operative Technique

#### Stage 1: Posterior Approach

Patient was positioned prone on the Jackson table with head fixation in a Mayfield head clamp to minimize the risk of a facial pressure ulcer [40]. Continuous

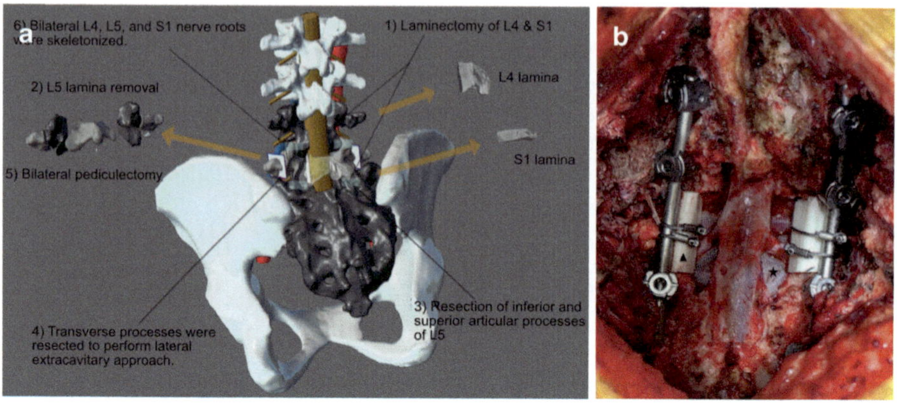


**Fig. 10.3** (**a**) Illustration of stage 1 posterior approach of L5 total en bloc spondylectomy (TES) with removal of the posterior elements of L4, L5, and S1. (**b**) The intraoperative photo showed the silastic sheet (star) was placed between thecal sac and L4 to S1 vertebral body as well as L4, L5, and S1 nerve roots. The structural fibular allografts (triangle) were used to manage the defect between L4-S1

neuromonitoring was used throughout the case. The bony exposure was made from L3 to the pelvis. We used the Stealth navigational system, placing the navigational frame on the L2 spinous process to assist with pedicle screw insertion at L3, L4, and S1 as well as S2AI screws. The L4 and S1 laminectomies were performed followed by removal of the posterior bony elements at L5. The posterior element specimens were sent for pathological examination in order to confirm there was no tumor invasion (Fig. 10.3). Once the posterior elements were completely removed, the L4, L5, and S1 nerve roots were skeletonized until they were completely mobilized. The psoas muscles were then dissected away from the L4 and L5 vertebral bodies. The L4-L5 and L5-S1 disk spaces were disconnected up to the ALL. Once this was complete, we took the utmost care to separate the ventral epidural connection between the thecal sac and the L5 vertebral body to prevent a cerebrospinal fluid leak and to control epidural bleeding. We then placed a silastic sheet from L4 to S1 to provide a protective barrier to the thecal sac during the second stage (Fig. 10.4). The contoured lordotic rods were locked with screws into her current scoliotic position. The gap between L4 and S1 was stabilized by a fibula graft tied to the rods with cables. Morselized allogenic bone graft was applied to achieve the posterolateral arthrodesis from L3 to S1. The wound was closed by plastic surgery.

### Stage 2: Anterior Approach

The patient was set in the supine position. A midline laparotomy exposure from L4 to S1 was performed with the assistance of a vascular surgeon. Once the great vessels and anterior vertebral column were exposed, the psoas muscles were dissected down to the silastic sheet in order to communicate the previous lateral dissection planes while carefully avoiding injury to the L4, L5, and S1 nerve roots. The residual attachments of the ALL and anterior disks at L4-L5 and L5-S1, from the first stage, were then completely disconnected. Finally, the tumor was then delivered en

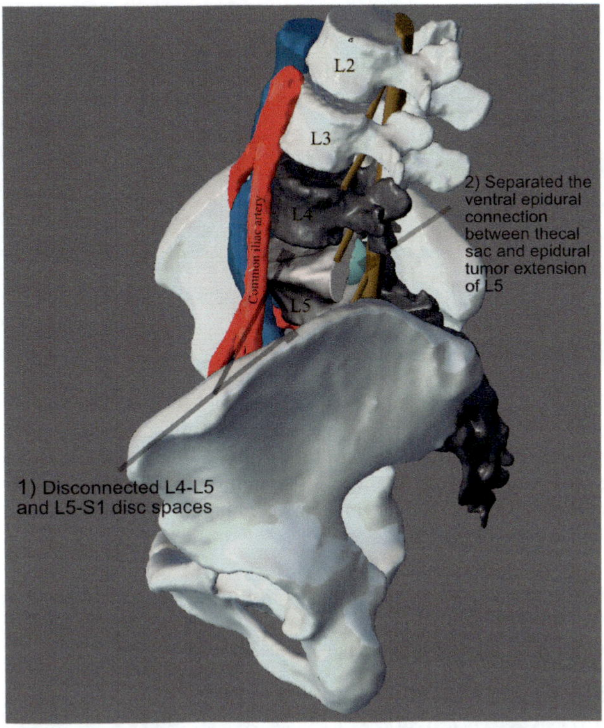


**Fig. 10.4** Illustration of a lateral extracavitary approach (LECA) in order to disconnect the L4-L5 and L5-S1 disk spaces as well as separate the ventral epidural connection between epidural tumor and the thecal sac

bloc with no breach and sent for permanent pathology (Fig. 10.5). The silastic sheet was removed. A TMC was cut according to the pre-planned CT measurement with 46 degrees of lordosis and 11 degrees of coronal curve, in order to appropriately appose the endplates. The cage was inspected to ensure a good fit across L5. Unfortunately, due to a high sacral slope, we could not put the anterior plate across the whole construct. Thus, we fixed the anterior lumbar plate superiorly to two 26 mm screws into the L4 vertebral body. Inferiorly, the L5-S1 junction was secured with a washer plate and screws (Fig. 10.6). The appropriate alignment of the implants was confirmed by intraoperative radiographs. Finally, the vascular surgeon closed the wound.

## Postoperative Follow Up

Postoperative CT scan demonstrated well-aligned anterior-posterior robust constructions in her scoliotic position (Fig. 10.6). Surgical margins from the pathology review were negative for tumor. At discharge, she was able to ambulate with a rolling walker. At 6-month follow-up, she was ambulating independently without any assistive device.

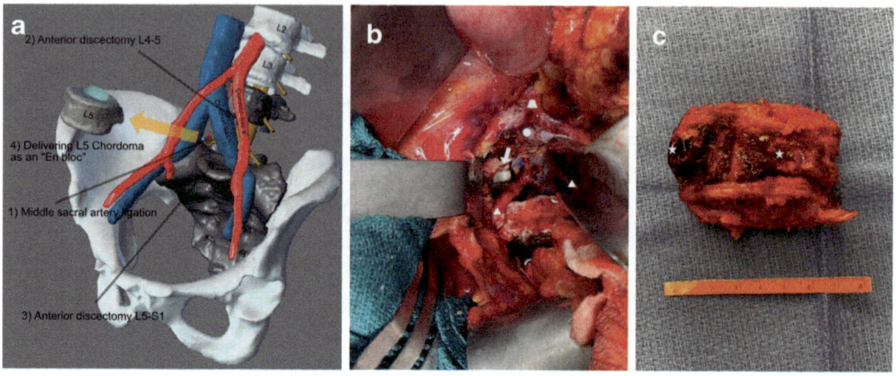


**Fig. 10.5** (**a**) Illustration of stage 2 anterior approach of L5 total en bloc spondylectomy (TES), delivering the tumor en bloc after detaching anteriorly at L4-5 and L5-S1. (**b**) The aortic bifurcation (trapezoid) as well as common iliac vein bifurcation (circle) were visualized and retracted. After the silastic sheet was removed, the thecal sac, lumbar nerve roots (triangle), and structural fibular allografts (arrow) were identified. (**c**) Demonstrating the en bloc specimen of fifth lumbar chordoma with the cut edge of pedicles (star)

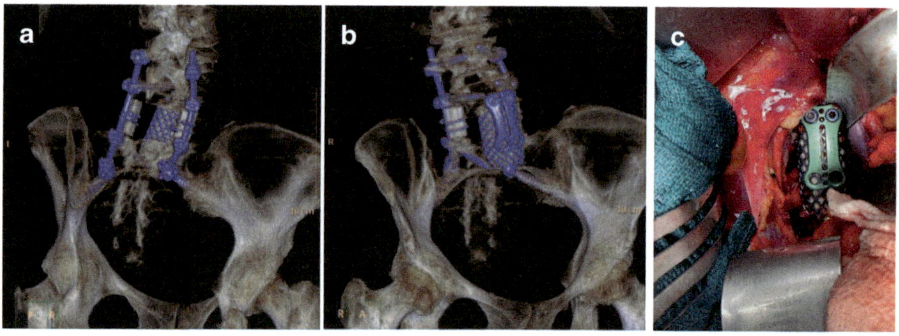


**Fig. 10.6** (**a**) Postoperative CT scan demonstrating the endplate apposition of the titanium mesh cage (TMC) and its anterior fixation. The fibula graft was well-aligned posteriorly between L4 and S1. Additionally, there was good placement of the rest of the hardware. (**b**) The intraoperative photo showed the fibular strut allograft indwelling titanium mesh cage. The anterior dislodgement was prevented by the anterior lumbar plate from L4 and traumatic screw with washer plate at L5-S1 junction

## Complications

1. Sciubba et al. reported that common perioperative complications of lumbar TES were wound infection and ileus (26.1%), deep vein thrombosis and pulmonary embolism (17.4%), and postoperative cerebrospinal fluid leak (13.0%). Vascular injuries occurred with 4.4% of anterior osteotomies [38].
2. Instrumentation failure after TES is a common postoperative complication. Park et al. reported rod fractures in 37.5% of patients at an average follow-up of

29.2 months after TES. The significant risk factors are TES at the lumbar level and a history of RT. [41] Matsumoto et al. reported 40% instrumentation failure in patients who underwent TES and survived for more than 1 year after surgery [36]. Sciubba et al. reported instrumentation failure in cases of TES of the lumbar spine in 39.1% of patients (9 out of 23 patients) [38].

## Conclusion

According to recent studies, TES of lumbar chordomas is preferred to reduce recurrence; however, the operation can lead to significant morbidity. Perioperative complications and instrumentation failure rates are quite high, even when performed by surgeons at the most experienced cancer centers. The standard surgical approach for lumbar TES is posterior-anterior; however, a modified TES with posterior-anterolateral and posterior-only approaches are potential options depending on the patients' anatomy and the tumor size and location.

## References

1. Yamazaki T, McLoughlin GS, Patel S, Rhines LD, Fourney DR. Feasibility and safety of en bloc resection for primary spine tumors: a systematic review by the Spine Oncology Study Group. Spine (Phila Pa 1976). 2009;34(22 Suppl):S31–8.
2. Fisher CG, Versteeg AL, Dea N, Boriani S, Varga PP, Dekutoski MB, et al. Surgical management of spinal chondrosarcomas. Spine (Phila Pa 1976). 2016;41(8):678–85.
3. Boriani S, Saravanja D, Yamada Y, Varga PP, Biagini R, Fisher CG. Challenges of local recurrence and cure in low grade malignant tumors of the spine. Spine (Phila Pa 1976). 2009;34(22 Suppl):S48–57.
4. Louis C, Louis R. Anatomy of the thoraco-lumbar facet joint. In: Vital JM, Cawley DT, editors. Spinal anatomy. Modern Concepts: Springer; 2020.
5. Weinstein JN, Rydevik BL, Rauschning W. Anatomic and technical considerations of pedicle screw fixation. Clin Orthop Relat Res. 1992;284:34–46.
6. Lee BC, Kazam E, Newman AD. Computed tomography of the spine and spinal cord. Radiology. 1978;128(1):95–102.
7. Vital JM. The spinal canal. In: Vital JM, Cawley DT, editors. Spinal anatomy: modern concepts. Springer; 2020.
8. Hoppenfeld S, deBoer P, Buckley R. Surgical Exposures in Orthopaedics : The Anatomic Approach. Philadelphia: Wolters Kluwer Health; 2009.
9. Shi J-G, Yuan W, Sun J-C. Surgical anatomy of the lumbar spine. In: Shi J-G, Yuan W, Sun J-C, editors. Anatomy atlas and interpretation of spine surgery. Singapore: Springer; 2018.
10. Baaj AA, Papadimitriou K, Amin AG, Kretzer RM, Wolinsky JP, Gokaslan ZL. Surgical anatomy of the diaphragm in the anterolateral approach to the spine: a cadaveric study. J Spinal Disord Tech. 2014;27(4):220–3.
11. Tribus CB, Belanger T. The vascular anatomy anterior to the L5-S1 disk space. Spine (Phila Pa 1976). 2001;26(11):1205–8.
12. Sciubba DM, Chi JH, Rhines LD, Gokaslan ZL. Chordoma of the spinal column. Neurosurg Clin N Am. 2008;19(1):5–15.
13. Ailon T, Torabi R, Fisher CG, Rhines LD, Clarke MJ, Bettegowda C, et al. Management of locally recurrent chordoma of the mobile spine and sacrum: a systematic review. Spine (Phila Pa 1976). 2016;41 Suppl 20(Suppl 20):S193–s8.

14. Chen YL, Liebsch N, Kobayashi W, Goldberg S, Kirsch D, Calkins G, et al. Definitive high-dose photon/proton radiotherapy for unresected mobile spine and sacral chordomas. Spine (Phila Pa 1976). 2013;38(15):E930–6.
15. Bilsky MH, Yamada Y, Yenice KM, Lovelock M, Hunt M, Gutin PH, et al. Intensity-modulated stereotactic radiotherapy of paraspinal tumors: a preliminary report. Neurosurgery. 2004;54(4):823–30; discussion 30–1.
16. Dea N, Fisher CG, Reynolds JJ, Schwab JH, Rhines LD, Gokaslan ZL, et al. Current treatment strategy for newly diagnosed chordoma of the mobile spine and sacrum: results of an international survey. J Neurosurg Spine. 2018;30(1):119–25.
17. Murakami H, Kawahara N, Tomita K, Demura S, Kato S, Yoshioka K. Does interruption of the artery of Adamkiewicz during total en bloc spondylectomy affect neurologic function? Spine (Phila Pa 1976). 2010;35(22):E1187–92.
18. Yoshioka K, Niinuma H, Ehara S, Nakajima T, Nakamura M, Kawazoe K. MR angiography and CT angiography of the artery of Adamkiewicz: state of the art. Radiographics. 2006;26 Suppl 1:S63–73.
19. Kawahara N, Tomita K, Murakami H, Demura S. Total en bloc spondylectomy for spinal tumors: surgical techniques and related basic background. Orthop Clin North Am. 2009;40(1):47–63, vi
20. Sangsin A, Murakami H, Shimizu T, Kato S, Demura S, Tsuchiya H. Surgical technique of vertebral body removal and anterior reconstruction in L5 sondylectomy. Spine Surg Relat Res. 2018;2(3):236–42.
21. Yang X, Yang J, Jia Q, Zhong N, Jiao J, Hu J, et al. A novel technique for total En bloc spondylectomy of the fifth lumbar tumor through posterior-only approach. Spine (Phila Pa 1976). 2019;44(12):896–901.
22. Foreman PM, Naftel RP, Moore TA 2nd, Hadley MN. The lateral extracavitary approach to the thoracolumbar spine: a case series and systematic review. J Neurosurg Spine. 2016;24(4): 570–9.
23. Bennett EE, Benzel EC. Operative Techniques: Spine Surgery. In: Baron EM, Vaccaro AR, editors. Operative techniques: spine surgery. 3rd ed; 2018. p. 311–6.
24. Steinmetz MPPR, Resnick DK. Anterior transperitoneal lumbar approach. In: Fundamentals of operative techniques in neurosurgery. 2nd ed. New York: Thieme; 2010. p. 502–5.
25. Dalle Ore CL, Lau D, Ames CP. Anterior lumbar and lumbosacral approach: transperitoneal. In: Sciubba DM, editor. Spinal tumor surgery: a case-based approach. Cham: Springer; 2019. p. 107–18.
26. Shah AA, Paulino Pereira NR, Pedlow FX, Wain JC, Yoon SS, Hornicek FJ, et al. Modified En bloc spondylectomy for tumors of the thoracic and lumbar spine: surgical technique and outcomes. J Bone Joint Surg Am. 2017;99(17):1476–84.
27. Disch AC, Schaser KD, Melcher I, Luzzati A, Feraboli F, Schmoelz W. En bloc spondylectomy reconstructions in a biomechanical in-vitro study. Eur Spine J. 2008;17(5):715–25.
28. Richardson B, Paulzak A, Rusyniak WG, Martino A. Anterior lumbar corpectomy with expandable titanium cage reconstruction: a case series of 42 patients. World Neurosurg. 2017;108:317–24.
29. Cardenas RJ, Javalkar V, Patil S, Gonzalez-Cruz J, Ogden A, Mukherjee D, et al. Comparison of allograft bone and titanium cages for vertebral body replacement in the thoracolumbar spine: a biomechanical study. Neurosurgery. 2010;66(6 Suppl Operative):314–8; discussion 8.
30. Li Z, Wei F, Liu Z, Liu X, Jiang L, Yu M, et al. Risk factors for instrumentation failure after total En bloc spondylectomy of thoracic and lumbar spine tumors using titanium mesh cage for anterior reconstruction. World Neurosurg. 2020;135:e106–e15.
31. Aliano KA, Agulnick M, Cohen B, Gonya G, Low C, Stavrides S, et al. Spinal reconstruction for osteomyelitis with free vascularized fibular grafts using intra-abdominal recipient vessels: a series of three cases. Microsurgery. 2013;33(7):560–6.
32. El Dafrawy MH, Raad M, Okafor L, Kebaish KM. Sacropelvic fixation: a comprehensive review. Spine Deform. 2019;7(4):509–16.

33. Cunningham BW, Sefter JC, Hu N, Kim SW, Bridwell KH, McAfee PC. Biomechanical comparison of iliac screws versus interbody femoral ring allograft on lumbosacral kinematics and sacral screw strain. Spine (Phila Pa 1976). 2010;35(6):E198–205.
34. Jain A, Kebaish KM, Sponseller PD. Sacral-alar-iliac fixation in pediatric deformity: radiographic outcomes and complications. Spine Deform. 2016;4(3):225–9.
35. Kuklo TR, Bridwell KH, Lewis SJ, Baldus C, Blanke K, Iffrig TM, et al. Minimum 2-year analysis of sacropelvic fixation and L5-S1 fusion using S1 and iliac screws. Spine (Phila Pa 1976). 2001;26(18):1976–83.
36. Matsumoto M, Watanabe K, Tsuji T, Ishii K, Nakamura M, Chiba K, et al. Late instrumentation failure after total en bloc spondylectomy. J Neurosurg Spine. 2011;15(3):320–7.
37. Clarke MJ, Hsu W, Suk I, McCarthy E, Black JH 3rd, Sciubba DM, et al. Three-level en bloc spondylectomy for chordoma. Neurosurgery. 2011;68(2 Suppl Operative):325–33; discussion 33.
38. Sciubba DM, De la Garza RR, Goodwin CR, Xu R, Bydon A, Witham TF, et al. Total en bloc spondylectomy for locally aggressive and primary malignant tumors of the lumbar spine. Eur Spine J. 2016;25(12):4080–7.
39. Kawahara N, Tomita K, Murakami H, Demura S, Yoshioka K, Kato S. Total en bloc spondylectomy of the lower lumbar spine: a surgical techniques of combined posterior-anterior approach. Spine (Phila Pa 1976). 2011;36(1):74–82.
40. Goodwin CR, Recinos PF, Omeis I, Momin EN, Witham TF, Bydon A, et al. Prevention of facial pressure ulcers using the Mayfield clamp for sacral tumor resection Technical note. J Neurosurg Spine. 2011;14(1):85–7.
41. Park SJ, Lee CS, Chang BS, Kim YH, Kim H, Kim SI, et al. Rod fracture and related factors after total en bloc spondylectomy. Spine J. 2019;19(10):1613–9.

# Surgical Management of Chordoma of the Sacrum

# 11

Peter S. Rose, Matthew T. Houdek, and Cory G. Couch

## Abbreviations

| | |
|---|---|
| CT | Computed tomography |
| MR | Magnetic resonance |
| SI | Sacroiliac |
| VRAM | Vertical rectus abdominus muscle |

## Introduction

The sacrum remains the most common location for chordoma, with roughly half of all tumors arising in this location. Interestingly, there appears to be a male predominance for sacral chordomas which is more striking than the male predominance of chordomas in other locations. In 437 chordomas reviewed by Unni and Inwards, 71% of sacral tumors occurred in males while only 55% of spheno-occipital tumors were in men. The reason for this remains unclear [1].

While chordomas have been recognized for over 150 years, the modern era of treatment for chordomas did not arise until the advent of computed tomography (CT) scanning in the late 1970s. This, coupled with magnetic resonance (MR) imaging becoming commonly available in the late 1980s allowed for accurate assessment of chordomas preoperatively. Coincident with improved imaging came an improved understanding of the biological behavior and high risk for local recurrence with inadequate surgery [2]. These advances in the evaluation and understanding initiated the common acceptance of en bloc excision of sacral chordomas.

P. S. Rose (✉) · M. T. Houdek · C. G. Couch
Department of Orthopaedic Surgery, Mayo Clinic, Rochester, MN, USA
e-mail: rose.peter@mayo.edu; Kleinhans.Valerie@mayo.edu



D. M. Sciubba, J. H. Schwab (eds.), *Chordoma of the Spine*,
https://doi.org/10.1007/978-3-030-76201-8_11

More recent work (covered elsewhere in this book) has focused on the potential for adjuvant radiation and medical treatments in conjunction with or in place of surgical resection. However, as of this writing, negative margin surgical resection remains the most established curative treatment for sacral chordoma [3–5].

A key aspect in the treatment of sacral chordomas remains proper diagnosis and preoperative imaging. In contemporary practice there is very little role for open surgical biopsies of sacral chordomas; transrectal biopsies should be avoided. Chordoma has a well-recognized propensity for seeding biopsy tracts, and all sampling should be designed to minimize tumor contamination in light of anticipated surgical resection. Appropriate and inappropriate biopsies of sacral chordomas are demonstrated in Fig. 11.1.

Once a chordoma is identified, patients are staged for evidence of distant metastatic disease. While institutional practice patterns will vary, most commonly this

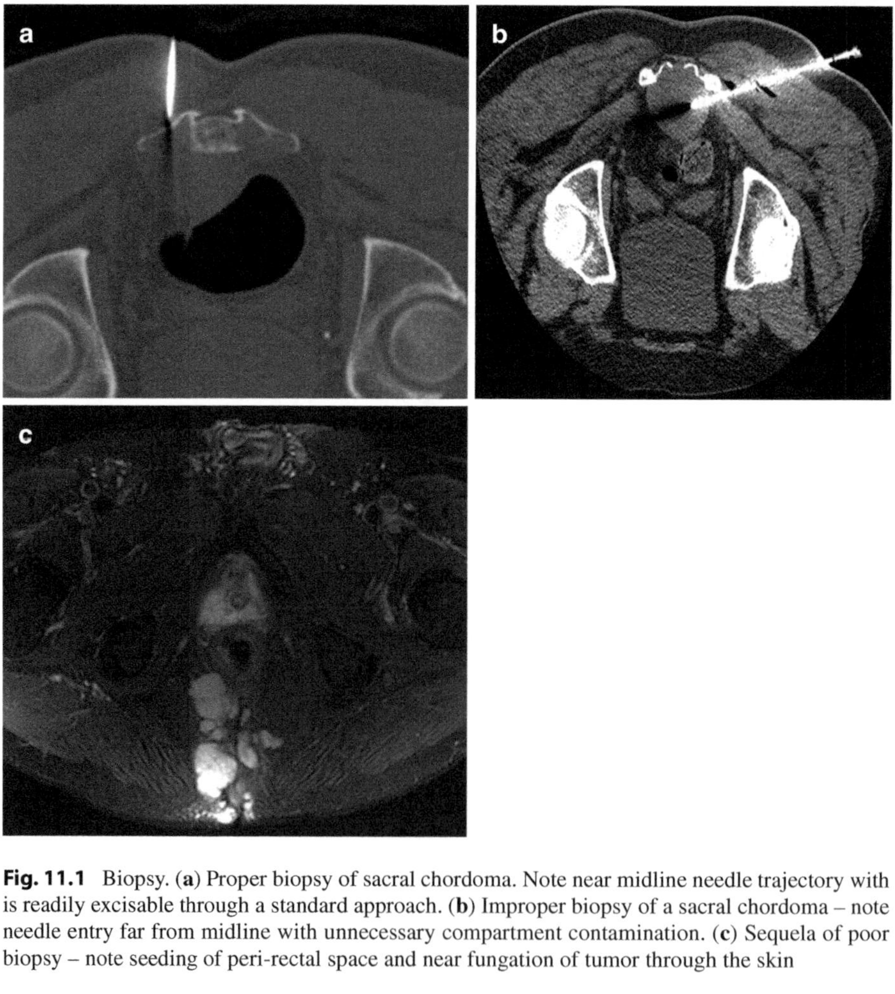

**Fig. 11.1** Biopsy. (**a**) Proper biopsy of sacral chordoma. Note near midline needle trajectory with is readily excisable through a standard approach. (**b**) Improper biopsy of a sacral chordoma – note needle entry far from midline with unnecessary compartment contamination. (**c**) Sequela of poor biopsy – note seeding of peri-rectal space and near fungation of tumor through the skin

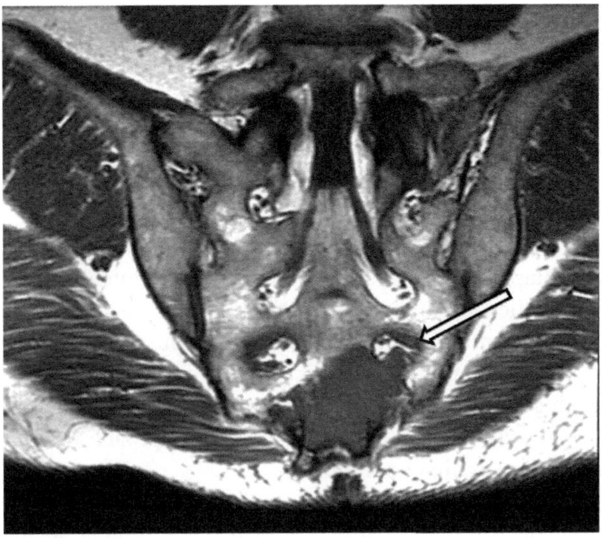

**Fig. 11.2** Coronal oblique images. T1-weighted coronal oblique MRI demonstrates subtle tumor extension into left S3 foramen

involves CT of the chest and CT and/or MR imaging of the pelvis. Our institution traditionally obtains technetium bone scans at presentation, although the yield of this study is low; some centers advocate for MR of the entire spinal axis as well [6]. In addition to detecting potential metastatic lesions, imaging of sacral chordomas defines the rostral extent of disease, extra-osseous soft tissue extension, and the relationship to the rectum. These all influence the surgical management of these tumors. Our team has found coronal oblique images (coronal images taken in the plane of the sacrum) to be particularly helpful in planning resections. These provide an "en foss" view of the sacrum which reproduces the surgeon's view at the time of resection and facilitates tracing of nerve root pathways with relation to the tumor (Fig. 11.2).

## Anatomy of the Sacrum

The sacrum provides the anatomic junction between the pelvis/lower extremity and the torso/mobile spine. As such, the sacrum must resist both axial and rotational loads with rotational forces centered at the posterior aspect of the L5/S1 disk [7]. The iliolumbar ligaments (spanning from the transverse processes of L5 to the inner table of the medial ilium) and the sacrospinous/sacrotuberous ligaments provide secondary restraints to motion beyond the sacroiliac joints.

Classically, the sacroiliac joints terminate just below the level of the S2 neuroforamina and serve as a valuable intraoperative landmark. However, surgeons approaching tumors in the sacrum should carefully scrutinize imaging for the possibility of a lumbarized S1 segment (present in approximately 2% of the population) or sacralization of L5 (present in 17% of the population either unilaterally or bilaterally) [8]. A similar percentage of patients will have some degree of spina bifida occulta [9]. Put in context, it is nearly twice as common for a patient to have transitional anatomy at the lumbopelvic junction and/or spinal bifida occulta than it is for them to be left handed, and these findings are relevant for the execution of an oncologic sacral resection.

The posterior anatomy of the sacrum is straightforward to surgeons. Standard posterior closure flaps for sacral resections include gluteal advancement flaps. These flaps are supplied by branches of the gluteal vessels (which arise from the internal iliac system). Tumors with lateral extension into the sciatic notches or proximal extension which require the sacrifice of the internal iliac vessels often are poorly closed with gluteal flaps. Surgeons should consider this anatomy when planning resections and may need to utilize an anterior approach to obtain proper flap coverage if gluteal flaps will not suffice.

Ventral to the sacrum is Waldeyer's fascia (separating the anterior sacral periosteum from the mesorectum). This structure provides a reliable anatomic barrier to tumor extension anteriorly. However, distally this structure fuses with the mesorectal fascia. Thus, in tumors with anterior extra-osseous extension, it is more reliable to dissect proximally to distally to ensure that the plane of dissection is anterior to Waldeyer's fascia. In patients undergoing a posterior-only approach for tumor delivery, this is facilitated by delivering the tumor from proximal (where the fascial planes are separate) to distal (where the fascial planes fuse and the proper plane is less distinct) (Fig. 11.3).

The pyriformis muscles begin on the anterior aspect of the sacrum; surgeons should be aware of the possibility of chordoma spread along the longitudinal fibers of this muscle and may wish to section it laterally through its tendon rather than through the muscle bellies. Branches of the internal iliac vessels lie over the sacral ala between S1 and the sciatic notch. Surgeons executing resections at this level should carefully consider the role of an initial anterior approach for vessel ligation or embolization to minimize the risk of hemorrhage from these structures during a

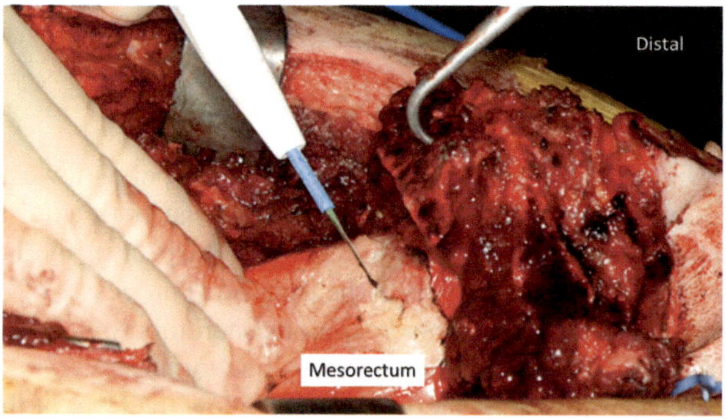


**Fig. 11.3** Tumor dissection proceeds proximal to distal through the mesorectum to maintain a plane strictly ventral to Waldeyer's fascia

posterior approach. If these vessels are ligated or embolized, gluteal advancement flaps rely on collateral perfusion only and are less reliable for wound closure.

The geometry of the sacroiliac joints is wider anteriorly than posteriorly. In tumors which extend above the level of the inferior sacroiliac joints, careful dissection and planning is necessary to ensure that osteotomies are of adequate width to obtain a clear margin. It is deceptive how wide an exposure is needed to perform osteotomies lateral to the sacroiliac joints from a posterior approach. In wide tumors of the upper sacrum, strong consideration of an anterior approach for initial osteotomies is recommended.

## Surgical Approaches

A major consideration a surgeon must make when planning a sacral resection for chordoma is whether to perform an all posterior approach or to perform an initial anterior approach. Anterior approaches have several benefits:

- Allow reliable mobilization of anterior pelvic structures (particularly in the setting of prior surgery, radiation therapy, diverticulitis, etc.).
- Allow ligation and division of the internal iliac vessels in high tumors or those with significant extra-osseous extension into the sciatic notch.
- Allow performance of a colostomy. This may be selected either for rectal invasion, anticipated rectal de-vascularization, or anticipated loss of bowel function for patient function and wound hygiene. In the case that a patient is "borderline" as to whether they will regain bowel function, a loop colostomy can be performed which may be easily reversed if a patient maintains/regains anal sphincter function or left permanent if they do not.
- Allow reliable osteotomy lateral to the sacroiliac joints in high, wide tumor presentations.
- Allows for the harvest of a pedicled rectus abdominus or omental flap if gluteal flaps are not anticipated to be viable or sufficient for posterior soft tissue coverage.

Anterior approaches do incur the morbidity of an additional surgical approach, however, and generally require the assistance of a general surgeon who is facile in this area. Different institutions have adopted different practice patterns as to when to perform anterior approaches and whether or not to combine them with posterior tumor resection in a single anesthetic or to stage them. While our group routinely performs anterior approaches in the circumstances outlined above, other centers have reported good outcomes with all posterior approaches [10]. Our group has additionally examined the role of staging these resections and found strong benefits in terms of patient morbidity and institutional cost [11]. Thus, at our institution most patients requiring combined anterior/posterior approaches are staged by 48 hours; a handful are staged 24 hours apart because of concern for rectal de-vascularization, and none are staged more than 72 hours apart. We will perform an anterior approach for nearly all tumors requiring an osteotomy at or above the S1 foramina (unless the bony cuts are very central with minimal anticipated risk to the internal iliac vessels) and also utilize it for lower tumors with large soft tissue extensions requiring extensive flap coverage or those in whom a colostomy is planned.

## Anterior Approach

Patients undergo placement of ureteral stents if prior surgery or tumor extension causes anatomic distortion. A midline laparotomy and trans-peritoneal approach is used to access the pelvis. In most cases a standard operating room table is used; if complex lateral osteotomies will be made which require antero-posterior fluoroscopy for localization, a flat radiolucent table is used. If the rectum is to be spared, it is mobilized off the sacrum and tumor with dissection through the mesorectum to guarantee that the plane of dissection is anterior to Waldeyer's fascia. If the rectum is to be resected with the tumor, it is transected above the level of the tumor in preparation for an end colostomy at closure. If the tumor abuts the rectum low in the pelvis and an abdominoperineal resection is planned, the plane between the rectum and vagina or prostate is developed. In most cases, this is not necessary as the terminal rectum can be dissected and stapled off below the tumor and above the anus (near the level of the anococcygeal ligament). If this is done during the anterior approach (stapling the rectum both above and below the tumor), we recommend resecting the tumor the same day to minimize the risk of perforation of a closed loop of rectum. More commonly the distal rectal stapling and transection at the level of the anococcygeal ligament is done during the final steps of posterior tumor delivery with 48-hour surgical staging at our institution.

The internal iliac vessels are identified and divided as indicated. Most chordomas are centered in the midline with symmetric involvement bilaterally. If asymmetric growth allows the preservation of unilateral internal iliac vessels, this is very valuable for two reasons. First, it preserves direct vascularity to one gluteus maximus flap. Second, once both internal iliac veins are ligated, the epidural veins (via Batson's plexus) provide the collateral pathway for blood return from the pelvis. Ligation of bilateral internal iliac veins can lead to dramatic epidural bleeding during the posterior approach [12].

Initial osteotomies are performed; localization of these is commonly based on distance from the midline, L5/S1 disk, and fluoroscopic guidance. Anterior osteotomies through the sacrum are typically unicortical to avoid the risk of nerve root avulsion or dural tear, and the level of osteotomy is marked with a small fragment screw (Fig. 11.4). This is readily visualized on lateral fluoroscopy during the posterior approach to join the anterior unicortical cut. Any far lateral osteotomies (lateral to the sacroiliac joints) are performed bicortically. Surgeons may choose a burr, long osteotome, or ultrasonic bone cutting device based on surgeon preference and the geometry of the cut at hand.

In almost all cases undergoing an anterior approach, a vertical rectus abdominus (VRAM) flap and/or omental flap is harvested and tucked into the pelvis to assist

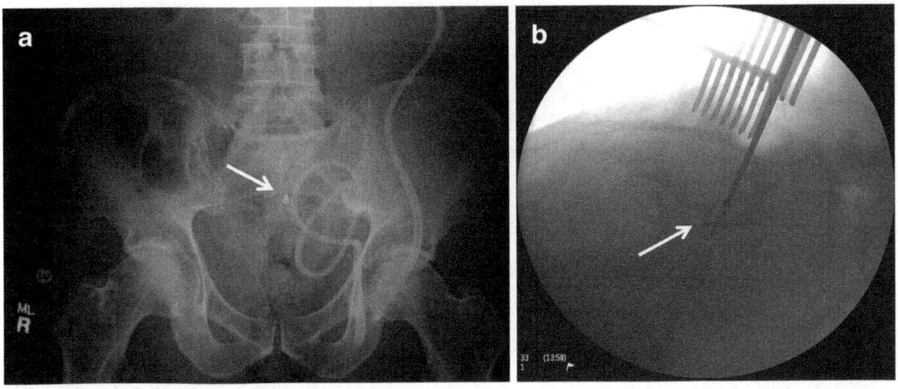

**Fig. 11.4** Localization. (**a**) Small fragment screw (arrow) is inserted at the level of the anterior osteotomy during anterior approach. (**b**) This screw is readily visible on lateral fluoroscopy during posterior tumor resection

with posterior wound management (Fig. 11.5). If a VRAM flap is planned, coordination between the assisting general surgeon and plastic surgeon is key to plan the anterior incision and ostomy placement. Prior to the closure of the laparotomy, a silastic sheet or sponge is placed between the tumor and the mobilized structures to mark the plane of dissection and protect against any errant deep dissection during tumor delivery. Once the laparotomy is closed, any colostomy is matured. Ureteral stents, if placed, are left in until after tumor delivery.

In patients undergoing total sacrectomies or resections proximal to the S1 neuroforamina, spinopelvic continuity is either disrupted or at risk of failure. Our group favors reconstruction of this junction with vascularized fibula grafts. If this is planned, the fibula grafts may be "pre-harvested" during an anterior approach to maximize efficiency during a posterior procedure. This involves in situ dissection and potential osteotomy of the fibulae without division of their vascular pedicles. If this is done it is important that these wounds be closed in a truly watertight manner so they may be re-prepped during the posterior approach without contamination of sterility.

Nearly all patients who undergo an initial anterior approach are extubated at the conclusion of the procedure and mobilized to chair between stages.

## Posterior Approach

Patients are positioned prone on a radiolucent spine table (Jackson table) with the abdomen allowed to hang free. If a prior anterior approach has been performed, the anterior abdomen is wrapped in several layers of adhesive drape ("Ioban") to minimize tension across the anterior incision. If no spinopelvic instrumentation is planned, patients are placed on a radiolucent Wilson frame to maximize sacral access and exposure. However, this frame places the lumbar spine in relative

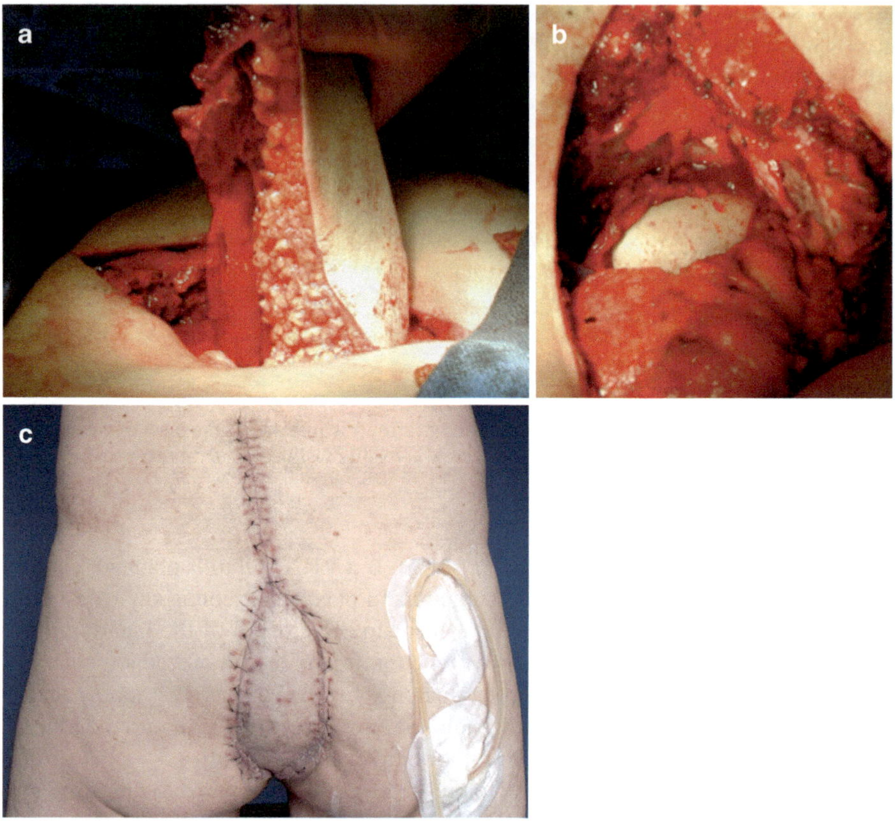


**Fig. 11.5** Vertical rectus abdominus flap. (**a**) Harvest of VRAM flap during anterior approach. (**b**) Flap is tucked into the presacral space prior to anterior wound closure. (**c**) Posterior inset of VRAM flap for high sacrectomy defect

kyphosis. If an instrumented spinopelvic resection is to be performed, the patient is placed on standard pads to maintain proper lumbar lordosis. If fibula grafts are planned the legs are prepped in; the buttocks are prepped widely to allow for gluteal advancement flaps. We temporarily sew the anus shut but do not drape it into the field unless felt necessary for concurrent resection with the tumor. In a prospective assessment, this protocol only resulted in positioning-related morbidity in cases >10 hours in length or in morbidly obese patients [13].

The biopsy tract is excised en bloc with the specimen; the standard incision for sacrectomy is a vertical midline incision with biopsy tract ellipse; this has the advantage of being extensile along the spine and readily accepts gluteal advancement or VRAM flap inset. It does have the disadvantage of terminating close to the anus. Other groups utilize a tri-radiate incision; this keeps a greater distance from the anus but does create a potentially ischemic epicenter. No studies have compared the relative merits of different incisions for sacral tumor resections.

Dissection initially establishes the proximal exposure and osteotomy level; this is typically verified with lateral fluoroscopy. In patients who are very heavy in which lateral fluoroscopy is unreliable at defining sacral landmarks and localization, a fiducial marker can be placed by interventional radiology prior to surgery at the planned level of osteotomy above the tumor, and this fiducial is viewable with lateral fluoroscopy to identify the site of osteotomy.

At the appropriate level, a laminectomy is performed and the cauda equina/dural tube is ligated and divided. This is performed early in the operation because of the risk of epidural bleeding during the time needed to complete the ultimate osteotomy. Laminectomy and division of the nerves are relatively rapid, and at this point, we will pack the sacral spinal canal with hemostatic agent ("Floseal," "Surgiflow," "Instat," or a similar hemostatic slurry). In the time it takes to complete the remainder of the tumor dissection this area will generally become hemostatic and prevent troublesome epidural bleeding during the sacral osteotomy and tumor delivery.

Subsequent dissection exposes the posterior sacrum and lateral para-sacral areas. In areas with contained tumor, the posterior sacrum may be exposed in an extraperiosteal manner. In any areas in which tumor extends to the dorsal cortex or has an extra-osseous extension, the paraspinal muscles are left in situ over the posterior sacrum. Lateral dissection must extend beyond the lateral aspect of tumor extension, including a margin of normal soft tissue. In the parasacral gutters, the sacrotuberous and sacrospinous ligaments are divided. Note that the pudendal nerve runs between these structures, and if appropriate may be spared to preserve sphincter function. The sciatic nerve runs through the greater sciatic foramen and all or part can usually be spared except in very proximal or lateral tumor presentations. Note that the superior gluteal vessels are located in the top of the greater sciatic foramen, typically ~1.5 cm lateral to the inferior sacroiliac joints. Significant bleeding can occur from these structures if they are injured and retract into the pelvis.

Very lateral tumors may require more complicated strategies for resection. For example, if tumor extends widely along the sacrospinous ligament, it may be necessary to osteotomize the ischial spine to prevent margin contamination. Rare very advanced tumors may require osteotomy of the posterior column of the pelvis. Extremely extensive tumors which involve the sciatic nerve and hip joint and/or femoral nerve may be considered for sacrectomy/hemipelvectomy. This is very rare for chordomas which typically arise in the midline and for which it would be unusual to have such lateral involvement at presentation but is seen with other sacropelvic tumors.

Once resection is performed, the margin is immediately analyzed. We perform this using three techniques:

1. Radiograph of the resected specimen to verify the planned resection was performed.
2. Direct inspection of the cut surface of the bony specimen (a band saw in the pathology suite is used to immediately section the bony specimen).
3. Frozen section analysis of soft tissue margins (paraspinal, pyriformis).

Our group ideally obtains a wide margin, operationally defined as

1. 1 cm of histologically normal bone.
2. A radial anatomic fascial barrier (e.g., Waldeyer's fascia ventrally).
3. 2 cm of longitudinal free tissue (e.g., pyriformis).

Different centers define a wide margin differently, and there is no standardized definition of a wide margin resection of the sacrum at this time. As well, the anatomic constraints of the sacrum and pelvis may make a margin by these criteria impossible or impractical to obtain. Significant effort, however, should be directed to obtaining a negative margin resection even if it is closer than these criteria specify. A negative margin is the single most predictive factor for disease-free survival in sacral chordoma surgery [3–5].

## Soft Tissue +/− Bony Reconstruction

Once the tumor is resected, all patients require soft tissue reconstruction and some will require bony reconstruction as well. The goal of soft tissue reconstruction is to obtain reliable healing of the wound and to prevent posterior visceral herniation [14]. If the gluteal vessels remain intact and relatively modest posterior soft tissue required resection for biopsy tract excision or tumor extension, bilateral gluteal V-Y advancement flaps are often a simple and reliable method of posterior wound closure (see Fig. 11.8d–f). However, if these flaps are not available or inadequate, pedicled VRAM and/or omental flaps can be brought into the wound following an anterior approach. VRAM flaps are typically myocutaneous flaps and assist with skin as well as muscle/fascia deficits (see Fig. 11.5). Omental flaps can bring well-vascularized tissue into the area and obliterate empty space but do not bring additional skin for closure or to mitigate wound tension.

In addition to skin closure and wound healing, soft tissue reconstruction seeks to reconstruct the posterior abdominal wall to minimize the risk of posterior visceral hernia (Fig. 11.8d, f). In patients who have preserved anal and/or urinary sphincter contraction, this is important to allow functional bowel and bladder capacity. Without a competent posterior abdominal wall, when patients Valsalva to evacuate stool or urine, the increased abdominal pressure of Valsalva merely displaces bowel posteriorly with less effective force given to evacuation and resultant voiding/defecating dysfunction. In patients without sphincter function, this is probably less important but may be a source of discomfort when sitting if bowel is directly under the posterior skin. As well, we have had a handful of cases of bowel obstruction from viscera herniated between spinal instrumentation rods who had an incompetent posterior abdominal wall reconstruction.

The technique of posterior abdominal wall reconstruction typically includes the use of a mesh reconstruction followed by gluteal advancement flaps in the case of posterior-based reconstruction. If a VRAM flap is used, the flap is carefully sewn to the fascia of the gluteus maximus muscles (and may require some gluteal advancement to accomplish this). In patients with spinal instrumentation, the VRAM flap is brought between the rods. Depending on the local geometry and flap fill, there may be a role to suture an additional mesh to the rods to help sequester bowel.

Bony reconstruction is strongly considered in cases in which the spinopelvic junction is disrupted. While it is theoretically possible to maintain some spinopelvic stability after total sacrectomy if the iliolumbar ligaments remain competent, in practice almost all resections this proximal involve osteotomies at or lateral to the sacroiliac joints that predictably remove the iliac insertion of the iliolumbar ligaments. Additionally, biomechanical studies and clinical experience have shown that resections above the S1 foramina have a high risk of ultimate bony failure [15].

Different options exist for the bony reconstruction of the spinopelvic junction. Our group favors the use bilateral fibula grafts in a "cathedral" reconstruction that seeks to recreate the anterior column function of the sacrum (Fig. 11.6) [16, 17]. Fibula grafts are docked proximally in the final remaining bone segment and distally in the supra-acetabular ilium (or rarely in the ischium). Grafts are spanned by rods extending from pedicle screws in the lumbar spine to pelvic screws and compressed into place. Our group typically places pedicles screws in the lower two or three lumbar vertebrae based on bone quality and patient body habitus. The use of fibula grafts has been shown biomechanically to double the load to failure in a cadaver model. Additionally, the use of four rod constructs has also been shown to significantly increase the stiffness of the reconstruction and removes the possibility of single rod breakage being catastrophic [18, 19].

Surgeons selecting this option may elect for vascularized or non-vascularized fibula grafts. While our group initially chose allograft fibula reconstructions, we

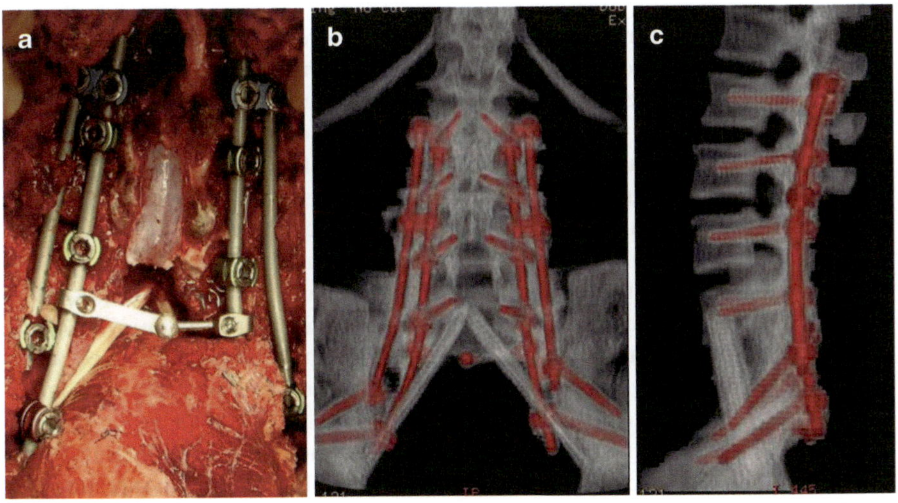


**Fig. 11.6** Cathedral reconstruction. (**a**) Intraoperative photograph of bilateral fibula reconstruction of the spinopelvic junction. (**b**) Postoperative coronal. (**c**) Sagittal CT reconstructions demonstrating reconstruction of the anterior column function of the sacrum by fibula grafts

have shifted our practice to favor vascularized grafts. While this does increase the length of the surgery, our group and others have shown much better healing with vascularized grafts [20, 21]. The vascular anastomosis is challenging in these cases, particularly the identification of donor vessels. We most commonly anastomose to branches of the gluteal vessels and are careful during tumor dissection and delivery to attempt to preserve vascular stumps as donor vessels. In the case of near total sacrectomy in which spinopelvic continuity is compromised but not disrupted, surgeons may elect to augment the area with spinopelvic instrumentation alone or to add additional strut grafts.

Other mechanisms of spinopelvic reconstruction have been reported. Custom sacral prostheses initially had poor results, but new developments in additive manufacturing ("3D printing") allow greater flexibility and have shown favorable initial results [22]. The transiliac bar technique is established in clinical practice [23] although recent biomechanical studies have questioned some of its utility [24]. Authors have reported the use of autoclaved specimen reimplantation for reconstruction as well [25]. At this time there are no comparative studies demonstrating the benefit of any one reconstruction technique over others, and individual surgeon preference and institutional practice patterns guide the selection of reconstruction.

Postoperatively patients are mobilized as rapidly as practical, but prolonged sitting is avoided during posterior wound healing. We will typically allow unlimited standing and walking but slowly advance sitting tolerance as the wound condition is monitored. For extensive closures, we will avoid hip flexion beyond 90 degrees to minimize wound tension.

## Complications/Outcomes

Sacrectomy surgery for chordoma unfortunately presents a high complication profile [26]. The most common complications encountered in the near postoperative period are wound healing difficulties and consequent infection. Surgeons recognized early the need for vascularized tissue to reconstruct defects in this area [27], and the VRAM flap is considered the standard flap for difficult sacrectomy wounds [28]. A recent meta-analysis of flap use in sacrectomy surgery demonstrated flap loss to be rare but an overall flap complication rate of 37% [14]. The use of radiation and high sacrectomies (with larger net tumor resections, greater risk of wound soilage from incontinence, and impaired patient mobility) were associated with an increased risk of complications. Similarly, an analysis of the role of radiotherapy in the care of sacral chordoma patients demonstrated radiation to be associated with a hazard ratio of increased wound complications of 2.76, but little if any benefit in local control (Fig. 11.7) [29]. Our group recently reported on 129 oncologic sacrectomy procedures (including 104 subtotal, 5 near total, and 20 total sacrectomies) for a variety of histologies with an infection rate of ~30% [30].

Sacral stress fractures are recognized after treatment for sacral chordoma [15]. The use of radiotherapy, particularly in high doses, is highly associated with an

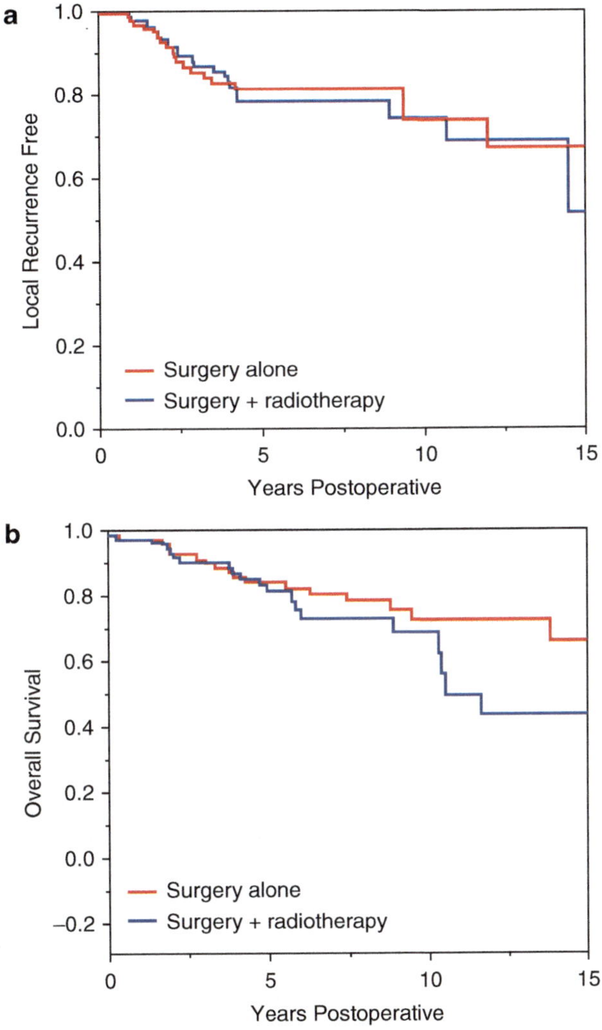


**Fig. 11.7** Radiation and outcomes in sacral chordoma. (**a**) Local recurrence-free survival and; (**b**) Overall survival in patients treated for sacrococcygeal chordoma with and without radiotherapy

increased risk of fracture [29, 31]. Once fracture occurs, treatment is challenging. It is not yet established whether or not prophylactic fixation is justified or beneficial in patients at high risk of fracture.

Patients undergoing total or near total sacrectomies generally benefit from bony reconstruction. Instrumentation failure is seen in approximately 25% of patients from either pseudarthrosis or infection [19, 30]. Our group has recognized the increased rate of failure with the use of allograft reconstructions and now favors vascularized autograft fibula struts; an internal analysis demonstrated a 17% non-union rate with vascularized fibula reconstruction used in oncologic sacral surgery compared to 55% non-union rate with allograft struts. Other authors have shown similar results [21].

Patient bowel and bladder function is frequently impacted by sacrectomy as a consequence of the operation rather than a complication. In patients in whom both S3 nerve roots can be preserved, the majority of patients will maintain or regain functional bowel, bladder, and sexual capacity provided the pudendal nerves are not involved by lateral soft tissue extension of tumor. Higher levels of sacrifice correlate with patient outcome, as expected [32–35].

Tumor recurrence and distant metastases create the primary oncologic outcomes of interest in this population. In a Sacral Study Group report of 193 patients treated for sacrococcygeal chordoma, 10-year disease-free and disease-specific survivals were 58 and 72 percent, respectively [29]. Other series have reported similar results [4, 5]. The use of adjunct radiotherapy has been postulated to increase local control after sacral chordoma surgery. However, radiotherapy was associated with increased complications without clearly improved oncologic outcomes in a series of 193 patients treated surgically with and without radiotherapy (see Fig. 11.7) [29].

Unfortunately, once tumor recurrence occurs, salvage is very difficult. However, clinicians should carefully tailor treatments to individual patients. In a large cohort of sacral chordoma patients, all-cause mortality increased with age, calling into question aggressive treatments of recurrent chordoma in elderly patients [36].

## Cases

### Case 1 – Mid Sacral Chordoma (Fig. 11.8)

A 34-year-old woman presented with increasing pain in the sacral region; imaging revealed an expansile, lobulated lesion which was confirmed on CT-guided needle biopsy as a chordoma. She staged negative for distant disease by CT chest, abdomen, and pelvis and bone scan. The patient's tumor was slightly asymmetric which allowed for the preservation of a single S3 nerve root and both S2 nerve roots.

The patient underwent resection through an all posterior approach through a midline incision with biopsy tract resection. Osteotomy was performed at the level of the S2 foramina to allow these nerves to be followed distally; additionally, a unilateral S3 nerve root was spared.

No bony reconstruction was necessary as the level of osteotomy was through S2. Soft tissue reconstruction was accomplished using bilateral gluteal V-Y advancement flaps over a posterior mesh reconstruction of the pelvis. The patient remains continually disease-free 8 years postoperatively with functional bowel, bladder, and sexual capacity.

### Case 2 – Total Sacrectomy for Chordoma (Fig. 11.9)

A 45-year-old man presented with an enlarging sacral chordoma with impending fungation through an incision through which he had undergone non-oncologic

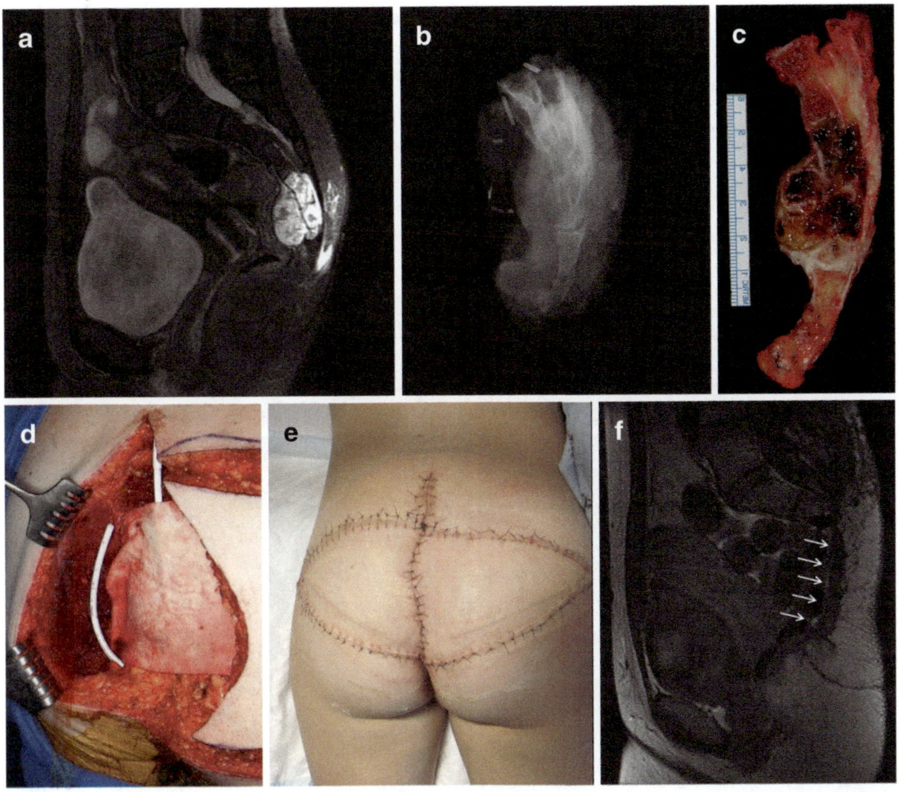


**Fig. 11.8** Case 1 (mid-sacral chordoma). (**a**) Chordoma extends to the caudal S3 segment on sagittal T2 fat saturated MRI. (**b**) Specimen radiograph. (**c**) Cut specimen demonstrating resection. (**d**) Posterior abdominal wall reconstruction. (**e**) Bilateral gluteal V-Y advancement flaps used for soft tissue reconstruction. (**f**) Sagittal T1-weighted MRI demonstrating posterior abdominal wall reconstruction (arrows)

manipulation of the tumor several months earlier. He staged negative for overt metastatic disease but had indeterminate lung nodules present.

The extent of the tumor is shown in Fig. 11.9a, b. The entire sacrum was involved, and significant soft tissue contamination was present. The patient underwent a total sacrectomy with osteotomy through the lower portion of L5 and osteotomies lateral to the sacroiliac joints. These surgeries were staged 48 hours apart.

Bony reconstruction was performed using bilateral vascularized fibula grafts. Because of extensive soft tissue contamination, the patient underwent soft tissue reconstruction using a pedicled transverse rectus abdominus myocutaneous flap to maximize bulk coverage capacity (Fig. 11.9e).

Initial healing was surprisingly uneventful. Because of concern for ill-defined soft tissue contamination from the patient's prior non-oncologic manipulation, postoperative proton beam radiotherapy was delivered despite negative surgical margins. The patient has subsequently undergone resection of a solitary pulmonary

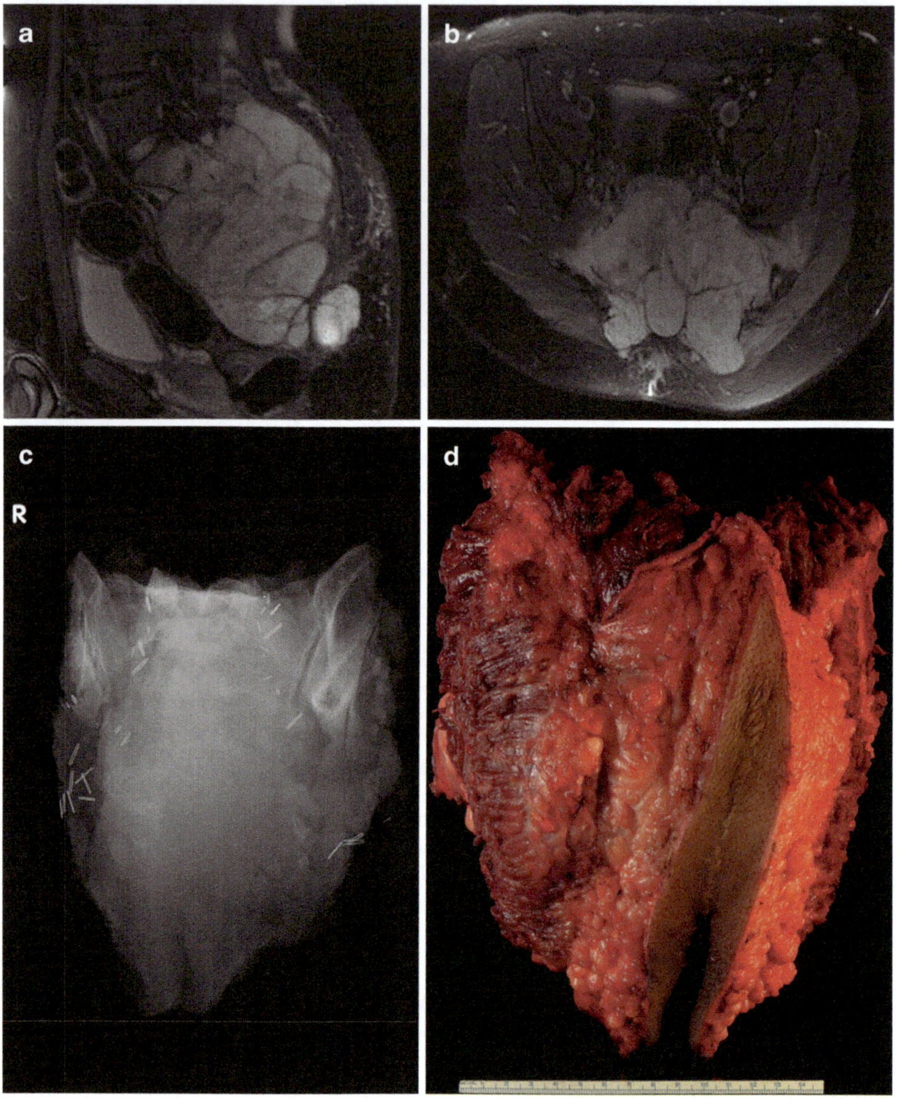


**Fig. 11.9** Case 2 (total sacrectomy for chordoma). (**a**) Sagittal and; (**b**) Axial T2 fat saturated images of locally advanced sacral chordoma. (**c**) Specimen radiograph. (**d**) Specimen gross photograph. (**e**) Use of transverse rectus abdominus flap for wound closure bulk over instrumentation. (**f**) Radiograph of spinopelvic reconstruction using bilateral vascularized fibula grafts. (**g**) CT demonstrating healed fibula graft reconstructions

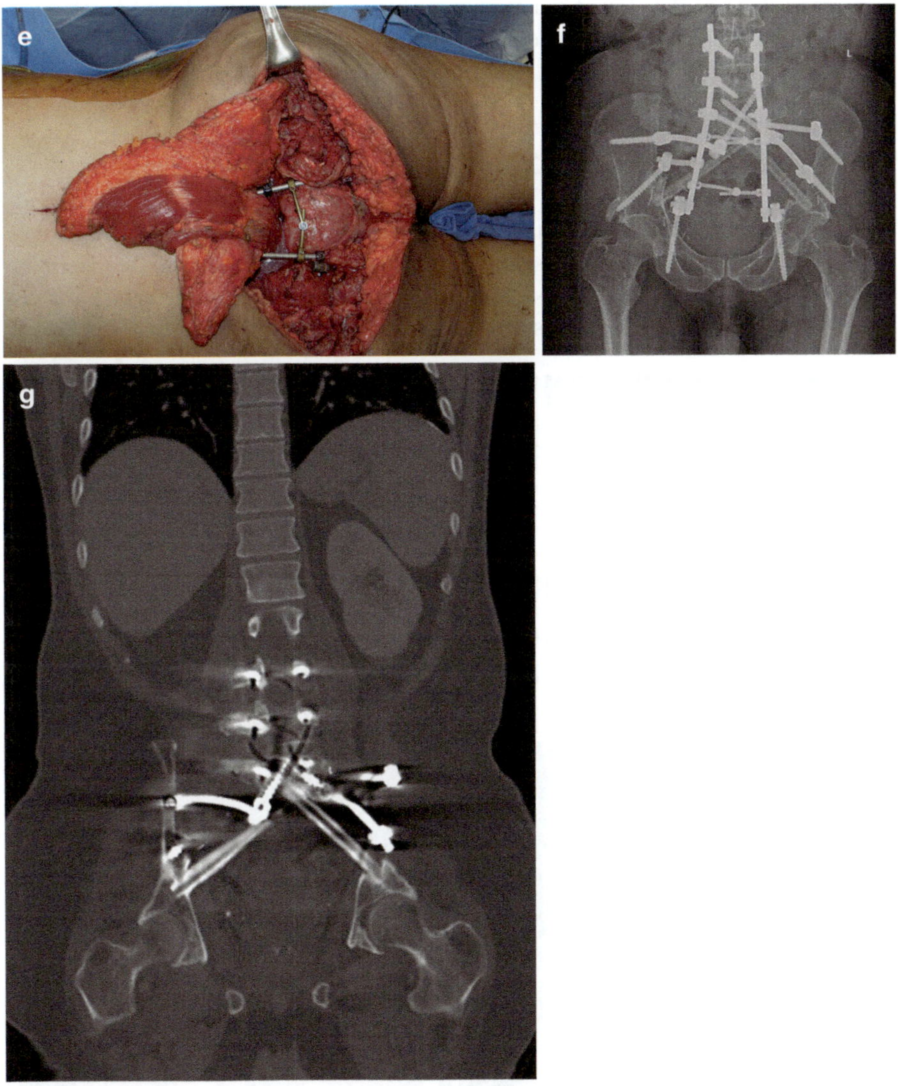


**Fig. 11.9** (continued)

metastasis and has developed radiation enteritis but has not developed local recurrence and has healed his bony reconstruction; he currently has no evidence of disease following pulmonary metastatectomy at 30 months postoperatively.

## **Case 3 – Locally Advanced Chordoma** (Fig. 11.10)

A 50-year-old man presented with obstipation and urinary retention and was diagnosed with a locally advanced sacral chordoma. While there was a concern for possible limited metastatic disease at presentation, he was felt to be at risk for visceral perforation and underwent surgical resection.

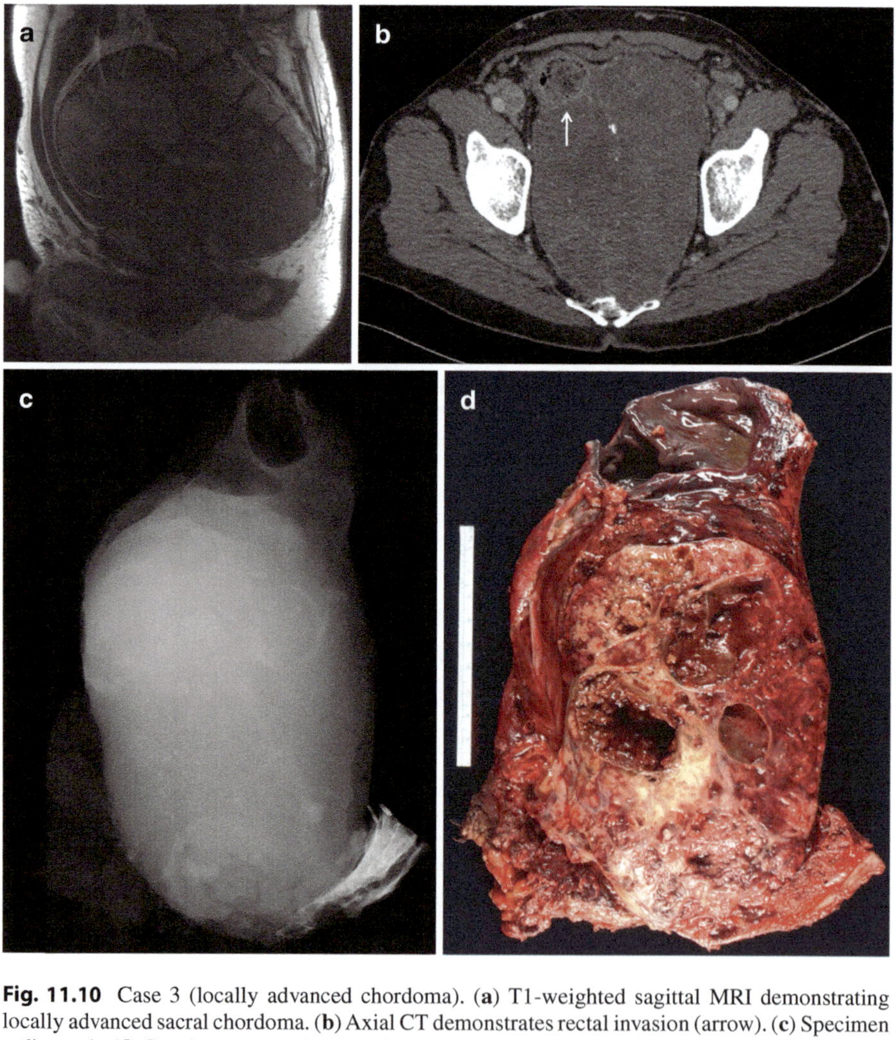


**Fig. 11.10** Case 3 (locally advanced chordoma). (**a**) T1-weighted sagittal MRI demonstrating locally advanced sacral chordoma. (**b**) Axial CT demonstrates rectal invasion (arrow). (**c**) Specimen radiograph. (**d**) Specimen gross photograph

While the bony involvement only extended to the S4 level, the anterior soft tissue extension was formidable (Fig. 11.10a). Additionally, tumor invaded the rectal wall (Fig. 11.10b). Because of the need to perform a colonic resection and the need for a large flap, the patient was approached initially in an anterior approach for colostomy and pre-sacral dissection. We were able to bluntly dissect between the tumor and the pre-sacral area to the S2/3 level. However, the tumor filled the pelvis and blocked dissection between the prostate and rectum from an anterior approach. Additionally, the bulk of tumor in the pelvis was too great to allow a VRAM flap to be tucked into the pelvis.

For this reason, the patient returned to the operating room 48 hours later. At that stage, a posterior approach was made with osteotomy of the sacrum at the S2/3 level to mobilize the specimen. The anus was excised with the specimen, and the plane between the rectum and prostate was developed from the posterior approach to free the specimen for final delivery. Once this was done, the patient was rolled into a lateral position to allow passage of a VRAM flap through the pelvis for wound closure.

The patient healed uneventfully but ultimately succumbed to hepatic metastases the following year.

## Conclusion

Surgical management of sacral chordomas consists of careful planning and execution to achieve a margin free en bloc tumor resection. Depending on the level of resection and tumor presentation, patients may benefit from an anterior/posterior approach or a single-stage posterior resection. Techniques of spinopelvic reconstruction have been developed for patients undergoing total or near total sacrectomies.

Unfortunately, complications in this practice are common, with wound dehiscence and infection being the most common surgical complications which are encountered. Preoperative radiotherapy is highly associated with an increase in wound and other complications without a clear oncologic benefit in patients undergoing surgical management. Patient outcomes center on neurologic function (a consequence of the level of tumor presentation) and recurrent disease. At present, a margin negative resection is the most proven treatment of sacral chordoma.

## References

1. Unni K, Inwards C. Chordoma. In: Dahlin's Bone Tumors. 6th ed. Philadelphia: Lippincott Williams and Wilkins; 2009.
2. Kaiser T, Pritchard D, Unni K. Clinicopathologic study of sacrococcygeal chordoma. Cancer. 1984;53:2574–8.
3. Angelini A, Pala E, Calabro T, Maraldi M, Ruggieri P. Prognostic factors in surgical resection of sacral chordoma. J Surg Oncol. 2015;112:344–51.
4. Fuchs B, Dickey ID, Yaszemski MJ, Inwards CY, Sim FH. Operative management of sacral chordoma. J Bone Joint Surg Am. 2005;87:2211–6.

5. Ruggieri P, Angelini A, Ussia G, Montalti M, Mercuri M. Surgical margins and local control in resection of sacral chordomas. Clin Orthop Relat Res. 2010;468:2939–47.
6. Sebro R, DeLaney TF, Hornicek F, Schwab J, Choy E, Nielsen GP, Rosenthal DI. Frequency and risk factors for additional lesions in the axial spine in subjects with chordoma: indications for screening. Spine. 2017;42:E37–40.
7. McCord D, Cunningham B, Shono Y, et al. Biomechanical analysis of lumbosacral fixation. Spine. 1992;17:S235–43.
8. Ucar D, UCar B, Coasr Y, et al. Retrospective cohort study of the prevalence of lumbosacral transitional vertebra in a wide and well-represented population. Arthritis. 2013;461425
9. Fidas A, MacDonald H, Elton R, et al. Prevalence and patterns of spina bifida occulta in 2707 normal adults. Clin Radiol. 1987;38:537–42.
10. Clarke MJ, Dasenbrook H, Bydon A, Sciubba DM, et al. Posterior-only approach for en bloc sacrectomy. Neurosurgery. 2012;71:357–64.
11. Brown MJ, Kor DJ, Curry TB, Warner MA, Rodrigues ES, Rose SH, Dekutoski MB, Moriarty JP, Long KH, Rose PS. Sacral tumor resection: the effect of surgical staging on patient outcomes, resource management, and hospital cost. Spine. 2011;26:1570–8.
12. Hata M, Kawahara N, Tomita K. Influence of ligation of the internal iliac veins on the venous plexuses around the sacrum. J Orthop Sci. 1998;3:264–71.
13. Sherman CE, Rose PS, Pierce LL, Yaszemski MJ, Sim FH. Prospective assessment of patient morbidity from prone sacral positioning. J Neurosurg Spine. 2012;16:51–6.
14. Asaad M, Rajesh A, Wahood W, et al. Flap reconstruction for sacrectomy defects: a systematic review and meta-analysis. J Plastic Reconstr Aesthet Surg. 2020;73:255–68.
15. Hugate RR Jr, Dickey ID, Phimolsarnti R, Yaszemski MJ, Sim FH. Mechanical effects of partial sacrectomy: when is reconstruction necessary? Clin Orthop Relat Res. 2006;450:82–8.
16. Dickey ID, Higate RR Jr, Fuchs B, Yaszemski MJ, Simg FH. Reconstruction after total sacrectomy: early experience with a new technique. Clin Orthop Relat Res. 2005;438:42–50.
17. Eck JC, Yaszemski MJ, Sim FH. Sacretomy and spinopelvic reconstruction. Semin Spine Surg. 2009;21:99–105.
18. Kelly B, Shen F, Schwab J, et al. Biomechanical testing of a novel four-rod technique for lumbopelvic reconstruction. Spine. 2008;33:E400–6.
19. Tang X, Yang R, Qu H, et al. Factors associated with spinopelvic fixation mechanical failure after total sacrectomy. Spine. 2018;43:1268–74.
20. Ackerman DB, Rose PS, Moran SL, Dekutoski MB, Bishop AT, Shin AY. The results of vascularized-free fibular grafts in complex spinal reconstruction. J Spinal Disord Tech. 2011;24:170–6.
21. Mericli A, Boukovalas S, Roubad M, et al. Restoration of spinopelvic continuity with the free fibula after limb-sparing oncologic resection is associated with a high union rate and superior functional outcomes. Plast Reconstr Surg. 2020;146:650–62.
22. Wei R, Guo W, Yang R, et al. Reconstruction of the pelvic ring after total en bloc sacrectomy using a 3D-printed sacral endoprosthesis with re-establishment of spinopelvic stability. Bone Joint J. 2019;101-B:880–8.
23. Gallia G, Haque R, Garonzik I, et al. Spinal-pelvic reconstruction after total sacrectomy for en bloc resection of a giant sacral chordoma: technical note. J Neurosurg Spine. 2005;3:501–6.
24. Macki M, De la Garza-Ramos R, Murgatroyd A, et al. Comprehensive biomechanical analysis of three reconstruction techniques following total sacrectomy: an in vitro human cadaveric model. JNS Spine. 2017;27:570–7.
25. Tomita K, Tsuchiya H. Total sacrectomy and reconstruction for huge sacral tumors. Spine. 1990;15:1223–7.
26. Zileli M, Hoscuskun C, Brastianos P, Sabah D. Surgical treatment of primary sacral tumors: complications associated with sacrectomy. Neurosurg Focus. 2003;15:1–8.
27. Loessin SJ, Meland NB, Devine RM, et al. Management of sacral and perineal defects following abdominoperineal resection and radiation with transpelvic muscle flaps. Dis Colon Rectum. 1995;38:940–5.

28. Glatt BS, Disa JJ, Mehrara BJ, et al. Reconstruction of extensive partial or total sacrectomy defects with a transabdominal vertical rectus abdominus myocutaneous flap. Ann Plast Surg. 2006;56:526–31.
29. Houdek M, Rose P, Hevesi M, et al. Low dose radiotherapy is associated with local complications but not disease control in sacral chordoma. J Surg Oncol. 2019;119:856–63.
30. Houdek M, Wellings E, Moran S, et al. Outcome of sacropelvic resection and reconstruction based on a novel classification system. J Bone Joint Surg Am. 2020;102(22):1956–65.
31. Bredella O, Hess K, Janssen S, et al. Sacral insufficiency fractures are common after high-dose radiation for sacral chordomas treated with or without surgery. Clin Orthope Relat Res. 2015;474:766–72.
32. Gunterberg B, Kewenter J, Petersen I, Stener B. Anorectal function after major resections of the sacrum with bilateral or unilateral sacrifice of sacral nerves. Br J Surg. 1976;63:546–54.
33. Gunterberg B, Norlen L, Stener B, Sundin T. Neurologic evaluation after resection of the sacrum. Investig Urol. 1975;13:183–8.
34. Todd LT Jr, Yaszemski MJ, Currier BL, Fuchs B, Kim CW, Sim FH. Bowel and bladder function after major sacral resection. Clin Orthop Relat Red. 2002;397:36–9.
35. Van Wulfften Palthe OD, Houdek MT, Rose PS, Yaszemski MJ, Sim FH, Boland PJ, Healey JH, Hornicek FJ, Schwab JH. How does the level of nerve root resection in en bloc sacrectomy influence patient-reported outcomes? Clin Orthop Relat Res. 2017;475:607–16.
36. Houdek M, Hevesi M, Schwab J, et al. Association between patient age and the risk of mortality following local recurrence of sacral chordoma. J Surg Oncol. 2019; epub ahead of print.

# Soft Tissue Reconstruction Following Surgery for Sacral Chordoma

# 12

Rachel Skladman, Zach Pennington, and Justin M. Sacks

## Abbreviations

| | |
|---|---|
| GM | Gluteus maximus |
| HADM | Human acellular dermal matrix |
| IOBL | Intraoperative blood loss |
| LD | Latissimus dorsi |
| VRAM | Vertical rectus abdominis muscle |

## Introduction

As en bloc resection of mobile spine [1] and sacral chordoma [2] has been demonstrated to improve local tumor control, most experts consider standard of care to be R0 resection, often accompanied by neoadjuvant or adjuvant radiotherapy [3]. The propensity of these lesions to be locally invasive [4, 5] means that such resection generally requires resection of a cuff of the healthy surrounding tissue. Consequently, oncologic resection of these lesions commonly produces large soft tissue defects that must be repaired to prevent wound breakdown and infection. This is especially important for sacral lesions, which often have profound soft tissue defects, given the

R. Skladman · J. M. Sacks (✉)
Division of Plastic and Reconstructive Surgery, Washington University in St. Louis School of Medicine, St. Louis, MO, USA
e-mail: jmsacks@wustl.edu

Z. Pennington
Department of Neurosurgery, Johns Hopkins University School of Medicine, Baltimore, MD, USA



D. M. Sciubba, J. H. Schwab (eds.), *Chordoma of the Spine*,
https://doi.org/10.1007/978-3-030-76201-8_12

proclivity of these indolent tumors to involve the gluteal muscles, presacral space, the sacral nerve roots, and even the sacroiliac joints.

Reconstruction therefore focuses on two key issues: (1) filling the soft tissue defect and (2) correcting the instability created by bony resection. As discussed in depth in Chap. 11, for sacral lesions, bony reconstruction is recommended for osteotomies made above the S1/2 junction [6]. Failure to restore the stability of the bony pelvis ultimately limits weightbearing and the ability to ambulate postoperatively [7]. Soft tissue reconstruction is required for all sacrectomy specimens though. The means of achieving correction is ultimately dictated by the size of the defect, the availability of local flap material, and the radiation history of the patient. In this chapter, we describe soft tissue reconstruction strategies following en bloc resection of chordoma, focusing specifically on sacral lesions. Additionally, we present a management algorithm employed by the senior author when selecting donor flaps and an approach for soft-tissue reconstruction.

## Previous Descriptions of Reconstructive Surgery Following En Bloc Spondylectomy and Sacrectomy

The goal of reconstructive surgery following sacrectomy is to restore the spinopelvic biomechanical stability necessary for physiologic loadbearing while sitting and standing (see Chap. 11) and to eliminate dead space that would preclude effective wound healing. Effective reconstruction may reduce the risk of wound breakdown and prolonged drainage, as well as prevent instrument-related pressure necrosis [8].

Several series have demonstrated that patients without spinopelvic reconstruction suffer higher rates of wound complications and reoperation than do those who undergo soft tissue reconstruction [9]. One notable series was published by Chang et al. In their series of 92 patients who underwent soft tissue reconstruction following spine tumor removal, the authors found those who underwent immediate, prophylactic soft tissue reconstruction had significantly lower odds of developing major complications requiring reoperation [10]. This benefit of prophylactic soft tissue reconstruction appeared greatest for those who underwent spinal instrumentation [10]. Additionally, in those requiring reoperation, debridement, and coverage with well-perfused soft tissue appeared to improve wound healing and maintain stability of the instrumentation [10].

The use of soft tissue reconstruction is especially important in patients who have undergone previous chemotherapy, radiation therapy, and prior surgery—all factors that independently increase the risk for wound healing complications. It may also be beneficial for those with poor preoperative nutritional status. In these patients, prior irradiation or manipulation of the soft tissues is associated with damage to the local microvasculature, which impairs wound healing potential. Transferring well-vascularized, nonirradiated tissue into the defect then provides protection of neural elements and coverage for instrumentation, well also providing a healthy vascular supply to promote wound healing [10]. When flaps are transferred into an irradiated field, the transferred tissue with its own blood supply provides a scaffold for neovascularization of the irradiated field. The healthy muscle transferred into the irradiated field thereby induces wound healing and decreases complications [11]. Furthermore, the transferred muscle obliterates the dead space created by sacral resection [7]. Dead space allows for local hematoma formation, which can become a secondary nidus for infection and chronic, nonhealing wounds. Consequently, failure to successfully eliminate dead space predisposes the patient to wound breakdown and infection [12].

Elimination of dead space with well-vascularized soft tissue has additionally been associated with lower rates of wound dehiscence, earlier pain-free mobilization, reduced length of hospital stay, and improved bone healing [9]. Support for this is provided by a systematic review by Reynolds et al., who analyzed 116 sacrectomy patients, of whom 92 underwent spinopelvic reconstruction. Rates of wound dehiscence (67% vs 23%) and reoperation were much higher in the group that did not undergo reconstruction. Additionally, the type of reconstruction appeared to influence outcomes, as reoperation rates were highest for those with no reconstruction (39%), intermediate (20%) for those with a local flap reconstruction (e.g., gluteus maximus, paraspinal), and lowest (0%) for those with a regional flap reconstruction (vertical rectus abdominis muscle) [9]. Similarly, mean length of stay was highest for those with no reconstruction and lowest for those with regional flap reconstruction, likely due to the lower complication and reoperation rates seen in patients who had reconstruction [9].

In this same review, the authors found that bony spinopelvic reconstruction was also associated with superior postoperative ambulatory outcomes. All patients with soft tissue reconstruction could walk, compared to only 88% of those with flap reconstruction. Of the ambulatory patients who had not received soft tissue reconstruction, only 26% were independently ambulatory [9]. While data is limited, when all stabilizers are sacrificed and subsequent reconstruction is not undertaken, patients are either bed or chair bound [13]. Thus for patients who have undergone total sacrectomy with complete sacrifice of iliolumbar ligamentous stability, experts strongly recommend spinopelvic reconstruction [9]. Thus to decrease length of stay, improve pain outcomes, and increase the likelihood of unassisted ambulation, experts recommend soft tissue coverage or spinopelvic reconstruction at the time of total en bloc sacrectomy [9, 10].

## Soft Tissue Reconstruction

Currently most experts recommend soft tissue reconstruction for spinopelvic defects following sacral resection. Soft tissue reconstruction has been found to decrease reoperation rates, wound dehiscence, and the length of hospital stay [7, 9]. Soft tissue reconstruction is the method of choice to eliminate dead space and reduce wound dehiscence by creating a barrier between the peritoneal space and the vertebral space. This prevents perineal herniation—a rare but major complication of pelvic diaphragm obliteration [7, 14, 15]. Dead space obliteration also reduces the risk of wound site hematoma, seroma, infection, fistula formation, and bowel obstruction [15]. Soft tissue reconstruction also helps decrease tension on the wound, which in turn reduces the risk of wound dehiscence. The donor, nonradiated, vascularized tissue additionally improves bone and soft tissue clearance, induces neovascularization, and protects against infection [8, 9, 11, 15–17]. There are several soft tissue reconstruction options: pedicled vertical rectus abdominis myocutaneous (VRAM) flap, gluteus-based flaps, posterior thigh flaps, paraspinous muscle flaps, and latissimus dorsi free flaps, and combinations of these methods. Each of these options will be discussed below.

## Vertical Rectus Abdominis Myocutaneous (VRAM) Flap

The gold standard for soft tissue reconstruction employs an inferiorly based, pedicled VRAM flap based on the deep inferior epigastric artery and vein [15]. The use of such a flap was first described by Mathes and Bostwick, who reported the use of a rectus abdominis muscle flap to reconstruct an abdominal wall defect in 1977. They found that the flap is dually vascularized by the superior epigastric artery and inferior epigastric artery. Importantly, the flap possesses numerous perforators that provide ample blood supply to the muscle and skin. Because of its dual vascularization, this myocutaneous flap can be based on the superior or deep inferior epigastric artery successfully [18].

Shukla and Hughes were the first to describe the use of an inferiorly based VRAM flap to close large perineal and pelvic defects [19]. The skin flap is raised in continuity with the anterior rectus sheath and rectus muscle. The rectus muscle is mobilized within the sheath. The deep inferior epigastric vessels are preserved, and the superior epigastric vessels are ligated. The rectus abdominis myocutaneous unit is passed through the perineum, into the pelvis. Such an application is directly applicable to soft tissue reconstruction post-sacrectomy. In the latter situation, advantages of the VRAM flap include ease of access following an anterior approach or direct transpelvic approach for sacrectomy; the presence of a reliable vascular pedicle; the availability of a large volume of vascularized muscle for filling extensive soft tissue defects; the presence of well-vascularized skin used for primary wound healing; and the ability to perform the reconstruction without an operating microscope [7, 8, 11, 17, 19, 20].

### Technique: Isolated VRAM Flap

The technique employed for staged cases can be broken down into flap harvest (anterior stage) and flap installation (posterior stage). During the anterior stage, a skin paddle is designed from the umbilicus to the xiphoid; the flap is based on the deep inferior epigastric vessels. The flap is designed such that the abdomen can be closed primarily and the anterior rectus fascia is preserved below the arcuate line for this repair. The insertion of the rectus muscle is maintained at the pubic ramus to prevent twisting of the vascular pedicle [12, 16]. After the flap is designed, the anterior aspect of the oncologic operation is performed. An anterior intraperitoneal approach is taken to expose the ventral aspect of the tumor, mobilize the rectum, and ligate the internal iliac arteries. The pedicled VRAM flap is then placed in the pelvis for pull-through during the second stage. We do not divide the insertion of the rectus abdominis muscle from the pubic ramus since we believe leaving the insertion avoids inadvertent twisting of the pedicle during transpelvic delivery of the pedicled VRAM flap into the sacrectomy wound. We perform a unilateral component separation to minimize tension on the closure. We advocate the use of a prosthetic mesh to reinforce the pedicled VRAM donor site, as necessary [16]. During the second stage, the entire sacrum is resected from a posterior approach, and the VRAM flap is passed retroperitoneally to recreate the pelvic diaphragm. We advocate placing a portion of the flap posteriorly to the rectum to prevent herniation [15]. The skin paddle is sufficient for primary closure over the sacral defect (Fig. 12.1a–d) [15].

## Pairing with Pedicled Fibular Free Flap

The VRAM flap can also be paired with vascularized bone graft reconstruction techniques, such as the free fibular transfer (see Chaps. 11 and 13), which often requires the use of additional soft tissue flaps [14, 20]. The senior author of this chapter has previously described the pairing of a VRAM flow-through flap anastomosed to a free fibula flap in three patients who underwent total sacrectomy followed by instrumented fusion and soft tissue reconstruction (Fig. 12.2a–g) [16]. In this technique, a staged anterior-posterior approach is employed, with the VRAM harvested in a

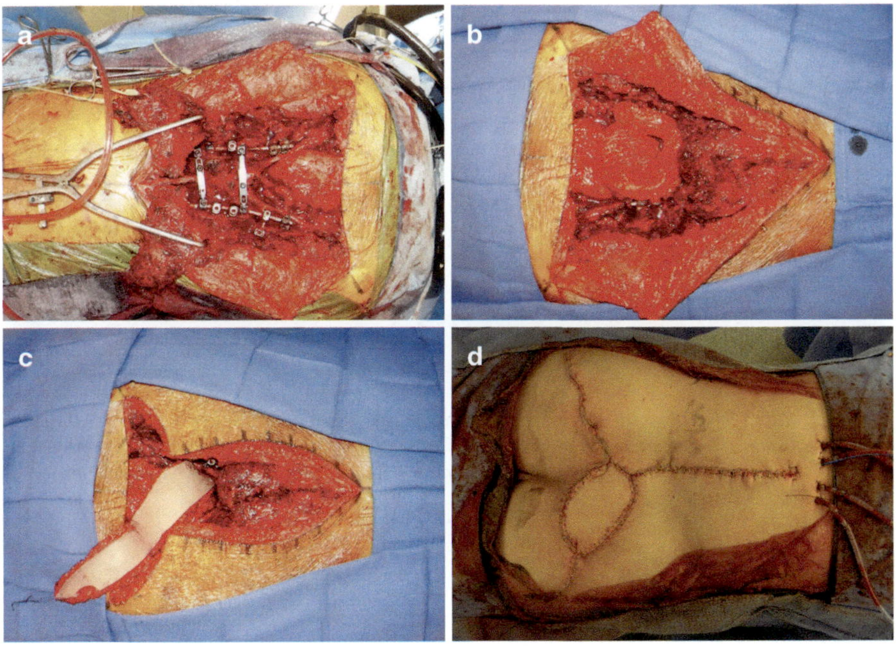


**Fig. 12.1** (**a**) Posterior approach, mobilization of sacral chordoma. (**b**) Posterior sacral defect, post en bloc sacrectomy. (**c**) Transpelvic vertical rectus abdominis myocutaneous (VRAM) flap. (**d**) Closure, VRAM, and local tissue rearrangement

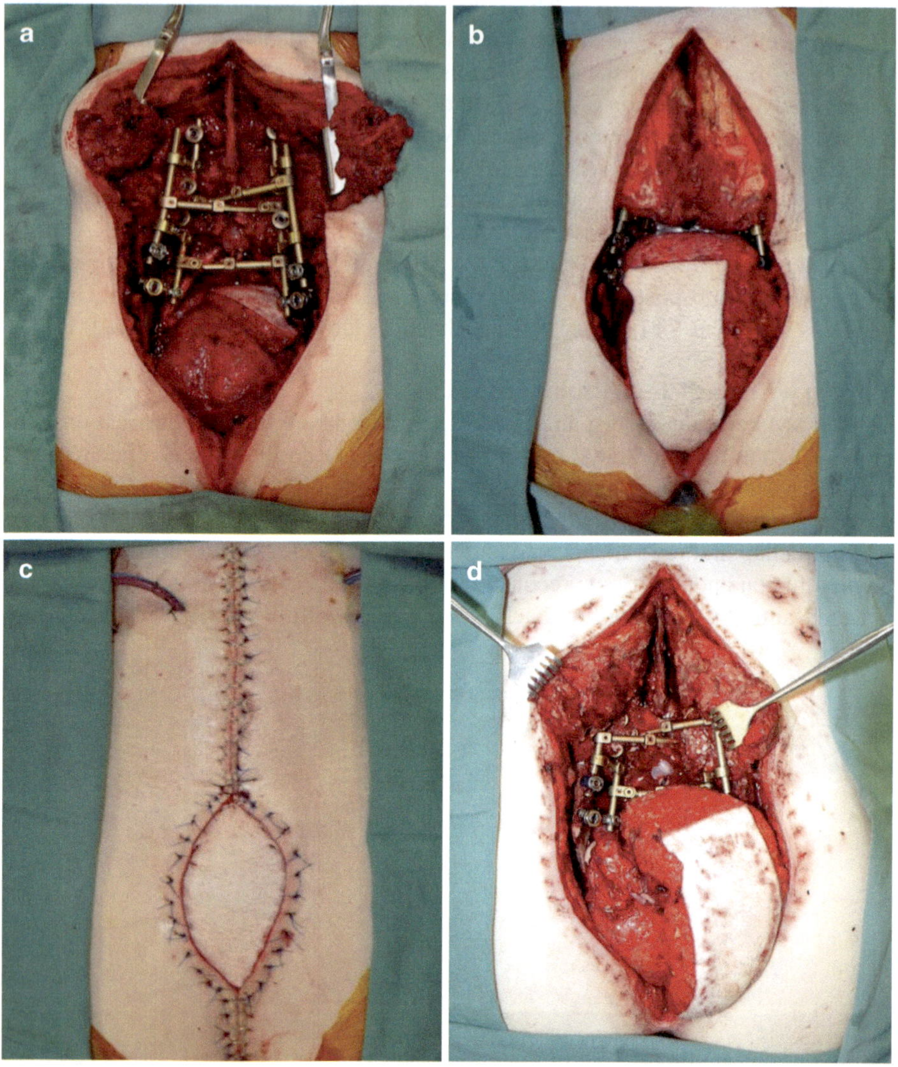


**Fig. 12.2** (**a**–**c**) VRAM, multistage approach, temporary inset of transpelvic VRAM. (**d**) Third stage illustrating anastomosis of peroneal vessels to deep inferior epigastric artery (DIEA) system. (**e**) Final flap construction. (**f**) Posterior incision at 3-month follow-up. (**g**) Anterior incision at 3-month follow-up

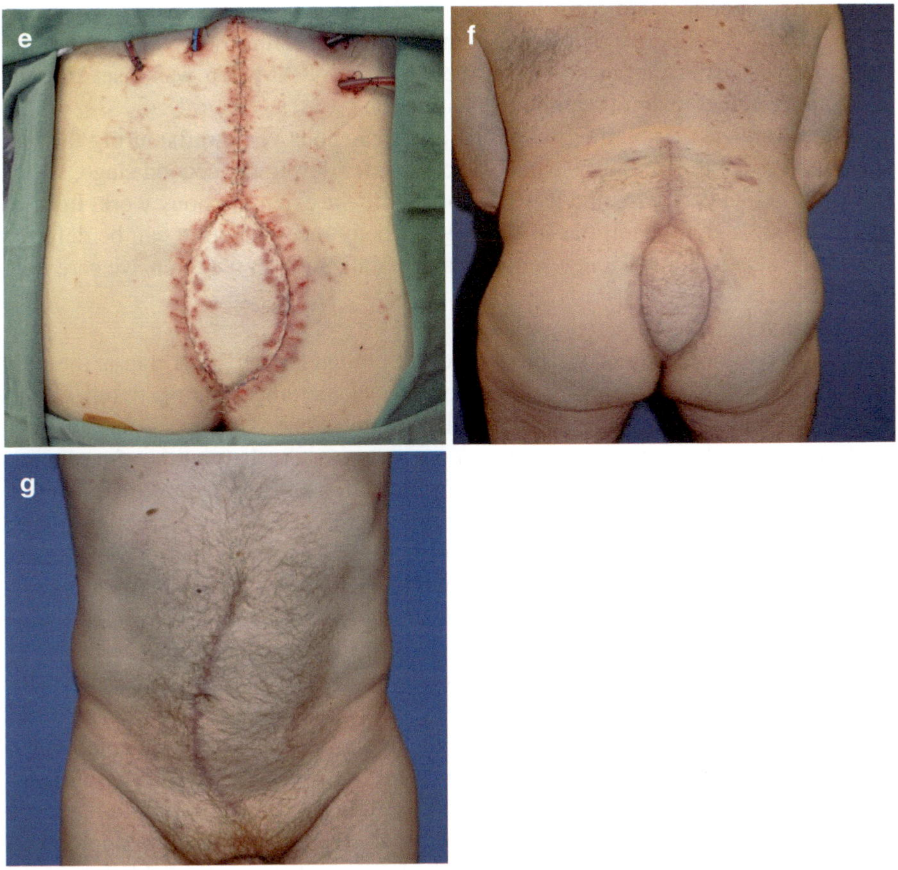


**Fig. 12.2** (continued)

manner as described previously. During the anterior stage, the plastic surgeons can isolate the prospective fibular graft in preparation for the second stage, the peroneal vessels just be left in continuity to keep the graft vascularized until transfer during the second stage. A length of saphenous vein below the knee is also isolated to serve as an interposition venous graft during the second stage. During this second, posterior stage, the fibular flap is harvested and installed ipsilateral to the pedicled VRAM flap. Installation in this orientation allows for optimal apposition of the donor VRAM vessels and recipient fibula flap pedicle. When harvesting the fibular flap, the peroneal vessels are left to serve as arterial recipients. During fibula harvest, the plastic surgeon creates an osteotomy in the middle of the free fibula to facilitate its placement between the body of the L5 vertebra and the ilia. Lag screws are used to affix the graft to the ilia above the sciatic notches. The distal branches of the deep inferior epigastric artery (DIEA) are dissected from the rectus abdominis muscle of the pedicled VRAM for microsvascular anastomosis with the peroneal artery. Where size and length discrepancies between the donor DIEA and recipient peroneal arteries exist, the isolated 3 cm segment of saphenous vein is extracted to serve as an interposition vein graft. The venae comitantes are anastomosed with venous coupling devices. After the anastomosis, the pedicled VRAM flap was inset into the sacrectomy defect to complete the reconstruction.

The advantage of isolating the fibular and saphenous vein grafts during the first stage is to make them readily available for transfer during the second stage, which is usually associated with high IOBL secondary to the extensive bony work. In cases where IOBL is significant, the soft tissue and bony reconstruction can be deferred to a third stage to allow for resuscitation and stabilization in the intensive care unit.

## Outcomes

In spite of the morbidity of the procedure, we contend the VRAM flap is the gold standard for soft tissue reconstruction after total sacrectomy. Relative to other operations, we find it to have a superior ability to obliterate dead space defects with well-vascularized soft tissue. It can also prevent posterior herniation of peritoneal contents. These advantages are probably greatest for patients with previous radiation that has damaged the gluteal vessels used for local flap reconstruction. Based on their series of 25 patients undergoing soft tissue reconstruction after total sacrectomy, Miles et al. concluded that a transpelvic VRAM flap is the ideal reconstructive option in this population [21]. However, the authors also argued that certain patient populations are poor candidates for VRAM flap reconstruction, specifically those with a history of laparotomy or ostomy. Based upon the experience of the senior author though, it is argued that prior abdominal surgery is not an absolute contraindication. We believe certain midline abdominal incisions may be compatible with VRAM flap use and recommend the use of preoperative CT angiography, which can visualize flap vascularity and the anatomy of the perforators to the skin paddle [15, 21]. Preoperative CTA also allows for preoperative recognition of abnormal DIEA anatomy and selection of the DIEA system most suitable for microvascular anastomosis.

The senior author has previously reported on VRAM flap usage for soft tissue reconstruction following total en bloc sacrectomy with lumbopelvic fixation [15]. In that series of nine patients, all had tumor involvement of the S2 and S3 levels with cephalad extension to or beyond the level of S1. Six patients underwent single-stage, posterior-only total en bloc sacrectomy with gluteal muscle flap closure (see *next section*), while three underwent multistage anterior-posterior approaches with VRAM flap reconstruction. Surgery was accomplished in two stages for two patients and in three stages for one patient who experienced intraoperative instability. One patient developed a pelvic hematoma during the anterior procedure which led to compression and venous congestion, so the VRAM flap was discarded. Reconstruction was performed with bilateral paraspinous muscle flap advancement, latissimus dorsi (LD) pedicled flap, and bilateral gluteus maximus muscle flaps (described in subsequent sections) [15]. In the series of three patients, the mean intraoperative blood loss (IOBL) for the multistage procedures was 7500 mL. However, neither patient who received a VRAM experienced postoperative wound complications, seroma, or hematoma by last follow-up [15]. No complications at the harvest site were observed; however, major complications were noted secondary to the extensive IOBL and hemodynamic instability. While the majority of blood loss occurred due to the prolonged tumor excision, it should be noted that the VRAM flap is associated with more numerous surgeries, longer operative times, and higher IOBL [15].

Another series reporting on the use of VRAM flap for post-sacrectomy soft tissue reconstruction was published by Glatt et al. [20]. VRAM reconstruction was performed either in one or two stages. Single-stage reconstruction performed VRAM flap reconstruction immediately following the extirpative procedure. In the two stage approaches, the technique was similar to that described above. Of the 12 patients, 3 suffered minor early flap complications, consisting of small areas of necrosis at the distal, superior portion of the flap. No late flap complications occurred, and all 12 completely healed by 20-month follow-up, even those having undergone prior abdominal surgery.

More recently, Garvey et al. reviewed their experience of 50 patients treated over 15 years. They found no difference in complication rates between patients treated with VRAM flaps and those treated with local gluteal muscle flaps. However, they noted that relative to those treated with local flap closure, patients who underwent VRAM reconstruction were more likely to have undergone preoperative radiation therapy and had larger defect volumes [22]. The authors did note a correlation between larger-volume defects and worse functional outcomes, including increased length of hospitalization, poorer likelihood of independent postoperative ambulation, higher likelihood of bowel and bladder incontinence, and worse oncologic prognosis [21]. As a result, any beneficial effect of VRAM flap closure was likely masked by the fact that it was employed in higher-risk patients. Consequently, we contend that more invasive, higher tissue volume flaps, such as the VRAM flap, may be advantageous for more radical resection defects. Other authors have made similar arguments, citing the advantages of the VRAM flap's arc of rotation, low morbidity, favorable complication rate, technical feasibility, and high success—especially for the reconstruction of large defects in an irradiated field [12, 15, 20–22]. For those with especially large defects, gluteal advancement flaps, omentum, or paraspinous flaps can be used to supplement the VRAM flap.

The senior author has also had good experience with the concomitant VRAM, pedicled fibular free flap technique [16]. In a series of three patients treated using this technique following total sacrectomy, no patients experienced postoperative wound complications, and all experienced bony union at a mean of $2.7 \pm 0.6$ months. The average length of hospitalization for the cohort was 79 days. By the time of discharge, all patient were ambulatory with the assistance of a walker, and all achieved independent ambulation by last follow-up. During the first 4 postoperative weeks, patients were maintained on an air-fluidized mattress in a non-weight-bearing state. Hip flexion and sitting were avoided for 2 months postoperatively.

## Local Flaps: Gluteus Muscle and Paraspinal Flaps

Partial sacrectomies (defined by a cranial osteotomy below S2) can feasibly be treated by a posterior-only approach. Accordingly, they do not require VRAM flap reconstruction; additionally, the sacral defect may be too small to allow for safe pass-through of the VRAM flap. For these partial sacrectomies, local flaps, such as gluteus maximus or posterior thigh flaps (Fig. 12.3a–c), or paraspinal muscle flaps may be used. Posterior-only approaches using these local flaps are advantageous relative to staged approaches as they avoid a laparotomy and reduce total operative time [23].

Paraspinous flaps are the easiest flaps to harvest, but are able to fill significantly lower-volume defects than VRAM or other flap types [22]. Gluteal flaps offer an intermediate level of coverage and have been recommended for reconstruction of partial or sacrectomy defects [22]. These flaps receive robust blood supply from the hypogastric, superior gluteal, and inferior gluteal arteries [15]. As such, they can be used in a variety of configurations to close sacrectomy defects, including rotation flaps, V-Y advancement flaps, and turnover or sliding flaps. Small defects can be covered with a gluteus muscle turnover or advancement flap; for moderate-volume defects, unilateral or bilateral gluteal rotation flaps may be employed [22]. It is also possible to use a superior gluteal artery perforator flap. The advantage of this flap is that it causes a lesser degree of damage to the gluteus maximus muscle which translates into less morbidity related to ambulation, less postoperative pain, and quicker functional recovery [22].

One point of debate surrounding the use of gluteal-based flaps is whether they are safe in patients who have been previously irradiated. Based on prior experiences [22], we contend that they are a reasonable option in this patient population if a superior or inferior gluteal artery remains intact. If all the gluteal vessels have been sacrificed, then it is possible to reconstruct smaller-sized defects using unilateral or bilateral sliding V-Y gluteus advancement flaps. These flaps receive perfusion from the medial circumflex and first perforating femoral arteries [22]. However, if a larger defect must be closed and both the superior and inferior gluteal arteries have been obliterated, it is appropriate to use a gluteal thigh flap may be a reasonable option [22]. The reverse turnover LD muscle flap can be also used with split thickness skin grafts to reconstruct lumbosacral defects when the gluteal vessels have been damaged or local muscles are insufficient to cover the damage [15]. An inferior gluteal artery-based gluteal thigh flap may also be used for large defects that are not amenable to VRAM reconstruction [22].

## Previous Experiences

Miles and colleagues at MD Anderson Cancer Center previously described the successful use of bilateral gluteal myocutaneous V-Y advancement flaps to repair large sacral defects [21]. The authors argued that such an approach is only reasonable where the bilateral superior and inferior gluteal vessels are intact, in order to provide complete vascularization of the gluteal flap. Additionally, they recommend the flap be contoured along the direction of the gluteal muscles, taking care to design the flap so that the upper and lower flap limbs are longer than the medial/midline limb. This helps to facilitate a tension-free closure.

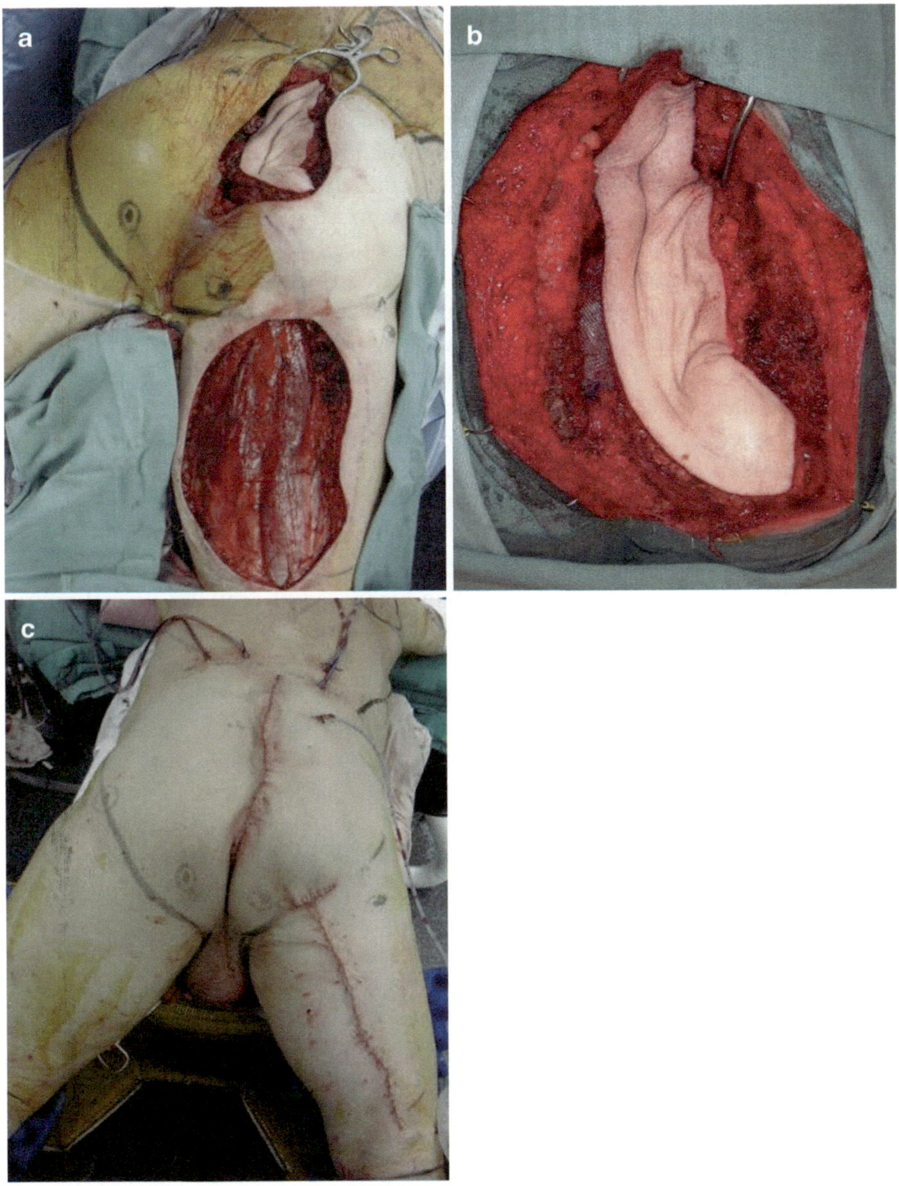


**Fig. 12.3** (**a**) Posterior thigh flap for en bloc sacrectomy reconstruction. (**b**) Posterior thigh flap. (**c**) Primary closure of defect and donor site

A subsequent series from Johns Hopkins described using a combination of human acellular dermal matrix (HADM) and GM flaps in a series of 34 patients who underwent posterior en bloc sacrectomy [23]. The HADM was used to recreate a pelvic diaphragm and to serve as a retaining wall that would prevent herniation of the rectosigmoid colon through the posterior wound opening [23]. The design of the GM flaps was based upon the extent of gluteal muscle resection. Where the superior gluteal artery was patent, the GM pedicle was based on this vessel. However, in cases where the superior gluteal artery was sacrificed with the sample or had been destroyed by prior radiation, an inferiorly pedicled GM flap was advanced into the defect. In both techniques, the gluteal muscles were freed from their origin along the posterior iliac crest, elevated, and positioned midline over the HADM placed in the sacrectomy defect. Skin flaps were then mobilized and closed in tension-free manner over the muscle flaps. Of the 34 patients, 20.6% experienced postoperative wound dehiscence, and 14.7% required operative debridement. Subsequently, 38.2% of patients underwent postoperative adjuvant radiation. Despite this, none of the patients experienced late-onset wound dehiscence [23].

In a subsequent series of nine patients from the same institution who underwent total sacrectomy, complex closure was accomplished in six using bilateral gluteus maximus flaps and a prosthetic rectal sling composed of acellular dermal matrix [15]. Four of these patients required additional mobilization of bilateral paraspinal muscle flaps or pedicled latissimus dorsi (LD) fasciocutaneous flaps [15]. For one patient initially treated with a VRAM flap reconstruction, a reoperation was required in which the residual defect was closed with a combination of bilateral paraspinal muscle advancement, pedicled LD flaps based on posterior intercostal perforators, and bilateral GM flaps. In line with this, for single-stage posterior approaches, we advocate for GM flap closure as the first choice to obliterate the dead space. If additional soft tissue bulk is needed, paraspinal muscle and LD flaps can be mobilized [15].

## Biological Matrix Use

There is ongoing debate regarding the use of biological matrices in oncologic spine surgery. Despite the positive results described above, the evidence for their use is mixed. Proposed benefits of biological matrices include protection of the flap from increases in intra-abdominal pressure; prevention of abdominal content herniation through the sacral defect; promotion of local tissue growth, angiogenesis, and cellular migration; creation of a bridge between the intra-abdominal contents and external hardware; and reconstruction of the posterior abdominal wall [23, 24]. However, work by our own group suggests that HADM use may be associated with increased complications. We examined 293 spine oncology surgeries on 260 unique patients in which plastic surgery was recruited for wound closure. We found patients receiving a biological matrix in their closure had an increased odds of postoperative wound complications in. Notably, patients undergoing closures with biological matrices were found to have higher rates of infection and seroma formation [25]. In spite of these higher wound complication rates, the rates of reoperation for wound revision or removal of infected hardware did not differ significantly between the groups [25]. The reason for this discrepancy is unclear, but it may be that more complicated defects required the use of biological matrices. Regardless, there appears to be no clear correlation of biological matrix use and wound complications. Therefore, the senior author advocates for the decision of whether to use an acellular dermal matrix during closure should be made on an individual patient basis.

## Latissimus Dorsi Free Flap

A third option for sacral defect reconstruction is the latissimus dorsi (LD) free flap. This option is generally employed in cases where both inferior gluteal arteries have been sacrificed and no other options for local or reginal flaps exist. One of the difficulties with employing the LD flap stems from the fact that recipient vessels for free tissue transfer are not readily accessible in the lumbosacral region. Consequently, a vein graft from distant perfusion sources must be harvested for anastomosis, which increases the chance for anastomotic thrombosis.

Several authors have noted poor outcomes following free tissue flap to the lumbosacral region, with complication rates up to 50% [22]. Therefore, we recommend free flap reconstruction only as a last resort, in cases where a regional or local flap is unavailable, such as in patients whose superior and inferior gluteal arteries have been damaged by radiation, surgery, or prior embolization. In general, when patients require a posterior flap reconstruction and GM or posterior thigh flaps are unavailable, we advocate for LD flaps pedicled on the posterior intercostal perforators [15, 16]. However, if a free flap is necessary, then we employ an LD flap anastomosed to the femoral, thoracodorsal, or iliac vessels which may be necessary [15, 21]. Anastomosis to these vessels requires long vein grafts though.

## Other Flap Types

One of the drivers that has led plastic surgeons to seek alternatives to the gluteal flaps is the potential functional limitations posed by such flaps. Several authors have noted that using gluteus maximus local rotation flaps may result in significant functional deficits when running, jogging, climbing stairs, or even walking [21, 26]. Furthermore, gluteal rotation flap reconstructions appear to have a higher incidence of partial loss and nonhealing wounds—particularly in the setting of preoperative radiation [21]. They may also be insufficient to obliterate large dead space defects. One series of nine patients treated for sacral malignancies at the University of Miami found local GM flaps to be insufficient to obliterate dead space in six patients. In these patients, a polyglactin 910 mesh and an omental flap based on the gastroepiploic vessels were required to completely obliterate the defect and prevent herniation of abdominal contents into the wound [26]. Advantages of this omental flap include its large size (mean area of 400 $cm^2$), thorough vascularization, antibacterial properties, and ability to absorb fluid from the tissue defect. Additionally in those requiring postoperative radiation, it may decrease enteritis and enteropathy [26].

However, harvesting the omental flap requires an anterior approach with its associated risk of wound-site seroma, wound infection, chyle leak, ileus, intra-abdominal abscess, and ventral hernia which should be assessed [15, 26]. We feel that these associated risks are disproportionate to the potential benefits and consequently advocate against the use of this flap type.

## Complications

En bloc sacrectomy and subsequent soft tissue reconstruction is a complicated, frequently multistage intervention. Complications include wound dehiscence, seroma, deep wound infection, distant infection, sepsis, sacral stress fracture, hernia, deep vein thrombosis, flap failure, and total flap loss. The rates of these complications vary, but reports place the occurrence of one or more postoperative complication in the range of 40–89% [8, 12, 15, 21, 22]. Risk factors associated with complications include vacuum-assisted closure, use of adjuvant radiotherapy, previous chemotherapy, and colostomy [15]. Wound-related complications are more prevalent among patients who have undergone prior radiation [22]. This is likely due to fibrosis of the irradiated tissue with accordant obliteration of the local tissue vasculature, which is essential for wound healing.

In the senior author's experience, 1/3 of patients with prior radiotherapy and 1/2 of patients with prior chemotherapy experience wound dehiscence [15]. Patients who undergo more extensive resections are additionally more likely to suffer postoperative complications, including unplanned reoperation. They also generally suffer poorer functional outcomes, including worse ambulatory function and higher rates of bowel and bladder incontinence [22, 27]. Other risk factors for postoperative wound complication include a history of diabetes mellitus, prior tobacco use, obesity, hypertension, hyperlipidemia, malnutrition (as assessed by a serum albumin <3.5 g/dL), and prior surgery [15, 20]. Though some of these factors are fixed, others (blood pressure, blood sugar levels) are modifiable and may be optimized in the preoperative setting to help optimize patient outcomes.

## Conclusion

The selection of a soft tissue reconstruction strategy following sacrectomy is not a strict science; however, donor tissue selection is dictated by the health of the locoregional vasculature, the surgical approach, and the post-resection defect. Our previously described surgical algorithm is presented in Fig. 12.4 [15]. Briefly, for those undergoing multistage anterior-posterior approaches, we advocate for the use of pedicled VRAM flap. This flap is well-vascularized, allows for a tension-free closure, and is able to obliterate the large dead space left by total sacrectomy. The VRAM also provides a skin paddle for primary closure that can be used for flap monitoring and does not require microvascular techniques. Even in the case of previous abdominal surgery, we believe the superior functional outcomes and

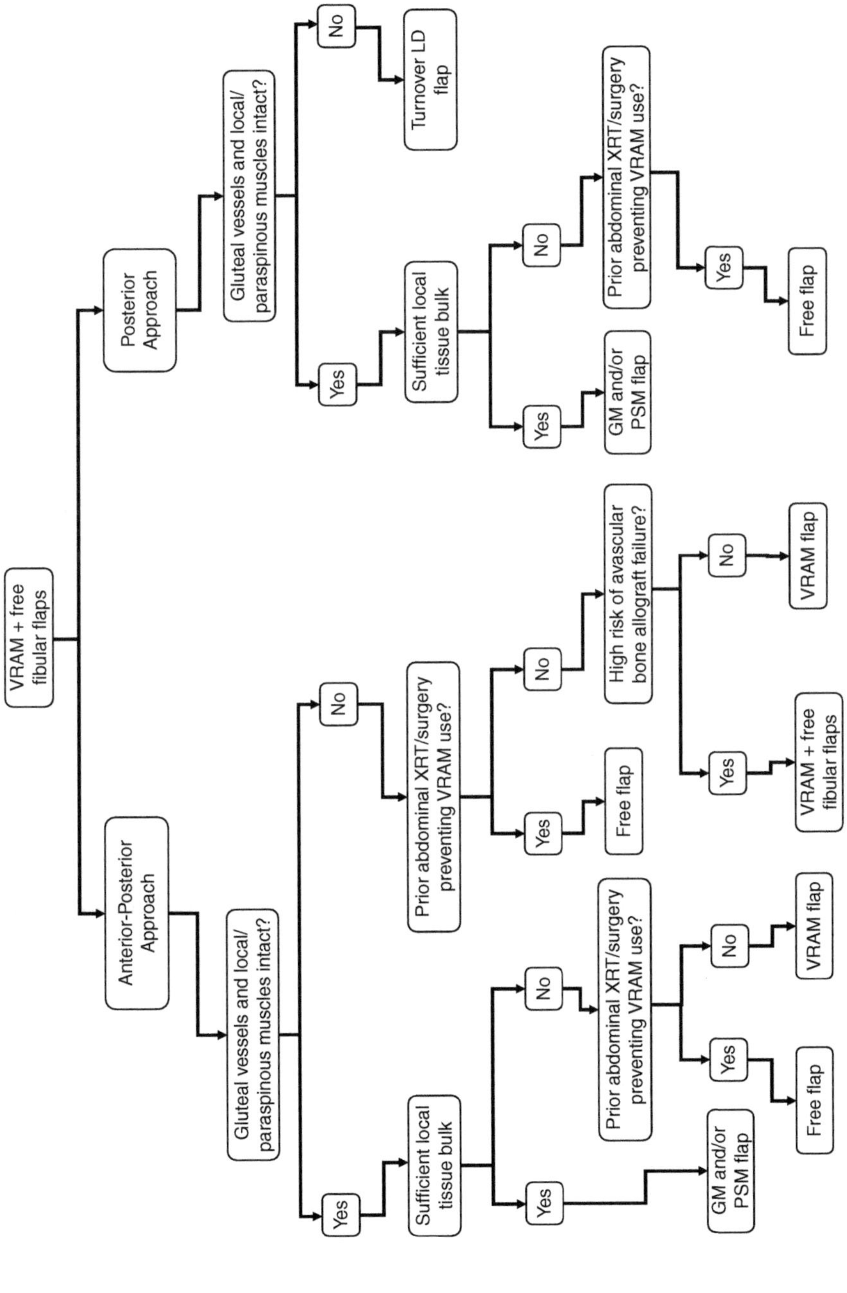


**Fig. 12.4** Operative algorithm for reconstruction after en bloc sacrectomy. (After Kim et al. [15])

ambulation rates afforded by the VRAM flap lead it to be the preferred closure technique. If additional bony support is required, a pedicled VRAM flow-through flap can be used, which allows for soft tissue reconstruction and vascularization of the free fibula used in the bony reconstruction. For single-stage posterior sacrectomies, gluteal and/or paraspinal muscle flaps are preferable as they allow for good soft tissue coverage with low associated morbidity. Lastly, if local gluteal flaps and VRAM flaps are infeasible, a latissimus dorsi free flap may be used, though we recommend only as a last resort. Further research is necessary on the safety and efficacy of biological matrices for enhancing soft tissue reconstruction.

## References


1. Gokaslan ZL, Zadnik PL, Sciubba DM, et al. Mobile spine chordoma: results of 166 patients from the AOSpine Knowledge Forum Tumor database. J Neurosurg Spine. 2016;24:644–51.
2. Varga PP, Szövérfi Z, Fisher CG, et al. Surgical treatment of sacral chordoma: prognostic variables for local recurrence and overall survival. Eur Spine J. 2015;24:1092–101.
3. Dea N, Fisher CG, Reynolds JJ, et al. Current treatment strategy for newly diagnosed chordoma of the mobile spine and sacrum: results of an international survey. J Neurosurg Spine. 2019;30:119–25.
4. Akiyama T, Ogura K, Gokita T, et al. Analysis of the infiltrative features of chordoma: the relationship between micro-skip metastasis and postoperative outcomes. Ann Surg Oncol. 2018;25:912–9.
5. Zuckerman SL, Bilsky MH, Laufer I. Chordomas of the skull base, mobile spine, and sacrum: an epidemiologic investigation of presentation, treatment, and survival. World Neurosurg. 2018;113:e618–27.
6. Gallia GL, Haque R, Garonzik I, Witham TF, Khavkin YA, Wolinsky JP, Suk I, Gokaslan ZL. Spinal pelvic reconstruction after total sacrectomy for en bloc resection of a giant sacral chordoma. Technical note. J Neurosurg Spine. 2005;3:501–6.
7. Asaad M, Mericli AF, Hanasono MM, Roubaud MS, Bird JE, Rhines LD. Free vascularized fibula flap reconstruction of total and near-total destabilizing resections of the sacrum. Ann Plast Surg. 2020; https://doi.org/10.1097/SAP.0000000000002562.
8. Zhang H-Y, Thongtrangan I, Balabhadra RSV, Murovic JA, Kim DH. Surgical techniques for total sacrectomy and spinopelvic reconstruction. Neurosurg Focus. 2003;15:1–10.
9. Reynolds JJ, Khundkar R, Boriani S, Williams R, Rhines LD, Kawahara N, Wolinsky J-P, Gokaslan ZL, Varga PP. Soft tissue and bone defect management in total sacrectomy for primary sacral tumors. Spine (Phila Pa 1976). 2016;41:S199–204.
10. Chang DW, Friel MT, Youssef AA. Reconstructive strategies in soft tissue reconstruction after resection of spinal neoplasms. Spine (Phila Pa 1976). 2007;32:1101–6.
11. Manrique OJ, Rajesh A, Asaad M, Bakri K, Tran NV, Houdek MT, Dozois EJ, Rose PS. Surgical outcomes after abdominoperineal resection with sacrectomy and soft tissue reconstruction: lessons learned. J Reconstr Microsurg. 2020;36:064–72.
12. Houdek MT, Bakri K, Tibbo ME, Wagner ER, Rose PS, Sim FH, Moran SL. Outcome and complications following vertical rectus abdominis myocutaneous flap surgery to reconstruct sacrectomy defects. Plast Reconstr Surg. 2018;142:1327–35.
13. Kiatisevi P, Piyaskulkaew C, Kunakornsawat S, Sukunthanak B. What are the functional outcomes after total sacrectomy without spinopelvic reconstruction? Clin Orthop Relat Res. 2017;475:643–55.
14. Moran SL, Bakri K, Mardini S, Shin AY, Bishop AT. The use of vascularized fibular grafts for the reconstruction of spinal and sacral defects. Microsurgery. 2009;29:393–400.

15. Kim JE, Pang J, Christensen JM, et al. Soft-tissue reconstruction after total en bloc sacrectomy. J Neurosurg Spine. 2015;22:571–81.
16. Garvey PB, Clemens MW, Rhines LD, Sacks JM. Vertical rectus abdominis musculocutaneous flow-through flap to a free fibula flap for total sacrectomy reconstruction. Microsurgery. 2013;33:32–8.
17. Radwan RW, Tang AM, Harries RL, Davies EG, Drew P, Evans MD. Vertical rectus abdominis flap (VRAM) for perineal reconstruction following pelvic surgery: a systematic review. J Plast Reconstr Aesthetic Surg. 2020; https://doi.org/10.1016/j.bjps.2020.10.100.
18. Mathes SJ, Bostwick J. A rectus abdominis myocutaneous flap to reconstruct abdominal wall defects. Br J Plast Surg. 1977;30:282–3.
19. Shukla HS, Hughes LE. The rectus abdominis flap for perineal wounds. Ann R Coll Surg Engl. 1984;66:337–9.
20. Glatt BS, Disa JJ, Mehrara BJ, Pusic AL, Boland P, Cordeiro PG. Reconstruction of extensive partial or total sacrectomy defects with a transabdominal vertical rectus abdominis myocutaneous flap. Ann Plast Surg. 2006;56:526–31.
21. Miles WK, Chang DW, Kroll SS, Miller MJ, Langstein HN, Reece GP, Evans GRD, Robb GL. Reconstruction of large sacral defects following total sacrectomy. Plast Reconstr Surg. 2000;105:2387–94.
22. Garvey PB, Rhines LD, Feng L, Gu X, Butler CE. Reconstructive strategies for partial sacrectomy defects based on surgical outcomes. Plast Reconstr Surg. 2011;127:190–9.
23. Dasenbrock HH, Clarke MJ, Bydon A, Witham TF, Sciubba DM, Simmons OP, Gokaslan ZL, Wolinsky J-P. Reconstruction of extensive defects from posterior en bloc resection of sacral tumors with human acellular dermal matrix and gluteus maximus myocutaneous flaps. Neurosurgery. 2011;69:1240–7.
24. Maricevich M, Maricevich R, Chim H, Moran SL, Rose PS, Mardini S. Reconstruction following partial and total sacrectomy defects: an analysis of outcomes and complications. J Plast Reconstr Aesthetic Surg. 2014;67:1257–66.
25. Coon D, Calotta NA, Broyles JM, Sacks JM. Use of biological tissue matrix in postneurosurgical posterior trunk reconstruction is associated with higher wound complication rates. Plast Reconstr Surg. 2016;138:104e–10e.
26. Diaz J, McDonald WS, Armstrong M, Eismont F, Hellinger M, Thaller S. Reconstruction after extirpation of sacral malignancies. Ann Plast Surg. 2003;51:126–9.
27. Vartanian ED, Lynn JV, Perrault DP, Wolfswinkel EM, Kaiser AM, Patel KM, Carey JN, Hsieh PC, Wong AK. Risk factors associated with reconstructive complications following sacrectomy. Plast Reconstr Surg Glob Open. 2018;6:e2002.

# 13 Vascular Reconstruction After En Bloc Resection

## Vascular Reconstruction

Daniel G. Tobert and Joseph H. Schwab

## Abbreviations

EBR En bloc resection
FVFG Free vascularized fibular graft

## Introduction

Successful oncologic resection of chordomas of the mobile spine and sacrum often creates a state of biomechanical instability in the spine. Therefore, following tumor removal, attention focuses on implementing a robust reconstruction of the defect. A thoughtful reconstruction plan with multiple contingency options is best developed in tandem with the resection. Variables to consider include the anatomical region as the biomechanical ramifications change considerably as a resection moves caudal. Additionally, the extent of resection is an important consideration as multilevel EBR may require a larger reconstruction than single-level EBR. Finally, the use of adjuvant or neoadjuvant radiotherapies (RT) can affect osseous integration of reconstruction components. The role of RT and emerging therapies within that field are discussed in subsequent chapters. Yet, the potential ramifications of RT on reconstructive efforts should not be underestimated. If a successful oncologic outcome is attained, the patient's quality of life can be significantly impacted by the mechanical complications surrounding reconstruction. The relative rarity of these tumors and rapid pace of device innovation creates a limited body of evidence for

D. G. Tobert (✉) · J. H. Schwab
Department of Orthopaedic Surgery, Massachusetts General Hospital, Harvard Medical School, Boston, MA, USA
e-mail: dotobert@mgh.harvard.edu



D. M. Sciubba, J. H. Schwab (eds.), *Chordoma of the Spine*,
https://doi.org/10.1007/978-3-030-76201-8_13

reconstruction that is confounded by heterogenous surgical technique. However, the biology that serves as the foundation for successful reconstruction remains the same. The purpose of this chapter is to discuss the role of vascularized reconstruction after EBR of chordoma tumors.

## Anatomical and Biomechanical Considerations

The forces applied to the axial skeleton throughout physiologic motion vary considerably and mirror the morphologic differences in anatomy. Although traditionally demarcated into cervical, thoracic, lumbar, and sacral regions, the biomechanical differences occur along a spectrum. The expected physiologic burden is an important consideration when planning a reconstruction. The cervical spine is the most mobile of the spine regions, with flexion/extension arc of motion averaging approximately 70° [1]. In contrast, the thoracic and lumbar spine display half the amount of flexion/extension, averaging approximately 30° and 35° throughout those regions [2, 3]. Depending on the size of the defect after EBR, the reconstruction will confer a significant amount of rigidity to otherwise mobile segments. The ability to withstand compressive loads increases substantially moving caudally in the spine. The L5 vertebral body is estimated to yield at 4500 N, which is more than twice the estimated that of T6 at approximately 2200N [4]. The increased load tolerance of the thoracolumbar and lumbar spine reflects the physiologic requirements of this region. Reconstructive efforts at the thoracolumbar junction and caudal must account for this if a vascularized autograft is chosen. The readily available options for vascularized reconstruction include the rib and fibula—both of which have biomechanical limits that can be exceeded in isolation.

The blood supply of the spinal cord is relevant to both resection and reconstruction [5]. Often, circumferential exposure and dissection are required to safely perform EBR with satisfactory margins. A chordoma involving a single vertebra in the thoracic or lumbar spine commonly requires dissection of the adjacent vertebrae and ligation of the accompanying radicular vessels. Using a dog model, researchers demonstrated that ligation of bilateral segmental vasculature in three levels did not lead to a change in transcranial motor-evoked (tcMEP) or somatosensory potentials (SSEP) [6, 7]. A case series of 15 patients in which the artery of Adamkiewicz was purposefully interrupted did not result in neurologic deterioration [8]. Despite the lack of clinical manifestations in these studies, the authors did report changes in blood flow in the adjacent vessels after ligation. Additionally, the authors note anecdotally that patients with existing neurologic dysfunction preoperatively can exhibit worsened neurologic status postoperatively after ligation of the artery of Adamkiewicz, presumably due to a tenuous existing blood supply. This underscores the importance of counseling patients thoroughly about the neurologic risks associated with tumor resection secondary to spinal cord ischemia.

Although this challenges long-held assertions about spinal cord perfusion, this is salient to the vascular reconstruction effort. Often, preoperative embolization of the segmental vessels can facilitate EBR of chordoma. Yet, a vascularized reconstruction that requires anastomosis relies on the presence of arterial and venous branches of acceptable length. Therefore, we make a concerted attempt to identify the segmental vessels as far laterally as possible and temporarily clamp them in sequence during the dissection. The benefit is twofold: it affords the possibility of releasing the clamp if tcMEP deteriorate and also allows the microvascular surgeon to evaluate the vessel as a possible anastomosis site before permanent ligation. It is important to note that this technique is not completely failsafe as ischemic changes can evolve in a delayed fashion. This phenomenon has long been reported in the vascular surgery literature, where the onset of paraplegia after abdominal aortic aneurysm repair ranges between 6 and 20 hours postoperatively [9].

## Radiotherapy Considerations

The use of RT and systemic therapies is discussed in full detail in Section IV of this textbook. However, RT drastically transforms the biologic environment in the tissue adjacent to the tumor. A successful reconstruction is reliant on the vitality of the tissue bordering the tumor and therefore deserves consideration. The rationale for RT utilization in chordoma is based on observations that approximately 50% of patients with wide surgical margins (R0) have local recurrence in the long term. A relatively large series of 99 patients with sacral chordoma from the Rizzoli Institute and National Cancer Institute of Milan reported a 49% disease-free survival at 15 years for patients with wide (R0) surgical margins [10]. Another series of 138 patients with sacral and mobile spine chordomas from the same institutions found a trend toward improved local control rates with wide margins but a 12-year, local recurrence-free survival of 56% even with wide surgical margins [11]. The discovery of micro- or "skip" metastases may explain the high local recurrence rate observed in chordoma despite adequate surgical margins. Akiyama et al. performed a histopathological study of 40 sacral chordoma resections and found skip metastases up to 20 millimeters away from the main lesion [12]. They reported that patients with skip metastases (clusters of tumor cells not recognizable on imaging) demonstrated significant association with local recurrence.

Although the results of conventional RT on chordoma outcomes were equivocal, updated data utilizing localized RT at higher doses indicates superior local control [13, 14]. The impact on higher-dose RT on osteology can have important functional ramification. Osler et al. reviewed 62 patients with sacral chordomas treated with high-dose radiation and reported a 47% rate of insufficiency fractures [15]. This indicates high-dose RT can have a detrimental impact on the viability of neighboring osteocytes. A separate study by van Wulfften Palthe et al. further characterized the impact of high-dose radiation on bone density using Hounsfield units measured by CT as a surrogate [16]. Patients with sacral chordoma were given 50.4 Gray (Gy) preoperatively and 19.8 Gy postoperatively via photon beam. Within weeks, the bone density within the field of radiation changed to values consistent with osteoporosis. However, bone outside of the field of radiation remained normal. These findings have important implications for reconstruction efforts. At our institution, high-dose RT is directed at a field that includes the chordoma visible on imaging but also to the vertebra above and below to account for the possibility of skip metastases. Although potentially beneficial from the standpoint of local control, it creates a penumbra of non-viable bone, which increases the possibility of nonunion and/or mechanical complications. With this set of physiologic circumstances, the surgeon often turns to a vascularized reconstruction option.

## Vascularized Reconstruction in the Cervical Spine

Anterior cervical surgery techniques became commonplace after the work of Robinson and Smith, Bailey-Badgley, and Cloward. While iliac crest graft was successful for interbody fusions, the structural properties were often insufficient for large defects encountered in traumatic or infectious settings. It is noteworthy that these techniques predate modern anterior and posterior instrumentation techniques and therefore the graft used in a corpectomy defect was necessarily used for both stabilization and fusion. Given the structural deficiencies of iliac crest over multilevel corpectomy defects, fibular strut grafts were often employed. The mechanical strength of differing types of autologous and allogenous grafts was studied by Wittenberg et al. who reported fibular strut graft mechanically favorable to iliac crest, rib, Bailey-Badgley, and Cloward grafts [17].

Yet, the osseous integration of fibular grafts often took a year or longer, required prolonged immobilization, and still could lead to nonunion. Although the free vascularized fibular graft (FVFG) was described for other clinical scenarios, Doi et al. described FVFG in 1988 for the cervical spine [18]. This retrospective case series served as proof-of-concept and described relatively rapid incorporation of the fibular graft within 4 months by anastomosing the peroneal vessels of the fibula to the superior thyroid vessels in the neck. EBR of chordoma of the cervical spine is undertaken with combined anterior and posterior approaches. A systematic review and expert opinion consensus was published in 2015 regarding reconstruction preferences after EBR [19]. For a single-level subaxial cervical corpectomy defect without postoperative radiation planned, 13/20 surgeons (65%) chose a cage reconstruction, 6/20 (30%) chose an autogenous or allogeneic strut graft, and 1/20 (5%) chose both. Although no surgeon chose a vascularized graft for a one-level cervical corpectomy defect, 10/20 (50%) of surgeons chose a vascularized graft for a three-level cervical corpectomy defect.

A fibular graft provides an ideal footprint and biomechanical support for the subaxial cervical spine and cervicothoracic region. As noted earlier, pre- and postoperative radiotherapy is increasingly utilized and confers an increased chance of nonunion. Furthermore, addressing nonunion after multilevel EBR through an irradiated soft tissue bed is best done by avoiding its occurrence altogether. Therefore, the authors recommend autogenous fibular strut graft or cage filled with iliac crest or morselized rib autograft for one-level EBR in the cervical spine. If two or more levels of EBR are planned, the authors advocate for FVFG. In both circumstances, robust posterior fixation is recommended as an adjunct with extension to the occiput or beyond the cervicothoracic junction if needed.

## Vascularized Reconstruction in the Thoracic Spine

This section covers the role of vascularized reconstruction in the thoracic spine after EBR but excludes the thoracolumbar junction, which is included in the following section. The physiologic burden in the thoracic spine is higher than that of the cervical spine, and the addition of the rib cage mitigates a portion of the burden on the thoracic spine. Yet, any stability conferred by the ribs may be reduced if multiple ribs are sectioned bilaterally during the posterior exposure.

The availability of reconstruction options is dependent on the planned approaches for resection (thoracic resections discussed in more detail in Chap. 9). Chordoma tumors that involve only portion of the vertebral body may be amenable to rotation dorsolaterally around the spinal cord through an isolated posterior approach. Although this saves the morbidity of multiple approaches, an isolated posterior approach limits the possible reconstruction options. Anterior reconstruction can be performed through the costotransversectomies, and options include autogenous (non-vascularized) or allogeneic fibular strut grafts. Alternatively, titanium static or expandable cages may be chosen for structural support. If synthetic cages are employed, osseous integration is limited to the cage/endplate interface. A vascularized graft is difficult in the anterior column given the limitations of an isolated posterior approach for the microvascular surgeon. However, in the case of posterior-only thoracic exposures, a vascularized rib can be utilized along the dorsal elements to provide a successful union across a defect. This technique has been described in detail by Dr. Alex Shin at the Mayo Clinic [20]. This technique can be used to span defects ranging from 4 cm to 25 cm. After anterior column reconstruction, the defect is measured with a planned rib length spanning two spinous processes above and below the defect. A vascular pedicle is identified at the costotransverse junction and preserved, while the rib is harvested. Multiple unicortical osteotomies can be made on the concave side to straighten the graft before it is rotated around its pedicle to span the defect. A monofilament suture is used to fix it to the spinous process. This technique followed a published series of 18 patients who underwent this procedure. The authors reported all formed union at an average of 6.8 months with an average rib graft length of 16.1 cm [21].

The vascular reconstruction options increase if multiple approaches are utilized. For EBR of chordoma, this often means a posterior approach to resect the dorsal elements, costotransverse joints, and free the tumor from the spinal cord followed by a thoracotomy to complete the spondylectomy and resect the tumor. Subsequently, a FVFG can be harvested and inserted to span the anterior column defect. The proximity to the aorta and the segmental vessels in the thoracic provides multiple options for the microvascular surgeon. If multilevel EBR is performed in the thoracic spine, there may be concern about long-term biomechanical stability.

Fresh-frozen humeral or femoral allografts are biomechanically favorable for anterior reconstruction in comparison to FVFG. Although using an allograft strut obviates the risk of graft fracture, it increases the risk of nonunion and subsequent instrumentation failure. Revision instrumentation and fusion operations in this population can be morbid and fraught with complications given the radiation and extensive fibrosis. Shinmura et al. reviewed 61 cases of EBR for oligometastatic disease and primary spine tumors and reported a 42.6% rate of instrumentation failure at an average of 32 months postoperatively [22]. This series performed anterior construction with a titanium cage filed with autograft but highlights the difficulty in achieving osseous union.

Capanna et al. described the use of an autograft intussuscepted within an allograft for spanning appendicular defects due to trauma or infection [23]. The same principle can be translated to reconstruction efforts in the spine. In the thoracic spine, the ribs that are separated from the spine for tumor resection provide ample autograft for reconstruction. These ribs can be dissected and harvested with their segmental vessels and rotated about their pedicle to be used for vascularized autograft. Figure 13.1 demonstrates a case performed by Dr. Joseph Schwab at Massachusetts General Hospital. A three-level EBR was performed, and a femoral graft was selected and shaped based on the measured defect. A notch was cut in the femoral

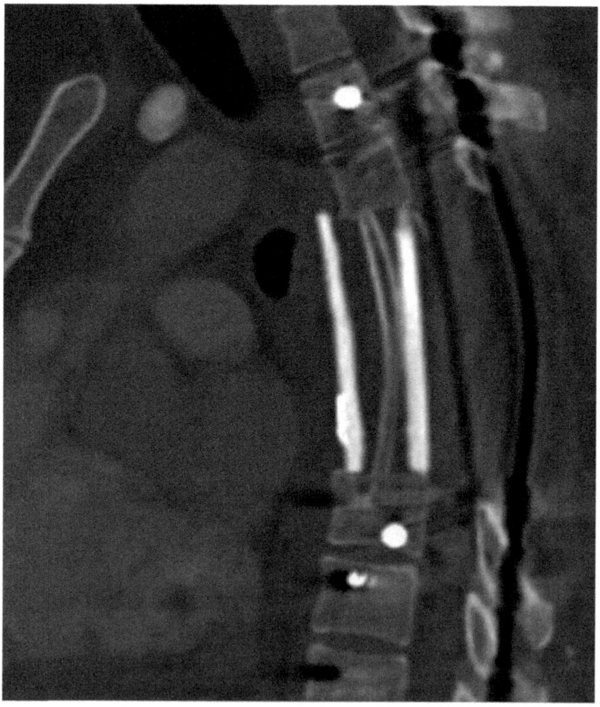

**Fig. 13.1** Parasagittal CT image of a 36-year-old male who underwent three-level EBR (T5-T7) with reconstruction using a vascularized rib intussuscepted into a femoral allograft

allograft to provide an untethered and unpressured passage for the rib's vessels. Additionally, the inner cortex of the femoral allograft was thinned with the help of a high-speed bur to allow successful intussusception of the vascularized rib. This unpublished technique provides direct endplate contact with a vascularized autograft source in addition to a customizable biomechanical support with use of a diaphyseal allograft. Furthermore, it avoids the morbidity of a separate graft harvest site if contrast to FVFG usage. Finally, by rotating the rib around the vascular source, it avoids the risk and time required by anastomosis of free vascularized autograft.

## Vascularized Reconstruction in the Lumbar Spine

The biomechanical demands of the lumbar spine require a more robust reconstruction effort after EBS. This is underscored by the results of a case series of 47 patients who had 1 year follow-up after EBR [24]. Yoshioka et al. reported the following rates of instrumentation failure: 0% (0/7) rate in the cervical/cervicothoracic region, 5.9% (1/17) rate in the thoracic spine, 25% (4/16) in the thoracolumbar spine, and 42.9% (3/7) in the lumbar spine. The Korean Spine Tumor Study Group reported instrumentation failure in 12 of 32 (37.5%) patients undergoing EBR for primary or oligometastatic tumors [25]. In this series, reconstruction was performed with non-vascularized autograft. They found a caudal location and a history of radiotherapy associated with instrumentation failure.

In a case series involving 39 patients (26 chordoma patients) who underwent vascularized reconstruction with FVFG after EBR, Bongers et al. reported a 33% implant failure rate with 26% of patients undergoing revision surgery for instrumentation failure [26]. Complete union was achieved in 76% of patients. Interestingly, there were examples in this series of instrumentation failure despite complete union and hypertrophy of the FVFG. This indicates that, despite union, there is an imbalance in the biomechanical load placed on the lumbar spine and the capacity of a FVFG with posterior instrumentation. The "double-barrel" vascularized fibula technique can be employed to increase the biomechanical support of the construct [27]. The challenges with this technique include correctly sizing both fibular struts after the osteotomy is made to create the second barrel. The periosteal hinge is important for maintaining the vascular supply but allows little opportunity to resize once the osteotomy is made.

A case report described the use of a FVFG within a femoral allograft sleeve for lumbar defects after EBR of a conventional chordoma at L3 [28]. Similar to the description in the previous section regarding vascularized rib within a femoral sleeve, this is modification of the Capanna technique. After the initial posterior approach with tumor and nerve root dissection along with instrumentation, an anterior approach is utilized to complete EBR of the chordoma. Simultaneously, a FVFG is harvested of a length based on preoperative measurements. After EBR, the defect is measured and femoral allograft cut to an appropriate length. Although EBR is often performed through the metaphysis of the vertebral bodies adjacent to the tumor, we advocate reconstruction from "endplate-to-endplate." Our center utilizes pre- and postoperative radiation for micrometastases control, which impairs the vertebral bodies adjacent to the tumor. This requires completing the vertebrectomy and discectomy after the tumor is removed and establishing docking sites for the graft on the endplates. A notch is then cut in the allograft, and the inner cortex is thinned with a high-speed bur until the FVFG can be easily inserted without undue pressure on the vascular leash (Fig. 13.2). An oscillating saw can finely resize the femoral allograft as needed until the appropriate fit is achieved. Beveled ends of the graft can help account for lumbar lordosis. Vascular anastomosis can then be performed by the vascular surgeon to branches of the aorta and vena cava. Figures 13.3 and 13.4 are illustrative of this technique. This combines the benefits of FVFG (rapid integration, resistance to infection) and structural allografts (favorable biomechanics). The drawbacks include increased operative time (up to an additional 3–4 hours) and increased donor site morbidity. We advocate the use of multiple surgical teams to allow simultaneous graft harvest and tumor resection. Further utilization and review of this technique is needed to determine if it represents an improvement on current techniques involving non-vascularized autograft or isolated FVFG.

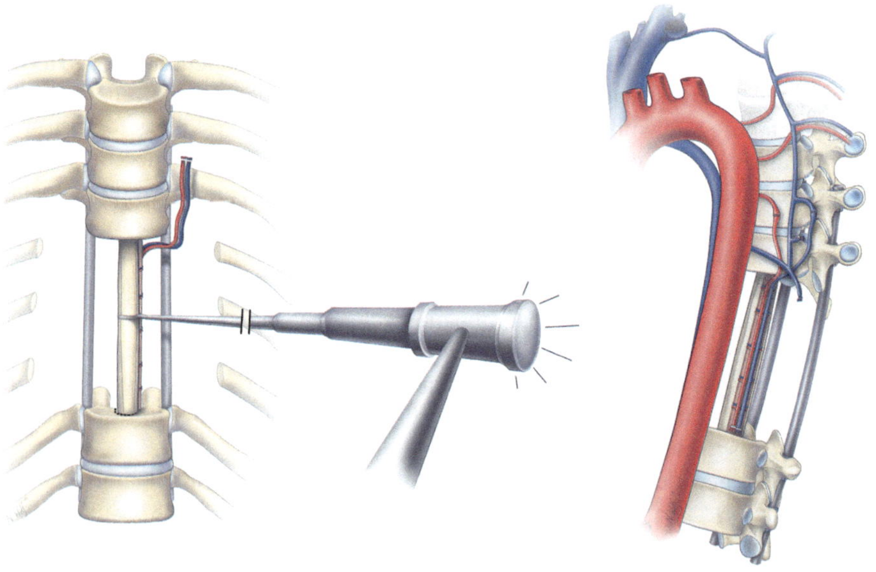

**Fig. 13.2** Illustration of a free vascularized fibular graft inserted within a femoral allograft after endosteal thinning. Note the notch in the femoral allograft, which prevents obstruction of the vascular leash. (Medical illustration courtesy of E.P. Trupia)

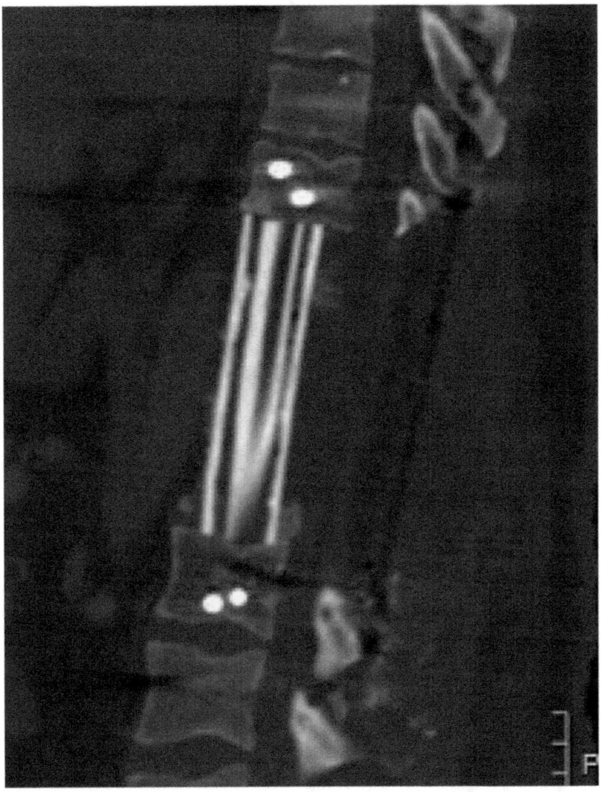

**Fig. 13.3** Parasagittal CT image of a 43-year-old male who underwent three-level EBR (T10-T12) for chordoma with reconstruction using a vascularized rib intussuscepted into a femoral allograft

## Vascularized Reconstruction in the Sacrum

The sacrum is a common region for chordoma to occur. En bloc sacrectomy is a morbid procedure that is recommended if successful resection can result in long-term oncologic control. EBR of the sacrum without reconstruction is an option that is described in the literature, yet it can result in permanent disability and immobility. Therefore, reconstruction is performed to improve a patient's physical function. The Galveston technique of lumbosacralpelvic fixation has been augmented in the decades since it was published to provide a durable construct [29]. Similar to the lumbar spine, instrumentation failure is a paramount concern for the surgeon and source of morbidity for the patient.

Tang et al. describe a series of 63 patients who underwent total sacrectomy and reported a 25% rate of instrumentation failure [30]. The authors identified use of anterior column support and four rod instrumentation (dual iliac fixation) as factors in successful reconstruction. Dickey et al. previously reported the use of fibular strut grafts along the anatomical force vectors as a successful technique [31]. From a biomechanical standpoint, strain is minimized utilizing a four-rod instrumentation and triangular fibular struts [32].

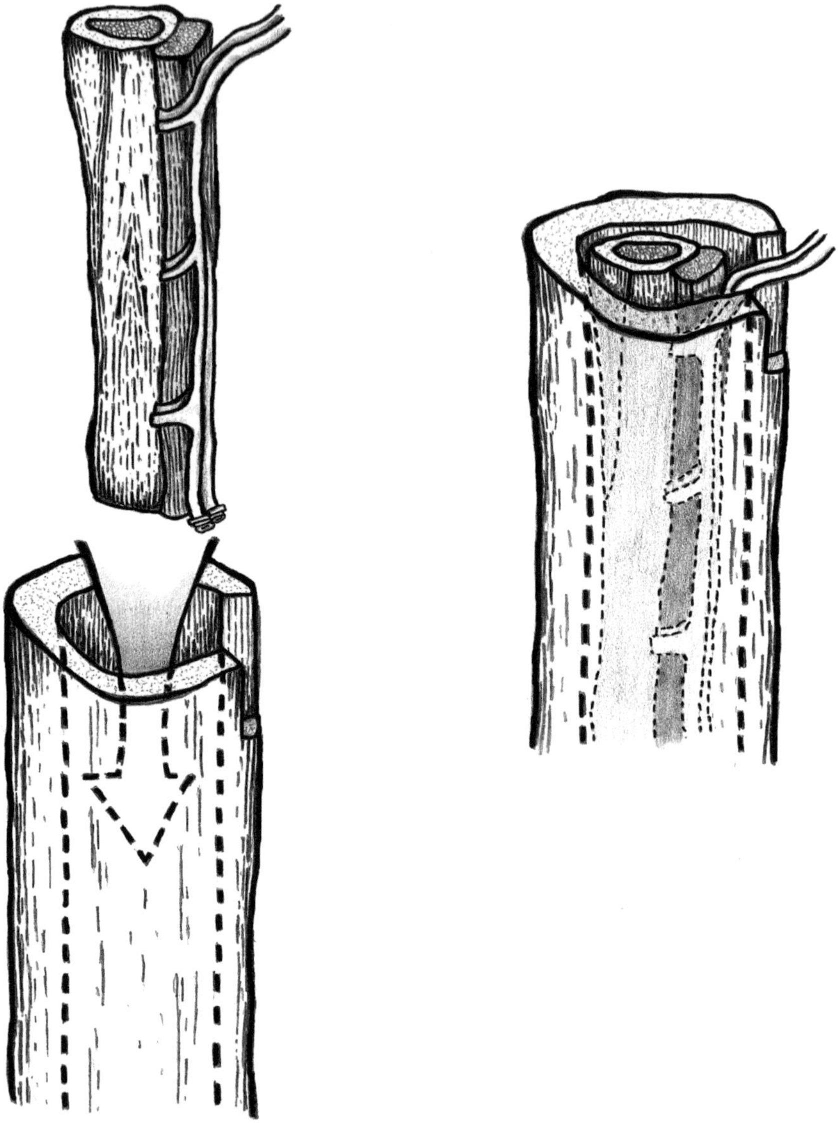

**Fig. 13.4** Illustration of a free vascularized fibular graft within a femoral allograft, anastomosed to the great vessels, and spanning a lumbar defect after en bloc resection. (Medical illustration courtesy of E.P. Trupia)

FVFG is the ideal graft choice after EBR of sacral chordoma as it provides more than 20 centimeters of structural, vascularized autograft. Furthermore, it can tolerate osteotomies, which can provide multiple struts from a single harvest. Despite this, even if sub-total sacrectomy is performed along with FVFG, instrumentation failure is still a concern as demonstrated in Fig. 13.5.

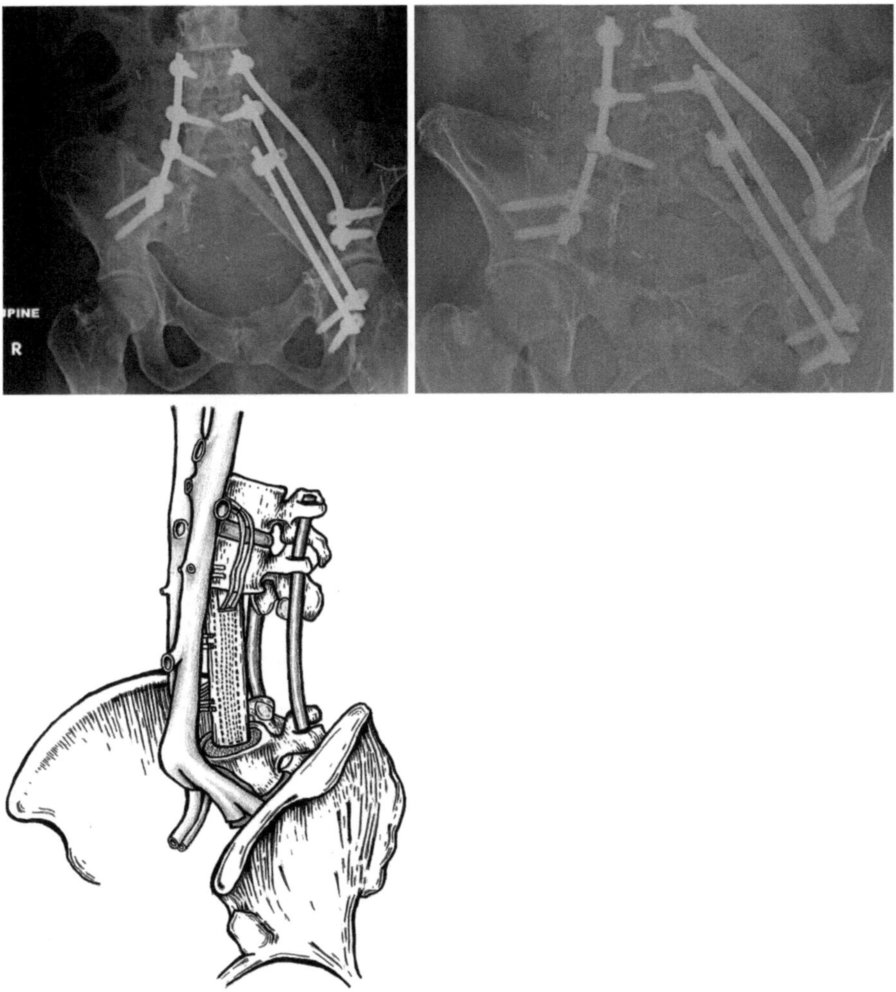


**Fig. 13.5** AP pelvis radiograph of a 36-year-old female who underwent staged EBR with partial sacrectomy and L5 vertebrectomy and FVFG reconstruction. Instrumentation failure and lucency around the L5-FVFG interface noted at approximately 10 months postoperatively

## Conclusions and Future Directions

Reconstruction after EBR of chordoma is a challenging endeavor. There is a high rate of surgical complications and instrumentation failure, in particular. The rate of instrumentation failure is directly related to the physiologic stress placed on the reconstruction. Therefore, EBR of lumbar and sacral chordoma leads to instrumentation failure in up to 50% of patients, in contrast to less than 10% in the cervical spine. Vascularized reconstruction options include FVFG, vascularized rib, and vascularized iliac crest. Of these, FVFG and vascularized rib are suitable for vascular reconstruction in the spine and pelvis.

In the cervical spine, FVFG in addition to posterior instrumentation is the preferred vascularized option. In the thoracic spine, vascularized rib can be successfully used along a dorsal defect in conjunction with allograft or titanium support anteriorly. Alternatively, FVFG can be used anteriorly proximally in the thoracic spine. As the biomechanical requirements increase caudally in the thoracic spine, a vascularized rib can be intussuscepted into a femoral allograft to provide increased support. In the lumbar spine, we advocate using a FVFG within a sculpted femoral allograft to provide biomechanical support and long-term physiologic integration. Total sacrectomies are ideally treated with four-rod instrumentation and FVFG as struts between the lumbar spine and pelvis.

As surgical techniques improve, there will be an increasing desire to measure the impact on functional outcomes [33]. The rarity of these tumors creates challenges for the research community, but collaborative research efforts will help us better understand the optimal reconstruction techniques.

## References


1. Lind B, Sihlbom H, Nordwall A, Malchau H. Normal range of motion of the cervical spine. Arch Phys Med Rehabil. 1989;70:692–5.
2. Santoni B, Cabezas AF, Cook DJ, Yeager MS, Billys JB, Whiting B, Cheng BC. Comparison of intervertebral ROM in multi-level cadaveric lumbar spines using distinct pure moment loading approaches. Int J Spine Surg. 2015;9:32.
3. Morita D, Yukawa Y, Nakashima H, Ito K, Yoshida G, Machino M, Kanbara S, Iwase T, Kato F. Range of motion of thoracic spine in sagittal plane. Eur Spine J. 2014;23:673–8.
4. Bruno AG, Burkhart K, Allaire B, Anderson DE, Bouxsein ML. Spinal loading patterns from biomechanical modeling explain the high incidence of vertebral fractures in the thoracolumbar region. J Bone Miner Res. 2017;32:1282–90.
5. Colman MW, Hornicek FJ, Schwab JH. Spinal cord blood supply and its surgical implications. J Am Acad Orthop Surg. 2015;23:581–91.
6. Nambu K, Kawahara N, Kobayashi T, Murakami H, Ueda Y, Tomita K. Interruption of the bilateral segmental arteries at several levels: influence on vertebral blood flow. Spine (Phila Pa 1976). 2004;29:1530–4.
7. Ueda Y, Kawahara N, Tomita K, Kobayashi T, Murakami H, Nambu K. Influence on spinal cord blood flow and function by interruption of bilateral segmental arteries at up to three levels: experimental study in dogs. Spine (Phila Pa 1976). 2005;30:2239–43.
8. Murakami H, Kawahara N, Tomita K, Demura S, Kato S, Yoshioka K. Does interruption of the artery of Adamkiewicz during total En Bloc Spondylectomy affect neurologic function? Spine (Phila Pa 1976). 2010;35:E1187–92.
9. Rosenthal D. Spinal cord ischemia after abdominal aortic operation: is it preventable? J Vasc Surg. 1999;30:391–7.
10. Radaelli S, Stacchiotti S, Ruggieri P, et al. Sacral Chordoma: long-term outcome of a large series of patients surgically treated at two reference centers. Spine (Phila Pa 1976). 2016;41:1049–57.
11. Stacchiotti S, Casali PG, Lo Vullo S, et al. Chordoma of the mobile spine and sacrum: a retrospective analysis of a series of patients surgically treated at two referral centers. Ann Surg Oncol. 2010;17:211–9.

12. Akiyama T, Ogura K, Gokita T, et al. Analysis of the infiltrative features of Chordoma: the relationship between micro-skip metastasis and postoperative outcomes. Ann Surg Oncol. 2018;25:912–9.
13. DeLaney TF, Liebsch NJ, Pedlow FX, et al. Long-term results of phase II study of high dose photon/proton radiotherapy in the management of spine chordomas, chondrosarcomas, and other sarcomas. J Surg Oncol. 2014;110:115–22.
14. Rotondo RL, Folkert W, Liebsch NJ, et al. High-dose proton-based radiation therapy in the management of spine chordomas: outcomes and clinicopathological prognostic factors. J Neurosurg Spine. 2015;23:788–97.
15. Osler P, Bredella MA, Hess KA, Janssen SJ, Park CJ, Chen YL, DeLaney TF, Hornicek FJ, Schwab JH. Sacral insufficiency fractures are common after high-dose radiation for sacral Chordomas treated with or without surgery. Clin Orthop Relat Res. 2016;474:766–72.
16. van Wulfften PO, Jee K-W, Bramer JAM, Hornicek FJ, Chen Y-LE, Schwab JH. What is the effect of high-dose radiation on bone in patients with sacral Chordoma? A CT study. Clin Orthop Relat Res. 2018;476:520–8.
17. Wittenberg RH, Moeller J, Shea M, White AA, Hayes WC. Compressive strength of autologous and Allogenous bone grafts for thoracolumbar and cervical spine fusion. Spine (Phila Pa 1976). 1990;15:1073–8.
18. Doi K, Kawai S, Sumiura S, Sakai K. Anterior cervical fusion using the free vascularized fibular graft. Spine (Phila Pa 1976). 1988;13:1239–44.
19. Glennie RA, Rampersaud YR, Boriani S, Reynolds JJ, Williams R, Gokaslan ZL, Schmidt MH, Varga PP, Fisher CG. A systematic review with consensus expert opinion of best reconstructive techniques after osseous En Bloc spinal column tumor resection. Spine (Phila Pa 1976). 2016;41:S205–11.
20. Wilden JA, Moran SL, Dekutoski MB, Bishop AT, Shin AY. Results of vascularized rib grafts in complex spinal reconstruction. Surgical technique. J Bone Jt Surg. 2007;89:128–41.
21. Wilden JA, Moran SL, Dekutoski MB, Bishop AT, Shin AY. Results of vascularized rib grafts in complex spinal reconstruction. J Bone Jt Surg. 2006;88:832–9.
22. Shinmura K, Kato S, Demura S, et al. Revision surgery for instrumentation failure after total en bloc spondylectomy: a retrospective case series. BMC Musculoskelet Disord. 2020;21:591.
23. Capanna R, Bufalini C, Campanacci M. A new technique for reconstructions of large metadiaphyseal bone defects. A combined graft (Allograft shell plus vascularized fibula). Orthop Traumatol. 1993;2:159–77.
24. Yoshioka K, Murakami H, Demura S, Kato S, Yokogawa N, Kawahara N, Tomita K, Tsuchiya H. Risk factors of instrumentation failure after multilevel total en bloc spondylectomy. Spine Surg Relat Res. 2017;1:31–9.
25. Park S-J, Lee C-S, Chang B-S, Kim Y-H, Kim H, Kim S-I, Chang S-Y. Rod fracture and related factors after total en bloc spondylectomy. Spine J. 2019;19:1613–9.
26. Bongers MER, Ogink PT, Chu KF, Patel A, Rosenthal B, Shin JH, Lee S-G, Hornicek FJ, Schwab JH. The use of autologous free vascularized fibula grafts in reconstruction of the mobile spine following tumor resection: surgical technique and outcomes. J Neurosurg Spine. 2020:1–10.
27. Jones NF, Swartz WM, Mears DC, Jupiter JB, Grossman A. The "Double Barrel" free vascularized fibular bone graft. Plast Reconstr Surg. 1988;81:378–85.
28. Bongers MER, Shin JH, Srivastava SD, Morse CR, Lee S-G, Schwab JH. Free vascularized fibula graft with femoral allograft sleeve for lumbar spine defects after Spondylectomy of malignant tumors: a case report. JBJS Case Connect. 2020;10:e20.00075.
29. Allen BL, Ferguson RL. The Galveston technique of pelvic fixation with L-rod instrumentation of the spine. Spine (Phila Pa 1976). 1984;9:388–94.
30. Tang X, Yang R, Qu H, Cai Z, Guo W. Factors associated with spinopelvic fixation mechanical failure after Total Sacrectomy. Spine (Phila Pa 1976). 2018;43:1268–74.
31. Dickey ID, Hugate RR, Fuchs B, Yaszemski MJ, Sim FH. Reconstruction after Total Sacrectomy: early experience with a new surgical technique. Clin Orthop Relat Res. 2005;NA:42–50.

32. Yu Y, Zhu R, Zeng Z-L, Jia Y-W, Wu Z-R, Ren Y-L, Chen B, Ding Z-Q, Cheng L-M. The strain at bone-implant interface determines the effect of spinopelvic reconstruction following total sacrectomy: a strain gauge analysis in various spinopelvic constructs. PLoS One. 2014;9:e85298.
33. Houdek MT, Rose PS, Bakri K, Wagner ER, Yaszemski MJ, Sim FH, Moran SL. Outcomes and complications of reconstruction with use of free vascularized fibular graft for spinal and pelvic defects following resection of a malignant tumor. J Bone Jt Surg. 2017;99:e69.

# Part IV

# Radiation and Chemotherapeutic Adjuvants for Chordoma

# Conventionally Fractionated and Hypofractionated Photon Radiation Therapy in the Management of Chordoma

14

Photon Therapy

Chunzi Jenny Jin and Yoshiya Josh Yamada

## Abbreviations

| | |
|---|---|
| CI | Confidence interval |
| CT | Computed tomography |
| CTCAE | Common Terminology Criteria for Adverse Events |
| DNA | Deoxyribonucleic acid |
| Gy | Gray |
| HR | Hazard ratio |
| IGRT | Image-guided radiation therapy |
| IMRT | Intensity-modulated radiation therapy |
| LRFS | Local relapse-free survival |
| MSKCC | Memorial Sloan Kettering Cancer Center |
| OS | Overall survival |
| P32 | Phosphorus-32 |
| PFS | Progression-free survival |
| PTV | Planned tumor volume |
| RT | Radiotherapy |
| SBRT | Stereotactic body radiation therapy |
| SRS | Stereotactic radiosurgery |

C. J. Jin
Division of Radiation Oncology, The Ottawa Hospital Cancer Centre, Ottawa, ON, Canada

Y. J. Yamada (✉)
Department of Radiation Oncology, Memorial Sloan Kettering Cancer Center, New York, NY, USA
e-mail: yamadaj@mskcc.org



D. M. Sciubba, J. H. Schwab (eds.), *Chordoma of the Spine*,
https://doi.org/10.1007/978-3-030-76201-8_14

## Introduction

Classically, chordoma was considered a disease not amenable to radiation therapy (RT) due to the high off-target toxicities that occurred when delivering therapeutic doses to the tumor. However, with the advent of modern advanced photon radiation modalities, it is now recognized that adjuvant RT plays a key role in local control for chordoma [1]. Additionally, modern photon-based RT has also been utilized successfully in the following settings: definitive therapy for unresectable tumors, neoadjuvant therapy prior to resection, adjuvant therapy post-subtotal resection for positive margins, palliative therapy for metastatic disease, and salvage therapy for local recurrence (Tables 14.1, 14.2, and 14.3).

In the neoadjuvant and adjuvant settings, it is now suggested that RT may improve local control and progression-free survival (PFS) irrespective of surgical margin. In other words, the combination of RT with any surgery will likely result in better patient outcomes than surgical resection alone. This is a crucial finding, for while the quality of the surgical margin is the most important determinant of local control and overall survival [2–4], recurrence rates can approach 67% even after R0 resection [5]. Thus, patients are often offered a combination of resection and RT or definitive RT for inoperable tumor locations [6].

Key to the increased role for RT have been technological advances in RT that increase the biological effective dose of radiation. This can be accomplished by either increasing the number of fractions delivered or by increasing the radiation dose per fraction. Higher radiation doses increase the likelihood of tumor cell death, but also increase the probability of radiation-related complications. As opposed to chordoma, this trade-off is manifest as the desire to deliver a therapeutic dose that can improve tumor control (≥70Gy) while minimizing irradiation of the spinal cord. Recommendations are that the spinal cord does not exceed 50Gy delivered over 25 fractions, which is associated with a <5% probability of myelitis within 5 years of treatment [7]. Similar constraints also exist for the cauda equina (thoracolumbar lesions), the esophagus (cervicothoracic lesions), the brainstem and cranial nerves (skull base lesions), and the bowel and lumbosacral nerve plexus (sacral lesions). Technological advancements in photon radiation have by and large allowed such constraints to be met, enabling the safe delivery of escalated radiation doses to tumor targets in close proximity to sensitive normal tissue to maximize the therapeutic ratio. Here we review the technological advancements that have enabled these gains and highlight paradigms for photon RT in the neoadjuvant, adjuvant, definitive-intent, and salvage roles.

## Photon-Based Intensity-Modulated Conventionally Fractionated Radiation Therapy

In the modern era, intensity-modulated radiation therapy (IMRT) is the most commonly used modality to deliver high-dose photon radiation to chordomas of the spine and skull base. IMRT provides radiation doses that tightly conform to the

**Table 14.1** Systematic literature review for adjuvant radiation therapy for primary/de novo spinal and sacral chordoma

| Authors | *N* | Treatment/ radiation modality | Median radiation dose | Local control | Survival rate |
|---|---|---|---|---|---|
| Catton C et al. [10] | 19 | Conventional RT | <60 Gy | <10% 5-year LC rate | ≈54% 5-year OS rate; 20% 10-year OS rate |
| Rich TA et al.[a, b] [9] | 19 | Conventional RT | >40 Gy | 54% 5-year LC rate[a] | ≈50% 5-year OS rate[a,c] |
| Zabel-du Bois A et al. [11] | 17 | IMRT (± surgery) | >60 Gy (14 pts); <60 Gy (3 pts) | ≈47% 5-year LC rate | ≈74% 5-year OS rate |
| Terezakis SA et al. [28] | 6 | Conventional RT | 66 Gy in a median of 33 fractions | Not reported for the 6 pts with primary chordomas (65% 2-year LC rate for all tumors within this study) | Not reported for the 6 pts with primary chordomas (79% 2-year OS rate for all tumors within this study) |
| Thieblemont C et al. [29] | 10 | Conventional RT | 43.6 Gy | 16% 5-year LC rate | 68% 5-year OS rate |
| Fuchs B et al. [3] | 22 | Conventional RT | 47 Gy | No reported for 22 patients who received adjuvant RT (59% 5-year LC rate for entire cohort including patient you received surgery alone) | No reported for 22 patients who received adjuvant RT (74% 5-year LC rate for entire cohort including patient you received surgery alone) |
| Berson et al. [30] | 25 | Conventional RT | 72 GyRBE | 78% 2-year LC rate; 55% 5-year LC rate | 62% 5-year OS rate |
| Romero J et al.[a] [31] | 10 | Conventional RT | 50.1 Gy in >30 fractions | Not reported for 10 pts with primary chordomas | Not reported for 10 pts with primary chordomas (38% 5-year OS rate & 17% progression-free survival rate for all tumors within this study) |

(continued)

**Table 14.1** (continued)

| Authors | *N* | Treatment/ radiation modality | Median radiation dose | Local control | Survival rate |
|---|---|---|---|---|---|
| Yamada Y, et al. [32] | 8 pts received true adjuvant therapy | Single Fraction Photon RT/ SRS | 24 Gy in 1 fraction | >95% 2-year LC rate (only 1 patient had a recurrence but unclear if this patient was *de novo* disease vs a previous recurrence) | >67% 2-year OS rate (8 of total 24 patients (33%) in this study died at a median follow-up of 24 months) |

*Key: Gy* gray, *LC* local control, *OS* overall survival, *RBE* relative biological equivalent, *RT* radiotherapy
[a]mixed cohort of skull-base and spine/sacral chordoma
[b]Nine of the 48 patients also received proton therapy in addition to photon RT
[c]Includes patients with chondrosarcoma

three-dimensional characteristics of the target volume by manipulating or modulating the intensity of multiple beams of radiation that approach the target volume from multiple angles. When coupled with image-guided treatment techniques, which help increase the geometric accuracy of treatment, it is possible to deliver radiation doses in excess of 70Gy to a chordoma while maintaining spinal cord doses less than 50Gy with a high degree of confidence. A dose falloff of approximately 10% per millimeter of distance between the target and organ at risk is feasible with IMRT, so a 3 mm separation between the spinal cord and tumor edge could make high-dose treatment of a spinal chordoma feasible while not exceeding the radiation dose tolerance of the spinal cord.

In the pre IMRT era, the majority of older publications that used conventional photon RT did not exceed 60 Gy owing to the normal tolerance of the spinal cord. Several series have demonstrated poor long-term local control of spinal and sacral chordomas with radical surgery and conventional RT at doses below 60 Gy, although palliation of symptoms is often achieved [8, 9]. The use of photon RT with doses less than 60 Gy has shown eventual recurrence rates of 50% to 100% and 5-year progression-free survival (PFS) rates of less than 25% [10]. This poor local control is due to the relative radioresistance of chordoma and the limitations of available technology to deliver adequately high doses to the tumor without exceeding dose safety limits for nearby normal tissues.

Proton therapy has been able to improve local control, by taking advantage of the Bragg peak to accomplish dose escalation close to the spinal cord. Due to the steep dose falloff beyond the Bragg peak, the exit dose delivered to the spinal cord is limited. Dose-response relationships have been suggested in studies using protons [9]. Since proton facilities are not readily available, image-guided stereotactic systems have been investigated to deliver dose using photon RT to chordomas. Because modern IMRT often involves the use of arc trajectories that intersect in the tumor,

**Table 14.2** Systematic literature review for salvage radiation therapy for recurrent spinal and sacral chordoma

| Authors | Year | Number of patients (*n*) | Treatment/ radiation modality | Median radiation dose | Local control | Survival rate | Findings |
|---|---|---|---|---|---|---|---|
| Zabel-du Bois A et al. [11] | 2010 | 17 | IMRT (± surgery) | >60 Gy (14 pts); <60 Gy (3 pts) | ~24% 5-year LC rate | 74% at median follow-up of 4.5 years | LC rate drop significantly with IMRT as a salvage therapy for recurrent chordoma. However, OS rate are not statistically different. |
| Yamada Y, et al. [32] | 2013 | 4 | Single Fraction Photon RT/SRS | 24 Gy in 1 fraction | Not reported for the 4 patients with recurrent chordomas (>95% 2-year LC rate (only 1 patient in the entire study had a recurrence but unclear if this patient was *de novo* disease vs a previous recurrence)) | Not reported for the 4 patients with recurrent chordomas (>67% 2-year OS rate (8 of total 24 patients (33%) in this study died at a median follow-up of 24 months. However, it is unclear if these patients were part of the 8 pts that received true adjuvant therapy for *de novo* disease)) | Single-fraction SRS provided tumor control as a salvage therapy. |

*Key: Gy* gray, *IMRT* intensity-modulated radiotherapy, *LC* local control, *OS* overall survival, *RT* radiotherapy, *SRS* stereotactic radiosurgery

**Table 14.3** Systematic literature review for primary radiation therapy for primary/de novo spinal and sacral chordoma

| Authors | Year | Number of patients (*n*) | Treatment/ radiation modality | Median radiation dose | Local control | Survival rate | Findings |
|---|---|---|---|---|---|---|---|
| Catton C et al. [10] | 1996 | 17 | Conventional RT | <60 Gy | No report for 17 patient who underwent biopsy alone with primary/*de novo* disease | No report for 17 patient who underwent biopsy alone with primary/*de novo* disease | Higher definitive radiation dose needed to achieve LC with RT alone as primary treatment |
| Rich TA et al. [9] | 1985 | 15 | Conventional RT | 40 Gy | No report for 15 patient who underwent biopsy alone with primary/*de novo* disease | No report for 15 patient who underwent biopsy alone with primary/*de novo* disease | Survival does not appear to be better in the group treated with partial or subtotal excision and radiation (range, 2.5–7.5 years) compared to patients treated with radiation alone after biopsy (range, 2.5–10.5 years). |
| Zabel-du Bois A et al. [11] | 2010 | 4 | IMRT | >60 Gy (14 pts); <60 Gy (3 pts) | No report for 4 patient who underwent biopsy alone with primary/*de novo* disease | No report for 4 patient who underwent biopsy alone with primary/*de novo* disease | There was a trend towards higher LC in patients treated after surgery compared to those treated with primary radiotherapy (42% versus 20%, $p = 0.592$), as well as a trend towards higher overall survival in these patients (83% versus 60%, $p = 0.192$) |
| Yamada Y, et al. [32] | 2013 | 7 | Single Fraction Photon RT/ SRS | 24 Gy in 1 fraction | 54% 2-year LC rate | No report for 13 patient who underwent biopsy alone with primary/*de novo* disease | Single-fraction SRS provide a treatment option in patients who are not candidates for wide-margin excision. Also, when used preoperatively, it can improve local control rate for sacral tumors that often spread along soft-tissue planes toward the ischial spine. |

*Key*: *Gy* gray, *LC* local control, *RT* radiotherapy, *SRS* stereotactic radiosurgery the radiation is spread out over hundreds of beams of radiation. One advantage of IMRT is that the skin dose with IMRT is much lower than typical proton beam treatment plans, which often utilize only a few beams and thus result in higher doses to the skin where the beams enter the patient, an important consideration for surgical wound complications.

The photon IMRT dose escalation experience closely mirrors that which has been well reported in the proton experience. This is not surprising since it is thought that the biologic impact of protons and photons is similar. IMRT offers the possibility for an integrated boost concept for dose escalation. In one series, 34 patients with sacral chordoma were treated with IMRT for primary or recurrent disease in both postoperative and definitive settings, with a median total dose to the boost volume (PTV2) of 66 Gy with 2 Gy per fraction using an integrated boost concept20. Median dose to target volume (PTV1) was 54 Gy in 1.8 Gy. Local control was significantly higher in doses >60 Gy (median total dose 66 Gy) with only moderate side effects of radiotherapy, and patients receiving >60 Gy showed a significantly improved overall survival (85% versus 43%, $p < 0.049$) after a median follow-up of 4.5 years [11]. In this mixed cohort of 34 patients with primary and recurrent chordomas treated with IMRT, the group actuarial local control was projected to be 79%, 55%, and 27% after 1, 2, and 5 years, respectively; in addition, the overall survival was projected to be 97%, 91%, and 70% at 1, 2, and 5 years, respectively. Comparatively, the Princess Margaret Hospital reported a cumulative incidence of local failure of 34% at 5 years for chordomas when the dose was escalated to median of 76 Gy with IMRT treatment techniques [12]. These data indicate that local control after IMRT for chordomas is improved using sophisticated radiotherapy techniques that enable dose escalation regardless of resection status.

## High-Dose Single-Fraction or Hypofractionated Photon Therapy

With the emergence of image-guided radiation therapy (IGRT), it has become possible to ablate tumors with high radiation doses using stereotactic techniques to limited target volumes with less morbidity. While conventional fractionation refers to treatment schedules that provide RT in doses of 1.8-2Gy per fraction, high-dose per fraction RT (typically 6Gy or higher in a limited number of fractions) is termed hypofractionation. When stereotactic treatment techniques are used to deliver hypofractionated treatment, it is commonly referred to as stereotactic body radiation therapy (SBRT). The use of advanced image-guided technology has greatly improved the precision of treatment, reducing the amount of high-dose radiation given to normal tissues surrounding the tumor to 2 mm or less [13, 14]. For example, these steep dose gradients can now be applied to treating gross tumor to 24 Gy in a single fraction while maintaining the spinal cord dose to less than 14 Gy. Onboard cone beam CT technology provides near real-time information about organ and tumor position during treatment delivery, ensuring that the planned treatment is given to the right place in the intended way [13].

SBRT offers biologic advantages by delivering a high biologically effective dose, significantly increasing the probability of lethal damage to tumor cells, and rendering tumors relatively resistant to conventionally fractionated treatment very responsive to hypofractionated RT [13]. Additionally, SBRT causes increased endothelial cell apoptosis within the tumor, contributing to death of the tumor, a phenomenon only seen with high-dose per fraction therapy [13]. With ultrahigh-dose SBRT where doses per fraction exceed 8–9 Gy, the biologic effectiveness of the radiation may increase in an exponential fashion.

The application of SBRT in the form of stereotactic radiosurgery (SRS) (single fraction) or hypofractionated RT (<5 fractions) to the treatment of spine tumors has steadily increased in recent years. This has translated into durable local control outcomes in patients with spine metastases, even for conventionally radioresistant solid tumor histologies [14–17]. Chordomas are considered resistant to conventionally fractionated RT, which is thought to be due to its ability to repair radiation-injured DNA [18]. Applying high doses per fraction to the treatment of chordoma similarly offers biological advantages, by causing irreparable lethal DNA damage. There is a growing body of literature that supports the use of SRS and SBRT for the treatment of spinal and sacral chordomas in the definitive, preoperative, postoperative, and salvage settings.

## Definitive SBRT

In cases where surgery is not feasible or the sequelae of definitive surgery are not acceptable to patients, definitive RT is also able to provide durable tumor control. Single-fraction spine SRS can provide long-term local control in greater than 90% of cases for typically radioresistant metastatic tumors such as renal cell carcinoma and melanoma [15–17]. SRS for chordoma can also provide a similar likelihood of durable local control [19].

A clear pattern of improved local control with escalating doses is also apparent in SRS studies. Investigators at the Cleveland Clinic utilized a prescribed dose of 16Gy in a single fraction and found that 3 of 8 patients developed local relapse at a median follow-up of under 10 months [20]. A 10% improvement in local relapse-free survival was found when escalating the dose from 18Gy to 24Gy. In a study done at the Memorial Sloan Kettering Cancer Center, 35 patients with primary chordoma of the mobile spine ($n = 17$) and sacrum ($n = 18$) underwent single-fraction SRS with a median post-SRS follow-up of 38.8 months [19]. The median prescribed dose was 24Gy single fraction. Figure 14.1 is a representative dose distribution. Overall, 12 patients (33%) underwent definitive SRS, and 23 patients (66%) underwent surgery with either neo- or postoperative adjuvant SRS. Definitive SRS was selectively used to treat both sacral ($n = 7$) and mobile-spine ($n = 5$) chordomas. The median PTV volume was 156 mL (range: 29–904 mL). Dosimetrically, tumor coverage was excellent with the median PTV V95 of 99.5% (82–100%). Overall, the 1-, 3-, and 5-year local relapse-free survival (LRFS) rates were 97.1% [95% Confidence Interval (CI): 91.4–100], 86.2% [95% CI: 73.6–98.9], and 80.5% [95% CI:

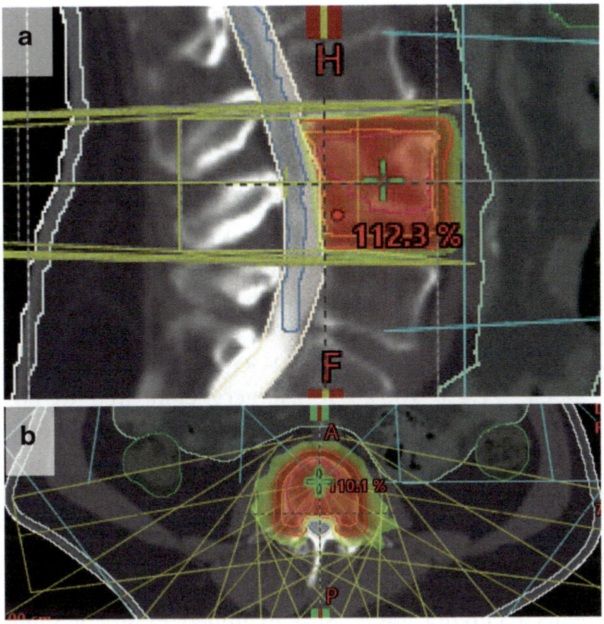


**Fig. 14.1** Stereotactic radiosurgery dose distribution for a L4 chordoma. The prescribe dose is 2400 cGy in a single fraction. (**a**) illustrates the plan in the sagittal plane and (**b**) illustrates the plan in the axial plane

64.4–96.5], respectively. In parallel, the 1-, 3-, and 5-year overall survival rates were 97.1% [95% CI: 91.4–100], 90.0% [95% CI: 79.1–100], and 84.3% [95% CI: 69.6–99.1], respectively. Among a subset of 32 patients receiving 24 Gy (91%), there were no recurrences in the first year. The 3- and 5-year LRFS were 10% higher than the overall cohort: 96.3% [95% CI: 89.2–100] and 89.9% [95% CI: 76–100], respectively. Three patients developed recurrence at the treatment site (9%) with a median time to local progression of 5.0 years [2.1–5.6]. Four patients developed metastatic disease (11%) to the lymphatics, lung, liver, and bone, at a median time to distant progression of 5.1 years (range 1.0–10.2), with no evidence of local disease recurrence in half of these cases. Regarding the relationship between tumor control probability and volume of disease, the three patients who had in-field disease recurrences had an average tumor volume of 110 mL, only slightly larger compared to 95 mL for the entire cohort [19].

The symptom response rate to treatment was 88% for pain and radiculopathy [19]. Extent or type of surgery was not associated with LRFS, overall survival, or symptom response rates ($p > 0.05$), but en bloc resection was associated with higher CTCAE v. 5.0 surgical toxicity compared to epidural decompression and curettage/intralesional resection ($p = 0.03$). The long-term ≥Grade 2 SRS toxicity rate was 31%, including 20% Grade 3 tissue necrosis, recurrent laryngeal nerve palsy, myelopathy, fracture, and secondary malignancy. These results illustrate that SRS represents an effective and durable treatment option for newly diagnosed chordomas.

## Preoperative SBRT

In a subset of 18 patients with sacral chordomas in the Memorial Sloan Kettering Cancer Center study, 15 patients were given neoadjuvant SRS with plans for surgery [19]. All 15 of these patients were treated with 24Gy single fraction. Four patients declined surgery after SRS because of rapid resolution of symptoms and early radiographic tumor response. Therefore, 11 received preoperative SRS, and 7 received SRS alone. Outcomes for neoadjuvant SRS followed by en bloc sacrectomy with the goal of achieving wide margins and SRS alone were not significantly different, although limited by the small number of events. The LRFS hazard ratio (HR) for surgery vs SRS alone was 0.28 [95% CI: 0.03–3.10], $p = 0.30$, and the overall survival HR was 0.56 [95% CI: 0.04–9.06], $p = 0.69$. The 3-year LRFS rate was 90% [95% CI: 71.4%–100%] for surgery compared to 68.6% [95% CI: 32.1%–100%] for SRS alone. Among the 11 sacral chordoma patients who were able to achieve en bloc resection with wide or marginal margins after preoperative SBRT, the local control rate was 100%. Three patients with sacral tumors were treated with definitive SRS alone, but were given lower doses (18, 20, and 21Gy), due to the proximity of bowel to meet dose constraints. There was one recurrence in the sacrum, and that patient was treated with definitive 18Gy SRS alone [19]. Chordoma patients receiving 24Gy SRS exhibited excellent tumor control outcomes, and lower doses are probably inadequate to control larger extent of disease. This data suggests that high-dose SRS given in the neoadjuvant setting results in excellent local tumor control, and one quarter of patients were able to avoid surgery.

## Postoperative SBRT

RT is often recommended after incomplete surgical intervention for the treatment of chordomas of the mobile spine and sacrum. Emerging long-term follow suggests that high-dose spine SRS provides durable local control for patients who undergo intralesional surgery [19, 21]. A cohort of 11 patients at MSKCC with mobile spine chordomas underwent adjuvant SBRT, following separation surgery ($n = 7$) and curettage, intralesional gross-total resection ($n = 4$) 27. Five of these patients underwent phosphorus 32 dural brachytherapy at the time of surgery, indicative of high-grade epidural disease at the time of presentation. The use of intraoperative phosphorus-32 (P32) plaques to deliver high doses superficially at the surgical margin where radiation treatment of dural tumor involvement would be complicated by tolerance of the spinal cord has previously been described [22]. Epidural decompression in these select cases was followed by intraoperative P32 brachytherapy. Flexible epoxy polymer plaques impregnated with the P32 isotope were placed on the surgical dural margin(s) identified at risk. A dose of 10 Gy was delivered to a 1 mm depth; the percent depth dose was <1% at 4 mm from the prescription depth. Among five patients with mobile spine chordomas treated with intraoperative P32 plaque brachytherapy following epidural decompression or curettage, the LC rate was 100% [19]. The two patients treated with 24Gy SRS following separation surgery, without P32 plaque brachytherapy, all developed local recurrence [19].

Overall, among the subset of 17 patients with mobile spine chordomas, when stratified according to the extent of surgery, the 3-year LRFS and OS rates were 75% [95% CI: 32.6%–100%] with separation surgery, 100% for curettage/intralesional resection, and 100% for SRS alone [19]. This data demonstrates that after separation surgery or intralesional surgery, a planned postoperative adjuvant approach provides hope of durable cure in patients who are unsuitable for en bloc surgery at diagnosis [19, 21].

## Salvage SBRT

Chordomas are known to have high rates of local recurrence and potential for metastases, with limited options for effective salvage. Spine SBRT outcomes support exploration of its role in the re-irradiation of these conventionally radioresistant tumors with or without combination surgery.

In one investigation, seven patients who had been treated at other institutions with surgery and prior radiation underwent salvage surgery and SBRT (salvage therapy) at Memorial Sloan Kettering Cancer Center [21]. The local control rate was 57.1%, and the median follow-up duration was 10.7 months. The mean actuarial estimations of overall survival were 68.6 months (95% CI 32–104.6 months). One patient required repeat irradiation. Major surgery- and radiation-related complications occurred in 18% and 27% of patients, respectively [21].

In another recent analysis from Memorial Sloan Kettering Cancer Center, 16 patients with recurrent chordomas of the mobile spine ($n$ = 6) and sacrum ($n$ = 5) underwent re-RT with SBRT in 1–5 fractions [19]. Three (19%) underwent definitive SBRT, seven (44%) underwent adjuvant SBRT postoperatively, and six (38%) were treated with palliative SBRT in the setting of metastatic disease with a median post-SBRT follow-up of 2.3 years. Overall, the median LRFS was 2.7 years (95% CI: 0.6–5.1), and the median overall survival was 3.2 y (0.6–6.4). The LRFS and overall survival rates were 75.0% (95% CI 53.8–96.2) at 1 year and 60.6% (95% CI 35.7–85.5) at 2 years. Among ten patients with localized disease, the LRFS/overall survival rates were 90.0% (95% CI: 71.4–100.0%) at 1 year and 80.0% (95% CI: 55.2–100.0%) at 2 years, respectively. No patients had >Grade 2 acute toxicity. The long-term ≥Grade 2 toxicity rate was 38%, including 19% Grade 3 neuropathy, fracture, and rectosigmoid ulceration. No patients had >Grade 3 late toxicities [19]. In this study, it was shown that re-irradiation with spine SBRT with or without combination surgery offers the chance of radiographic control and effective symptom relief.

## Toxicity

A gain in local tumor control with high-dose radiosurgery must be balanced with a higher rate of complications when considering whether ablative therapy should be employed. The patients reported by the Cleveland Clinic, with a median dose of 16Gy, reported no toxicity [20], whereas patients at Memorial Sloan Kettering

Cancer Center receiving a median dose of 24Gy experienced up to 31% long-term Grade 2–3 (CTCAE vs 5) complications, with 17% of patients experiencing Grade 3 toxicity [19]. The specific complications of SRS reflected tumor location, in relation to local organs at risk. The acute CTCAE Grade 2 toxicity rate was 40%, including dermatitis, myositis, mucositis, xerostomia, odynophagia, esophagitis, dysphagia, and nausea. No patients experienced acute ≥ Grade 3 RT toxicity. Long-term ≥ Grade 2 toxicity occurred in 11 patients (31%), including 7 (20%) with Grade 3 toxicity: soft tissue necrosis, osteonecrosis, recurrent laryngeal nerve palsy, myelopathy, spinal fracture, erectile dysfunction, and treatment-related secondary malignancy [19].

Although not specific to chordoma patients, long-term toxicity has been reported for high-dose spine radiosurgery. In a single institutional experience, 31 patients with 36 spinal segments were treated with high-dose SRS (24Gy) [16]. This cohort of patients survived at least 5 years after treatment and was followed up radiographically and clinically for a median of 6.1 years (maximum 102 months). Ten lesions (27.8%) were associated with acute Grade 1 cutaneous or gastrointestinal toxicity. Delayed toxicity ≥3 months after treatment included eight cases (22.2%) of mild neuropathy, two (5.6%) of gastrointestinal discomfort, eight (22.2%) of dermatitides, and three (8.3%) of myalgias/myositis. Thirteen treated levels (36.1%) in 12 patients demonstrated progressive vertebral body collapse or endplate fractures at a median of 25.7 months (range 11.6–76.0), of which 5 (14%) became symptomatic and subsequently required percutaneous cement augmentation or surgery [16]. Patients treated with SRS for primary and metastatic spinal tumors within the vicinity of the esophagus can suffer Grade 3 or higher esophageal complications, and care should be exercised when irradiating large thoracic chordomas that may involve the esophagus [23]. Long-term reports of spine SRS have reported spinal cord injury to be less than 1% [17].

## Future Directions

These data suggest promising trends for chordomas treated with high-dose regimens. SRS has emerged as an integral component of modern paradigms for the treatment of spinal tumors. Based on the experience of the Memorial Sloan-Kettering group using 24Gy as a single-fraction to treat chordoma, SRS may have a role as a neoadjuvant or adjuvant treatment in patients undergoing surgery or as the primary treatment for de novo chordomas [19]. Though this study has a mixed cohort of primary, metastatic, and recurrent chordomas, their report of a >95% 2-year local control rate after a median follow-up of 24 months should prompt further investigation on the use of single-fraction photon RT as a viable opt for recurrent chordoma [19]. SRS remains to be evaluated in comparison with proton and carbon ion treatments. Future studies will fully assess long-term SRS outcomes in recurrent chordomas, which are managed differently and likely have more unfavorable tumor biology. Given the aggressive tumor biology, even after optimal local control is obtained, the propensity for metastases must also be addressed to substantially change survival in the treatment of chordoma. In a study by Bergh et al., local control was significantly associated with an increased risk of metastasis and tumor-related death; thus as local control improves, better methods to control systemic disease become more significant [24]. Currently, a phase I/II trial of combined immunotherapy (nivolumab) and SBRT is ongoing. This trial is studying the effect of immunotherapy and high-dose per fraction radiation therapy on patients with recurrent and previously irradiated chordoma (NCT02989636). Additionally, a phase II trial combining a yeast-brachyury vaccine and radiation has completed accrual (NCT02383498).

The success of radiation may lead to a modification of the role of surgery. Data on marginal recurrence rates despite aggressive and frequently technically challenging operations indicate that a less morbid modality of chordoma treatment that provides more consistent tumor control is needed. Risks of en bloc resection include gait disturbance, bladder/bowel dysfunction, structural instability, prolonged hospital length of stay, and increased rate of complications [25–27]. With the growing body of literature supporting dose-escalated SBRT, en bloc resection may no longer be necessary to achieve tumor control, and surgery can be limited to spinal stabilization and epidural decompression in many cases to limit significant morbidity without sacrificing local control. Patients who present with surgically incurable disease may still have an opportunity for curative treatment when given high-dose IMRT or radiosurgery.

## References

1. van Wulfften Palthe ODR, Tromp I, Ferreira A, Fiore A, Bramer JAM, van Dijk NC, DeLaney TF, Schwab JH, Hornicek FJ. Sacral chordoma: a clinical review of 101 cases with 30-year experience in a single institution. Spine J. 2019;19:869–79.
2. Chen KW, Yang HL, Lu J, Liu JY, Chen XQ. Prognostic factors of sacral chordoma after surgical therapy: a study of 36 patients. Spinal Cord. 2010;48:166–71.
3. Fuchs B, Dickey ID, Yaszemski MJ, Inwards CY, Sim FH. Operative management of sacral chordoma. J Bone Joint Surg Am. 2005;87:2211–6.
4. Osaka S, Kodoh O, Sugita H, Osaka E, Yoshida Y, Ryu J. Clinical significance of a wide excision policy for sacrococcygeal chordoma. J Cancer Res Clin Oncol. 2006;132:213–8.
5. Hulen CA, Temple HT, Fox WP, Sama AA, Green BA, Eismont FJ. Oncologic and functional outcome following sacrectomy for sacral chordoma. J Bone Jt Surg. 2006;88:1532–9.
6. Di Maio S, Al Zhrani GA, Al Otaibi FE, Alturki A, Kong E, Yip S, Rostomily R. Novel targeted therapies in chordoma: an update. Ther Clin Risk Manag. 2015;11:873.
7. Rotondo RL, Folkert W, Liebsch NJ, et al. High-dose proton-based radiation therapy in the management of spine chordomas: outcomes and clinicopathological prognostic factors. J Neurosurg Spine. 2015;23:788–97.
8. Bjornsson J, Wold LE, Ebersold MJ, Laws ER. Chordoma of the mobile spine. A clinicopathologic analysis of 40 patients. Cancer. 1993;71:735–40.
9. Rich TA, Schiller A, Suit HD, Mankin HJ. Clinical and pathologic review of 48 cases of chordoma. Cancer. 1985;56:182–7.
10. Catton C, O'Sullivan B, Bell R, Laperriere N, Cummings B, Fornasier V, Wunder J. Chordoma: long-term follow-up after radical photon irradiation. Radiother Oncol. 1996;41:67–72.

11. Zabel-du Bois A, Nikoghosyan A, Schwahofer A, Huber P, Schlegel W, Debus J, Milker-Zabel S. Intensity modulated radiotherapy in the management of sacral chordoma in primary versus recurrent disease. Radiother Oncol. 2010;97:408–12.
12. Sahgal A, Chan MW, Atenafu EG, et al. Image-guided, intensity-modulated radiation therapy (IG-IMRT) for skull base chordoma and chondrosarcoma: preliminary outcomes. Neuro-Oncology. 2015;17:889–94.
13. Katsoulakis E, Kumar K, Laufer I, Yamada Y. Stereotactic body radiotherapy in the treatment of spinal metastases. Semin Radiat Oncol. 2017;27:209–17.
14. Yamada Y, Lovelock DM, Yenice KM, Bilsky MH, Hunt MA, Zatcky J, Leibel SA. Multifractionated image-guided and stereotactic intensity-modulated radiotherapy of paraspinal tumors: a preliminary report. Int J Radiat Oncol. 2005;62:53–61.
15. Yamada Y, Bilsky MH, Lovelock DM, Venkatraman ES, Toner S, Johnson J, Zatcky J, Zelefsky MJ, Fuks Z. High-dose, single-fraction image-guided intensity-modulated radiotherapy for metastatic spinal lesions. Int J Radiat Oncol. 2008;71:484–90.
16. Moussazadeh N, Lis E, Katsoulakis E, Kahn S, Svoboda M, DiStefano NM, McLaughlin L, Bilsky MH, Yamada Y, Laufer I. Five-year outcomes of high-dose single-fraction spinal stereotactic radiosurgery. Int J Radiat Oncol. 2015;93:361–7.
17. Yamada Y, Katsoulakis E, Laufer I, et al. The impact of histology and delivered dose on local control of spinal metastases treated with stereotactic radiosurgery. Neurosurg Focus. 2017;42:E6.
18. Cheng EY, Özerdemoglu RA, Transfeldt EE, Thompson RC. Lumbosacral Chordoma: prognostic factors and treatment. Spine (Phila Pa 1976). 1999;24:1639.
19. Jin CJ, Berry-Candelario J, Reiner AS, et al. Long-term outcomes of high-dose single-fraction radiosurgery for chordomas of the spine and sacrum. J Neurosurg Spine. 2020;32:79–88.
20. Jung EW, Jung DL, Balagamwala EH, Angelov L, Suh JH, Djemil T, Magnelli A, Chao ST. Single-fraction spine stereotactic body radiation therapy for the treatment of Chordoma. Technol Cancer Res Treat. 2017;16:302–9.
21. Lockney DT, Shub T, Hopkins B, et al. Spinal stereotactic body radiotherapy following intralesional curettage with separation surgery for initial or salvage chordoma treatment. Neurosurg Focus. 2017;42:E4.
22. Folkert MR, Bilsky MH, Cohen GN, Zaider M, Dauer LT, Cox BW, Boland PJ, Laufer I, Yamada Y. Intraoperative 32P high-dose rate brachytherapy of the dura for recurrent primary and metastatic intracranial and spinal tumors. Neurosurgery. 2012;71:1003–11.
23. Cox BW, Jackson A, Hunt M, Bilsky M, Yamada Y. Esophageal toxicity from high-dose, single-fraction Paraspinal stereotactic radiosurgery. Int J Radiat Oncol. 2012;83:e661–7.
24. Bergh P, Kindblom L-G, Gunterberg BB, Remotti F, Ryd W, Meis-Kindblom JM. Prognostic factors in chordoma of the sacrum and mobile spine: a study of 39 patients. Cancer. 2000;88:2122–34.
25. Fourney DR, Rhines LD, Hentschel SJ, Skibber JM, Wolinsky J-P, Weber KL, Suki D, Gallia GL, Garonzik I, Gokaslan ZL. En bloc resection of primary sacral tumors: classification of surgical approaches and outcome. J Neurosurg Spine. 2005;3:111–22.
26. Guo Y, Palmer JL, Shen L, Kaur G, Willey J, Zhang T, Bruera E, Wolinsky J-P, Gokaslan ZL. Bowel and bladder continence, wound healing, and functional outcomes in patients who underwent sacrectomy. J Neurosurg Spine. 2005;3:106–10.
27. Sciubba DM, Nelson C, Gok B, McGirt MJ, McLoughlin GS, Noggle JC, Wolinsky JP, Witham TF, Bydon A, Gokaslan ZL. Evaluation of factors associated with postoperative infection following sacral tumor resection. J Neurosurg Spine. 2008;9:593–9.
28. Terezakis SA, Lovelock DM, Bilsky MH, Hunt MA, Zatcky J, Yamada Y. Image-guided intensity-modulated photon radiotherapy using multifractionated regimen to paraspinal chordomas and rare sarcomas. Int J Radiat Oncol Biol Phys 2007;69(5):1502–8.
29. Thieblemont C, Biron P, Rocher F, Bouhour D, Bobin JY, Gérard JP, Blay JY. Prognostic factors in chordoma: role of postoperative radiotherapy. Eur J Cancer 1995;31A(13-14):2255–9.

30. Berson AM, Castro JR, Petti P, Phillips TL, Gauger GE, Gutin P, Collier JM, Henderson SD, Baken K. Charged particle irradiation of chordoma and chondrosarcoma of the base of skull and cervical spine: the Lawrence Berkeley Laboratory experience. Int J Radiat Oncol Biol Phys 1988;15(3):559–65.
31. Romero J, Cardenes H, la Torre A, Valcarcel F, Magallon R, Regueiro C, Aragon G. Chordoma: results of radiation therapy in eighteen patients. Radiother Oncol 1993;29(1):27–32..
32. Yamada Y, Laufer I, Cox BW, Lovelock DM, Maki RG, Zatcky JM, Boland PJ, Bilsky MH. Preliminary results of high-dose single-fraction radiotherapy for the management of chordomas of the spine and sacrum. Neurosurgery 2013;73(4):673–80; discussion 680.

# Heavy Particle Therapy for Chordoma

15

## Heavy Particle Therapy

David J. Konieczkowski, Reiko Imai,
and Thomas F. DeLaney

## Abbreviations

| | |
|---|---|
| CI | Confidence interval |
| CIRT | Carbon ion radiotherapy |
| CTV | Clinical target volume |
| DFS | Disease-free survival |
| DS | Double scatter |
| Fx | Fraction |
| GTV | Gross tumor volume |
| Gy | Gray |
| IMRT | Intensity-modulated RT |
| LC | Local control |
| LR | Local recurrence |
| NCDB | National Cancer Database |
| OER | Oxygen enhancement ratio |
| OS | Overall survival |
| PBS | Pencil-beam scanning |

D. J. Konieczkowski
Department of Radiation Oncology, Arthur G. James Cancer Center and Richard J. Solove Research Institute, The Ohio State University Comprehensive Cancer Center, Columbus, OH, USA

R. Imai
QST Hospital, Quantum Medical Science Directorate, National Institute for Quantum and Radiological Sciences and Technology, Chiba, Japan

T. F. DeLaney (✉)
Department of Radiation Oncology, Massachusetts General Hospital, Harvard Medical School, Boston, MA, USA
e-mail: tdelaney@mgh.harvard.edu



D. M. Sciubba, J. H. Schwab (eds.), *Chordoma of the Spine*,
https://doi.org/10.1007/978-3-030-76201-8_15

| | |
|---|---|
| PFS | Progression-free survival |
| PTV | Planning target volume |
| RBE | Relative biological effectiveness |
| RFS | Recurrence-free survival |
| RT | Radiotherapy |
| VMAT | Volumetric arc therapy |

## Introduction

Surgery has been the foundation of curative-intent treatment for localized chordoma of the spine and sacrum [1], but local control following surgery alone remains unsatisfactory, with rates of local recurrence reported between 30 and 40% [2–4]. Local failure is in turn a risk factor for distant metastatic recurrence [5], and for this reason, radiation therapy (RT) as a surgical adjuvant has been explored with the goal of increasing local control (reviewed in [6]). Of particular interest are heavy particle therapies—proton beam and carbon ion beam radiotherapy—which have the potential of delivering high, therapeutic doses to the oncologic target while minimizing irradiation of adjacent healthy tissues. Here we review the science behind charged particle therapy, highlight the current evidence for its use in both the surgical adjuvant and curative-intent roles, and identify areas for continued investigation.

## Basis for Adjuvant Radiotherapy in the Treatment of Chordoma

The relative rarity of chordoma has precluded the evaluation of RT in a randomized prospective study, yet evidence from large retrospective studies and single-arm prospective studies show promising results. For example, a National Cancer Database (NCDB) analysis demonstrated an OS benefit to adjuvant RT for patients with R1 (i.e., microscopically positive) margins [7], and a multi-institutional analysis likewise showed a trend toward improved local control (LC) in patients treated with adjuvant RT $\geq$ 70 Gy. Importantly, this difference was significant for patients with an R1 margin, suggesting that there is a clinically significant difference for those with potentially contaminated margins [8]. Most strikingly, multiple prospective studies of perioperative RT have demonstrated LC rates of around 80% at 5 years [9–11]. RT is also attractive as a curative-intent treatment for patients not undergoing surgery, with multiple series demonstrating promising local control in this context [11–13].

Despite the promise of radiotherapy to improve LC, RT for spinal chordomas is challenging because the radiation doses necessary for tumor killing exceed the radiation tolerance of nearby organs at risk. For example, while conventional spinal cord radiation tolerance is set at 45 Gy, doses of approximately 70 Gy are required in the perioperative setting; still higher doses are needed for unresected disease [7,

8]. Thus, the fundamental challenge in radiotherapy of chordomas is how to deliver an oncologically adequate dose of RT while respecting normal tissue radiation tolerance.

New advanced radiation modalities, such as stereotactic body RT (SBRT), proton therapy, and carbon ion radiotherapy (CIRT), may overcome this challenge. In addition to the promising outcomes from individual studies described below, a recent NCDB analysis has suggested that these techniques yield markedly superior outcomes in chordoma compared to conventional RT. [7] SBRT, which is discussed in Chap. 14, fundamentally relies on technological advancements including improved dose conformality and target localization to enable successful RT for chordomas using photons [14]. In contrast, proton and carbon ion RT leverage the physical properties of charged particles to limit RT dose to spinal cord and other organs at risk. This chapter will discuss the role of charged particle therapy in the management of spine and sacral chordomas.

Because of the complexities of care for this tumor, which may require very technically demanding surgery, high radiation doses in close proximity to critical normal tissues, and complex and prolonged rehabilitation, the Chordoma Foundation recommends that all chordoma patients seek care at a medical center with a multidisciplinary team of experts who have substantial experience treating chordoma patients (https://www.chordomafoundation.org/). Due to the potential magnitude of the impact of treatment on the patient's life and quality of life, the Chordoma Foundation also states that "every chordoma patient should be able to make informed decisions that will lead to the best possible outcomes."

## Protons and Carbon Ions

Charged particles such as protons and carbon ions have a fundamental physical advantage over photons for RT. In simplest terms, charged particles deliver dose to the target volume and then stop, whereas photons continue through the patient. More formally, photons deliver dose along the entire beam path—from patient entrance to exit—according to an exponential decay function. While modern technologies such as intensity-modulated RT (IMRT) or volumetric arc therapy (VMAT) can limit high doses to an area highly conformal to intended target volume, a significant volume of tissue is still exposed to medium and low doses of radiation (i.e., <50% of the target dose) [15]. In contrast, charged particles lose energy continuously in tissue; when their energy is reduced to zero, they stop and deposit nearly all of their dose at this point. This "Bragg peak" phenomenon means that charged particles deliver no "exit dose" beyond the target volume, sparing distal uninvolved tissues and reducing integral dose to the patient by up to 50–60% (Fig. 15.1) [16].

There are two fundamentally different technologies for conforming the proton or carbon ion dose to the target volume. The first, and original, technology is passive scattering. Here, a narrow proton beam is scattered in the x and y dimensions via two scattering foils in the beam path (hence, "double scattering" (DS)) into a wide and uniform beam, then conformed to the target volume in these same dimensions

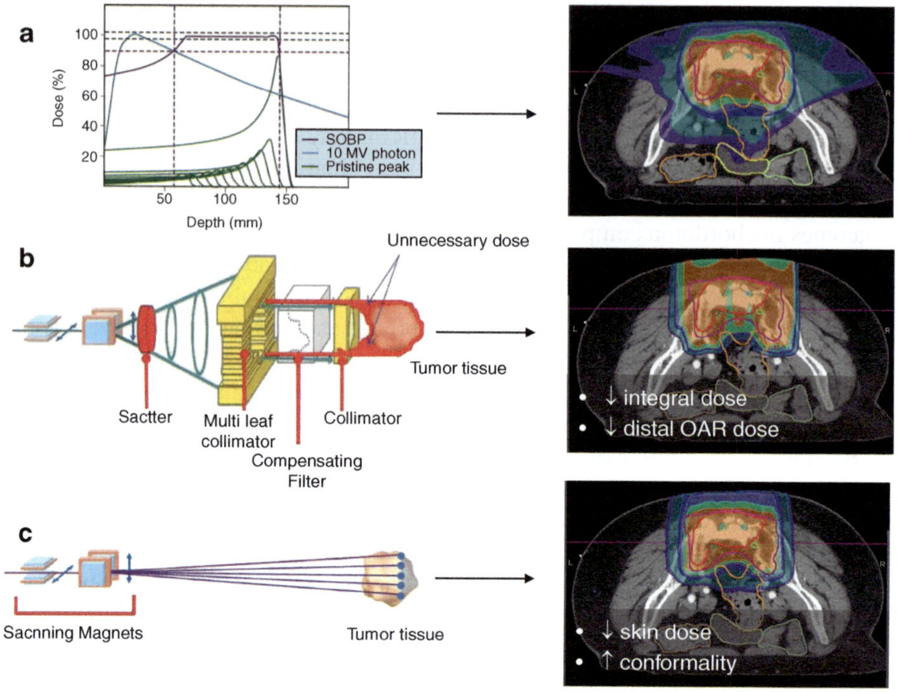


**Fig. 15.1** Photon and proton RT for chordoma. (**a**) Photons deposit dose throughout the beam path (left), leading to low-dose bath around the target volume (right). In contrast, protons deposit dose up until the Bragg peak and then stop (left). (**b**) In double scatter (DS) proton therapy, the proton beam is passively scattered by primary and secondary scattering foils in the X and Y directions, given lateral conformality by a collimation device and given distal conformality by a range compensator. Compared to photon therapy, DS protons reduce integral dose to the patient, particularly to organs at risk distal to the target volume in the beam path. (**c**) In pencil beam scanned (PBS) proton therapy, the proton beam is actively steered by magnets in the X and Y directions. Each voxel of the tumor at a given depth is "painted" before the beam energy is stepped and the next layer treated. Compared to DS protons, PBS protons improve conformality of the high dose to the target volume, particularly proximally, which reduces skin dose [6]

via a collimation device (aperture or multi-leaf collimator), then conformed to the distal contour of the target volume by a range compensator [17]. However, DS is unable to conform dose to the proximal contour of the target volume; thus, its ability to spare normal tissue proximal to the target, such as skin or spinal cord, is very limited.

The second, more modern, technology is pencil-beam scanning (PBS). Here, the narrow ("pencil") beam is not passively scattered but rather actively scanned with magnets in the x and y dimensions, "painting" each voxel of tumor at a given depth [18]. The beam energy is then modulated to treat the next depth layer. Compared to DS, PBS achieves much improved conformality of dose to the proximal aspect of the target volume; conformality of the high-dose region in other dimensions is also somewhat superior.

Within charged particle therapies, carbon ions have certain further physical advantages over protons. Carbon ions are approximately 12 times more massive than protons; this leads to a sharper lateral penumbra (due to reduced multiple coulomb scattering) at the expense of some increased dose beyond the Bragg peak (due to greater downstream fragmentation of the carbon nucleus) [19]. In addition to these physical properties, however, carbon therapy also has potential biological advantages [20]. Compared to both proton and photon therapy, carbon ions have a higher linear energy transfer (LET); that is, they create more ionization events per given length of beam path. This in turn leads to more tightly clustered DNA breaks, causing more tumor cell killing for a given physical radiation dose (i.e., higher relative biological effectiveness [RBE]), and less dependence of tumor cell killing on oxygenation (i.e., lower oxygen enhancement ratio [OER]). Because chordomas are both hypoxic and radioresistant, these properties may be particularly advantageous in this setting.

## Technical Aspects of Heavy Particle RT

### Simulation and Treatment Planning

RT for chordomas requires careful attention to technical details of simulation, target delineation, treatment planning, and radiation delivery.

Pre- and postoperative MRI are required, including T1 post-contrast images (to delineate gross tumor) and T2 (STIR or similar) images (to delineate peri-tumoral edema suspicious for subclinical/microscopic spread, as well as the thecal sac and spinal cord). Ideally, these sequences should be acquired in axial, sagittal, and coronal planes.

All patient should undergo CT simulation with IV contrast. For those with tumors at spinal cord level (L2 or above), contrast myelography at simulation is also helpful to define both the thecal sac (which is typically a barrier to tumor spread and can be excluded from the target volume) and the spinal cord (which is typically the most critical organ at risk). Where available, MR simulation (i.e., MR obtained in the treatment position with the immobilization devices that will be used during treatment) may be a promising alternative to CT simulation with myelography.

Immobilization should aim to achieve (a) rigidity (i.e., minimal motion during each fraction), (b) reproducibility (i.e., minimal motion between fractions), and (c) patient tolerability. While there are many reasonable approaches, our institutional practice is as follows. Cervical and upper thoracic spine tumors are simulated supine under a shoulder-length thermoplastic mask. Lower thoracic and lumbosacral tumors can be simulated either supine or prone; while supine offers a generally more stable setup, prone allows direct clinical alignment to the spine/sacrum and reduces the air gap between the patient and the proton beam treatment nozzle, which has dosimetric advantages. Daily image guidance is mandatory. While cone-beam CT can be helpful, since the target is located in close association with a bony structure, even daily orthogonal plain films provide excellent setup. A six degree-of-freedom treatment couch is helpful to optimize alignment.

Imaging artifacts due to metallic surgical hardware pose a serious challenge to postoperative RT because they (a) make it difficult for the radiation oncologist to accurately define the target volume at risk, (b) scatter the radiation during delivery, and therefore (c) interfere with the ability of the treatment planning algorithms to accurately calculate dose delivered to the affected volume. The magnitude of these effects is such that the presence of surgical hardware during RT may even be associated with inferior outcomes [21]. Thus, every available technique must be used to minimize artifacts. This begins at the time of surgery with reconstruction/stabilization approaches that generate fewer artifacts, for example, favoring allograft or cage reconstructions, using titanium or carbon fiber where rods are required [22], and avoiding rod cross-links at the tumor level. At the imaging and simulation phase, artifact reduction algorithms are critical. Finally, as photons are robust than charged particles to the dosimetric uncertainties associated with hardware artifact, delivering some of the treatment course with photons may help mitigate these issues.

A final technical aspect of chordoma RT is dose constraints. There is significant institutional variability in these constraints, particularly for spinal cord. In most cases, limiting the spinal cord to the conventional tolerance of 45 Gy would significantly underdose tumor and risk local failure. For conventionally fractionated proton therapy, our institution has adopted different dose constraints based on the cord level and surface vs center of cord: C spine, 67 GyRBE surface/55 GyRBE center; T/L spine, 63/54 GyRBE; and cauda 77.4/70.2 GyRBE, S1-S3 nerve roots 77.4/77.4 GyRBE. Data supporting the safety of such constraints are discussed below.

## Fractionation and Field Design

The proton and carbon treatment communities have generally taken different approaches to target volume and design and treatment fractionation (Table 15.1). The proton community has typically focused on doses of >70 Gy delivered in conventional fractionation (i.e., 1.8–2.0 Gy per day), yielding biologically equivalent doses of 66–76 GyRBE. In addition to the gross tumor volume (GTV), proton treatments generally include a generous elective clinical target volume (CTV) expansion to account for subclinical/microscopic spread beyond GTV. While institutional approaches vary, our approach is as follows.

**Table 15.1** Particle therapy for chordomas of the spine and sacrum

| Approach | Fractionation | Total physical dose | Total biologically equivalent dose (EQD2) | CTV expansion |
|---|---|---|---|---|
| Proton | Conventional fractionation (1.8–2.0 GyRBE/day) | 70–77.4 GyRBE | ≈70 GyRBE | Generous |
| Carbon Ion | Moderate hypofractionation (3–4 GyRBE/day) | 64–70 GyRBE | ≈105 GyRBE | Limited |

*Key: CTV* clinical tumor volume, *GyRBE* gray relative biological effectiveness

For chordomas of the sacrum being treated preoperatively or with radiation alone, CTV1 included a 2 cm uniform expansion on GTV. This volume is anatomically constrained out of structures not at risk of spread (visceral organs, subcutaneous tissues, pelvic bones, etc.—presuming they are grossly uninvolved). However, it is specifically allowed to expand into the parasacral soft tissues, particularly the gluteus, piriformis, and sacrococcygeus muscles and the sacrospinous ligaments. Typically, the latter three structures are nearly entirely included in this expansion, and it is reasonable to slightly further extend the CTV1 to fully cover these structures depending on tumor location. The rationale for this generous expansion is that these structures, particularly the muscles, have been shown to harbor micro-metastases out to at least 2 cm from the primary tumor [23]. Coverage generally extends 2 cm superiorly and inferiorly in the spinal canal and the sacral segment above and below the involved sacral segment; if S1 is involved, we generally extend coverage superiorly to at least the middle (superiorly/inferiorly) of L5 and adjacent spinal canal as the basivertebral veins/epidural venous plexus represent an additional potential route of spread.

For chordomas of the mobile spine being treated preoperatively or with radiation alone, CTV1 likewise includes a uniform anatomically constrained expansion from the GTV. In cervical and thoracic tumors, we typically use 1 cm and in lumbar tumors 1.5 cm; these expansions are smaller than in the sacrum as clinical experience has shown a somewhat smaller volume at risk of micro-skip metastases for chordomas of the spine. Like for sacral tumors, spinal CTV1 expansions are constrained out of uninvolved OARs but allowed to extend into paraspinal muscles. Analogous to coverage of L5 for sacral tumors, the CTV1 is extended superiorly and inferiorly to include the epidural venous plexus and basivertebral veins in the adjacent vertebral bodies (one each in the superior and inferior direction) to account for potential spread along this route.

If no preoperative RT was delivered, then, in addition to the above volumes, the postoperative CTV1 further aims to encompass all surgically manipulated tissues, hardware, drain sites, etc. to sterilize tumor cells that may have been seeded in these locations intraoperatively. Such comprehensive coverage is regrettably not possible for thoracolumbar tumors removed by anterolateral approaches, since these approaches violate the pleural and peritoneal cavities, which cannot be treated in their entirety to a tumoricidal dose.

Regardless of whether CTV1 is treated preoperatively, postoperatively, or without surgery, CTV2 is defined as the preoperative GTV plus a 5 mm anatomically constrained margin and treated with a sequential boost. If present after surgery (or in definitive-intent RT-only cases), any gross residual disease plus a 5 mm anatomically constrained margin is further boosted as a separate CTV3. In general, our dosing strategy is to treat CTV1 to 45–50.4 GyRBE in 25–28 fractions (preoperatively if at all possible), CTV2 postoperatively to 64.8–73.2 GyRBE total (depending on risk of residual subclinical/microscopic disease: 64.8 GyRBE for tumors with an R0 en bloc resection after only a core biopsy; 70.2 GyRBE for tumors with an R0 resection after a prior open biopsy or with limited intraoperative tumor spill or cut-through; 73.8 GyRBE for piecemeal or R1 resection), and CTV3 (if present) to 77.4–79.2 GyRBE total.

In contrast, the CIRT community has typically adopted moderate hypofractionation (3–4 GyRBE/day) to a total dose of 60–70 Gy, yielding biologically equivalent doses of 85–105 GyRBE—i.e., a substantial dose escalation from the standard proton approach. CIRT studies have also typically used smaller CTV expansion (e.g., 5 mm anatomically constrained).

## Timing of RT

An additional consideration is the timing of RT relative to surgery. In extremity soft tissue sarcoma, preoperative vs postoperative RT are oncologically equivalent approaches, albeit with different toxicity profiles. It is hazardous, however, to adopt this approach uncritically in an unrelated tumor such as chordoma. In both STS and chordoma, iatrogenic seeding of cells in the operative field is common, even during oncologic en bloc R0 resections. Therefore, postoperative RT is oncologically sound only when it is possible (a) to accurately define the surgically contaminated field (including all surgically manipulated tissues, hardware, drains, incision sites, etc.) and (b) to cover this volume to a tumoricidal dose. In extremity STS, these conditions are easily met, as the surgical field is well-defined and the required dose of RT is 60–66 Gy. In chordoma, these assumptions are more dubious, both because the surgical field is much more extensive (multilevel spinal hardware, violation of the pleural/peritoneal cavities in case of an anterior approach, etc.) and because such a large volume cannot be covered to a tumoricidal dose. Thus, in patients undergoing surgery, we favor use of at least some preoperative RT whenever possible. Even in patients with epidural disease with imaging evidence of mass effect on the spinal cord, we favor a short course of preoperative radiation of 19.8 Gy in 11 fractions +/− steroids followed by immediate surgery and the remainder of the usual RT dose (determined based on margin status) postoperatively, as even this low preoperative dose is sufficient to mitigate the risk of intraoperative iatrogenic tumor seeding [24]. If, however, the patient has clinical evidence of sensory, motor, or autonomic nerve dysfunction, immediate decompression should be done.

Finally, as illustrated below, substantial carbon and proton literature supports the efficacy of RT alone as a definitive-intent treatment option for chordoma. This is particularly important for tumors that are technically resectable but only with significant morbidity—for example, proximal sacral tumors in which a total sacrectomy would mean loss of upper sacral nerve roots and permanent incontinence or cervical spine tumors in which occipital-cervical fixation would risk unacceptable loss of range of motion and pharyngeal or laryngeal dysfunction. In such cases, RT alone may offer a curative-intent treatment approach with significantly less up-front morbidity.

## Proton Literature

Four prospective and nine main retrospective studies describe outcomes following proton RT for spine/sacral chordomas.

## Postoperative RT

In the postoperative setting, there are two prospective and several retrospective studies (Table 15.2). Indelicato et al. reported a prospective study (NCT00797602) of 51 patients from the University of Florida Jacksonville [25]. Eligible patients included those with chordomas (66.6%) or chondrosarcomas (33.3%) of the sacrum (41.2%) or spine (58.8%), treated either in the postoperative setting or in the definitive-intent setting (distribution not reported). 52.9% had gross disease at the time of RT, and 23.5% had recurrent disease. Median RT dose was 70.2 GyRBE (range 64.2–75.6). At a median follow-up of 3.7 years, LC4 (LC at 4 years) was 58%, DFS4 86%, and OS4 72%. Recurrent disease was associated with markedly inferior LC (19% vs 71%, $p < 0.01$), highlighting the importance of optimal management at initial presentation.

Baumann et al. reported a Phase I/II trial (NCT01449149) of 20 patients from the University of Pennsylvania [26]. Eligible patients included those with chordomas (90%) or chondrosarcomas (10%) of the skull base (60%) or spine (40%). 85% received adjuvant RT after surgery (of whom 76.5% had gross residual disease); 15% were treated with RT alone. Median RT dose was 73.8 GyRBE (range 68.4–79.2). The primary outcomes of feasibility and safety were met ($n = 2$ acute Grade 3 toxicity); one late Grade ≥3 toxicity (carotid blowout) was also reported. At a median follow-up of 37 months, secondary outcomes included LC3 of 86% (95% CI 77–96%) and PFS3 81% (70–90%); no deaths or subset outcome differences were reported.

Retrospectively, Murray et al. reported outcomes from 155 patients with spine (66%) or sacral chordomas (75%) or chondrosarcomas treated at the Paul Scherrer Institute in Switzerland between 1997 and 2016 [21]. Except for two who had biopsy only, all were treated with resection followed by postoperative RT. Only 46% had a GTR, and of those, only 39% were en bloc resections. Median RT dose was 74 GyRBE (range 48.6–77). At a median follow-up of 64.7 mo, LC5 was 64.9% (95% CI 56.3–73.5%), DFS5 59.4% (50.6–68.2%), and OS5 77.9% (70.6–85.2%). Rates of late Grade ≥3 RT toxicity were 7.7%. This study illustrates several key principles of proton RT. First, in this study, presence of stabilization hardware was associated decrement in all outcomes (e.g., OS5 66.8% vs 84.8%, $p = 0.002$), underlining the critical importance of thoughtful stabilization selection and management of the associated imaging artifact and treatment effects. Second, in this study, earlier patients were treated with very modest CTV expansions and later patients with more generous expansions (surgical bed plus one vertebral body above and below the tumor); the latter approach was associated with significantly improvement in all outcomes (e.g., OS5 91.1% vs 65.6%, $p = 0.05$), which is among the strongest evidence for the importance of generous CTV expansions in proton RT for this disease. Finally, as in numerous other studies, presence of gross residual disease was associated with inferior OS (OS5 70.4% vs 89.8%, $p = 0.001$), confirming that R2 procedures should be avoided whenever possible in this disease.

Youn et al. describe 58 patients treated between 2007 and 2015 in South Korea, either postoperatively or with RT alone, for skull base (59%) or spine/sacral (41%) chordomas [27]. 86.2% had gross residual disease at the time of RT. Median dose was 76.6 GyRBE (range 64.8–79.2); unlike other proton studies, modest

**Table 15.2** Postoperative proton therapy studies

| Study | Design | Center and years enrolled | Number of Pts | Location | Histology (% chordoma) | % Surgery | Margins | Median RT dose (range) | Median f/u | Disease outcomes | Key subsets | Grade≥3 toxicity |
|---|---|---|---|---|---|---|---|---|---|---|---|---|
| Indelicato et al. [25] | Prospective | UF Jacksonville 2007–2013 | 51 | 59% spine 41% sacrum | 67% | N.R. | N.R. | 70.2 GyRBE (64.2–75.6) | 3.7 yr | LC4: 58% PFS4: 57% OS4: 72% | Primary vs recurrent: LF 29% vs 81%; $p = 0.01$ | 8 pts |
| Baumann et al. [26] | Prospective | UPenn 2010–2014 | 20 | 60% skull base 15% spine 25% sacrum | 90% | 85% | 24% R0/1, 76% R2 | 73.8 GyRBE (68.4–79.2) | 37mo | LC3: 86% PFS: 90% OS: N.R. | – | Acute: 2 pts Late: 1 pt |
| Murray et al. [21] | Retrospective | PSI 1997–2016 | 155 | 66% spine 34% sacrum | 75% | 98.7% | R0/1 46%, R2 54% | 74 GyRBE (48.6–77) | 64.7mo | LC5: 64.9% DFS5: 59.4% OS5: 77.9% | GTR vs not: OS5 89.8% vs 70.4%; $p = 0.001$ Stabilization hardware present vs absent: OS5 66.8% vs 84.8%; $p = 0.002$ "Focal" CTV vs comprehensive CTV: OS5 65.6% vs 91.1%; $p = 0.05$ | 7.7% |

| | | | | | | | | | | | | |
|---|---|---|---|---|---|---|---|---|---|---|---|---|
| Youn et al. [27] | Retrospective | South Korea 2007–2015 | 58 | 59% skull base 12% spine 29% sacrum | 100% | N.R. | 14% R0/1, 86% R2 or biopsy only | 69.6 GyRBE (64.8–79.2) | 42.8mo | N.R. | Dose < vs ≥69.6 GyRBE (58% vs 95%; $p = 0.016$) | Late: 3 pts |
| Beddok et al. [28] | Retrospective | Curie Institute 2005–2018 | 41 | 100% sacrum | 100% | 73% | 50% R0/1, 50% R2 | N.R. (70–73.8 GyRBE) | 46mo | LF2/5: 11.4%/29% OS2/5: 91.4%/74% | – | – |

*Key: f/u* follow-up, *GTR* gross total resection, *GyRBE* gray relative biological effectiveness, *LC#* local control at # years, *LF#* local failure at # years, *mo* month, *N.R.* not recorded, OS# overall survival at # years, *PFS#* progression-free survival at # years, *PSI* Paul Scherrer Institute, *pt* patient, *yr* year hypofractionation (2.4 GyRBE daily) was employed. At a median 42.8 mo follow-up, LC5 was 87.9%, DFS5 86.7%, and OS5 88.3%. No Grade ≥3 acute toxicities were reported, but three patients had late Grade 3 toxicities. Consistent with the importance of dose escalation, dose ≥69.6 GyRBE was associated with improved LC5 (92.8% vs 63.5%, $p$ = 0.05) and distant metastasis-free survival at 5 years (95.0% vs 58.3%, $p$ = 0.016).

Finally, Beddok et al. describe 41 sacral chordoma patients treated between 2005 and 2018 at the Curie Institute in France [28]. 73% underwent surgery, of whom 50% had R2 resections. Dose range was 70–73.8 GyRBE by photon tomotherapy and/or proton therapy. At a median follow-up of 46 months, 2- and 5-year LR was 11.4%/29% and OS 91.4%/74%. Consistent with the known dosimetric advantages of proton therapy, rates of proctitis and cystitis were markedly lower with proton therapy.

## Preoperative RT

Two prospective and two retrospective studies, all from Massachusetts General Hospital, report outcomes in the preoperative setting (Table 15.3). The rationale for preoperative RT in this setting is to decrease the risk of iatrogenic tumor cell seeing by decreasing the number of viable clonogens at the time of RT; in this way, the postoperative course need not cover the entire surgical field but can be restricted to the tumor bed and areas at high risk for subclinical/microscopic residual disease based on the known patterns of local spread. An additional benefit is that patients can receive the majority of their radiation treatment without any spine hardware and associated imaging artifact and treatment effects.

DeLaney et al. have reported a Phase II trial of 50 spine sarcoma patients (48% chordoma, 52% sacral) treated with DS proton therapy at Massachusetts General Hospital between 1997 and 2005 [9, 10]. Patients could receive either (a) preoperative RT, resection, and postoperative RT (recommended), (b) postoperative RT alone, or (c) definitive-intent RT alone. 28% had recurrent disease. In total, 76% underwent surgery, of whom 68% achieved a GTR. Median RT dose was 76.6 GyRBE (range 59.4–77.41 GyRBE); 3 patients with tumor directly abutting dura received a 7.5–10 Gy boost via dural plaque brachytherapy. At a median 7.3-year follow-up, 5/8-year LC was 81%/74%, DFS 64%/52%, and OS 84%/65%. Cumulative Grade ≥3 toxicity at 5 and 8 years was 10% and 13%, respectively. Consistent with other studies, lower LR was seen in primary vs recurrent chordomas (0% vs 50% at 5 years, $p$ = 0.005), and there was a trend toward lower LR in R0 vs R1/2 resections ($p$ = 0.11).

A follow-up prospective study (NCT01346124) using PBS proton therapy has been reported but not yet published [11]. Here, 60 pts with chordoma (85%) or chondrosarcoma of the sacrum (55%) or spine were treated between 2013 and 2017. As in the prior study, patients could be treated pre- and postoperatively (preferred), postoperatively only, or with RT alone if not undergoing surgery. At a median 2.5-year follow-up, 2.5-year LC was 93%, PFS 81%, and OS 92%. While this study was

**Table 15.3** Preoperative proton therapy studies

| Study | Design | Center and years enrolled | Number of Pts | Location | Histology (% chordoma) | % Surgery | Margins | Median RT dose (range) | Median f/u | Disease outcomes | Key subsets | Grade ≥3 toxicity |
|---|---|---|---|---|---|---|---|---|---|---|---|---|
| DeLaney et al. [9, 10] | Pro-spective | MGH 1997–2005 | 50 | 48% spine, 52% sacrum | 58% | 74% | 22% R0 45% R1 32% R2 | 76.6 GyRBE (59.4–77.4) | 7.3 yr | LC5/8: 81%/74% PFS5/8: 64%/52% OS5/8: 84%/65% | Primary vs recurrent: LR5/8 0%/8% vs 50%/N.R.; $p = 0.005$ | 5y/8y = 10%/13% |
| Konieczkowski et al. [11] | Pro-spective | MGH 2013–2017 | 60 | 45% spine, 55% sacrum | 85% | 85% | 63% R0, 20% R1, 10% R0/1, 7% R2 | Surgical: 64.8 GyRBE (19.8–77.4) RT-only: 77.4 GyRBE (77.4–79.2) | 31mo | LC2.5: 93% PFS2.5: 81% OS2.5: 92% | Preop vs postop-only RT: RFS2.5 84% vs 62% ($p = 0.003$) | 26% at 2.5 yr (all in surgery + RT group) |
| Rotondo et al. [29] | Ret-rospective | MGH 1982–2011 | 126 | 44.1% spine, 55.9% sacrum | 100% | 93% | 27% R0 45% R1 24% R2 | 72.4 GyRBE (46.3–83.6) | 47mo | LC5: 62% OS5: 81% | Primary vs recurrent: LC5 68% vs 49%; $p = 0.058$ R0/1 vs R2 margin: OS5 88% vs 66%; $p = 0.017$ Preop RT vs not: LC5 85% vs 56%; $p = 0.019$ (1° only) En bloc vs intralesional resection: LC5 72% vs 55%; $p = 0.016$ | 50 pts |

(continued)

**Table 15.3** (continued)

| Study | Design | Center and years enrolled | Number of Pts | Location | Histology (% chordoma) | % Surgery | Margins | Median RT dose (range) | Median f/u | Disease outcomes | Key subsets | Grade ≥3 toxicity |
|---|---|---|---|---|---|---|---|---|---|---|---|---|
| Wagner et al. [24] | Ret-rospective | MGH 1982–2006 | 48 | 21% spine, 71% sacrum, 8% limbs | 52% | 100% | 44% R0<br>12% R1<br>44% R2 | Preop: 20 GyRBE (9–29.4)<br>Postop: 50.4 GyRBE (18–61.2)<br>Total: 70.4 GyRBE | 31.8mo | LC5: 72%<br>DFS5: 54%<br>OS5: 65% | Primary vs recurrent: LC5 89% vs 18%; $p = 0.001$<br>R0/1 vs R2: DFS5; $p = 0.07$ | 21% delayed wound healing "notable" late toxicity in 4 pt |

*Key: DFS#* disease-free survival at # years, *f/u* follow-up, *GTR* gross total resection, *GyRBE* gray relative biological effectiveness, *LC#* local control at # years, *LF#* local failure at # years, *MGH* Massachusetts General Hospital, *mo* month, *N.R.* not recorded, *OS#* overall survival at # years, *PFS#* progression-free survival at # years, *pt* patient, *RT* radiotherapy, *yr* year not designed to compare across treatment modalities, subset analysis was notable for improved RFS among surgical patients who received preoperative RT (85% vs 62%, $p = 0.003$) and no LF yet observed in the definitive-intent RT group ($p$ = ns vs surgical patients). Cumulative incidence of Grade 3 toxicity was 26% at 2.5 years, all in patients who underwent both surgery and RT.

Retrospectively, Rotondo et al. described 126 patients with spine (44%) or sacral chordoma treated between 1982 and 2011 [29]. 25.2% were recurrent after prior surgery. Treatment was generally with preoperative RT, surgery, and postoperative RT (median total dose 72.4 GyRBE, range 46.3–83.6). At a median follow-up of 47 months, LC5 was 62% and OS5 81%. A trend toward better LC5 was seen in patients with primary vs recurrent disease (68% vs 49%, $p = 0.058$). En bloc resection was associated with improved LC5 (72% vs 55%, $p = 0.016$) and GTR with improved OS5 (88% vs 66%, $p = 0.017$). Among primary tumors, five-year LC and locoregional control were higher with preoperative RT, 85% ($p = 0.019$) and 79% ($p = 0.034$), respectively, versus 56% and 56% if no preoperative RT was given. Intriguingly, no recurrences were observed among 28 patients with primary tumors treated by core biopsy, preoperative RT, and en bloc resection. Among all patients, 50 Grade ≥3 complications were observed.

In addition, Wagner et al. described 48 bone sarcoma patients treated with low-dose preoperative RT, resection, and postoperative RT, of whom 52% had chordoma and 29% had recurrent disease [24]. Median preoperative dose was 20 GyRBE (range 9–29.4), and median postoperative dose was 50.4 GyRBE (range 18–61.2). Fifty-six percent of patients achieved a GTR. The rationale for this approach is that even a low dose of preoperative RT sufficiently reduces the number of viable tumor cell clonogens present at the time of surgery to mitigate the risk of intraoperative seeding; thus, the postoperative RT course can be limited to the tumor bed and areas at high risk for subclinical/microscopic residual disease but need not cover all surgically manipulated tissues. At 32mo median follow-up, LC5 was 72%, DFS5 53.8%, and OS5 65%. LC and DFS were higher in primary disease ($p = 0.001$ for both) and trended higher in patients who underwent a GTR ($p = 0.07$). Twenty-one percent experienced delayed wound healing, and 4/37 evaluable in patients developed "notable" late toxicities.

## Definitive-Intent RT Without Surgery

In addition to the definitive-intent RT-only patients included in the above studies, two retrospective studies specifically describe results following definitive-intent proton RT (Table 15.4).

Kabolizadeh et al. described the Massachusetts General Hospital experience with 40 unresected sacral chordoma patients treated with proton RT alone between 1975 and 2012 [13]. Median dose was 77.4 GyRBE (64.7–79.2). At a median follow-up of 50.3 months, LC5 was 85.4% and OS5 was 81.9%. Underscoring the importance of dose escalation in this context, increased dose was associated with

**Table 15.4** Definitive-intent proton therapy studies

| Study | Design | Center and years enrolled | Number of Pts | Location | Histology (% chordoma) | % Surgery | Median RT dose (range) | Median f/u | Disease outcomes | Grade≥3 toxicity |
|---|---|---|---|---|---|---|---|---|---|---|
| Kabolizadeh et al. [13] | Retrospective | MGH 1975–2012 | 40 | 43% spine, 27% sacrum, 30% para-axial | 100% | 0% | 77.4 GyRBE (64.7–79.2) | 50.3mo | LC5: 85% DFS: N.R. OS5: 82% | 10 pts w/ sacral fractures; 6 sacral neuropathy; 1 bowel fistula |
| Aibe et al. [30] | Retrospective | Hyogo 2009–2015 | 33 | 100% sacrum | 100% | 0% | 70.4 GyRBE | 37mo | LC3: 89% DFS3: 82% OS3: 93% | Acute: 1 pt Late: 5 pt |

*Key: DFS#* disease-free survival at # years, *f/u* follow-up, *GyRBE* gray relative biological effectiveness, *LC#* local control at # years, *MGH* Massachusetts General Hospital, *mo* month, *N.R.* not recorded, *OS#* overall survival at # years, *PFS#* progression-free survival at # years, *pt* patient, *RT* radiotherapy improved OS ($p = 0.032$). Toxicity included ten sacral fractures, six sacral plexopathies, and one bowel fistula.

Aibe et al. reported a similar definitive-intent proton RT experience from Hyogo, Japan, in 33 sacral chordoma patients between 2009 and 2015 [30]. Median dose was 70.4 GyRBE in a modestly hypofractionated regimen of 2.2 GyRBE x 32 fractions. At 37-month median follow-up, LC3 was 89.6%, DFS3 88.2%, and OS3 92.7%. One acute and five late Grade ≥3 toxicities were reported.

## Toxicity

Three studies—one from Paul Scherrer Institute and two from Massachusetts General Hospital—describe neurologic toxicity outcomes in detail following proton RT.

Streib et al. reported on 76 patients with spine chordoma (78%) or chondrosarcoma treated between 2000 and 2014 at the Paul Scherrer Institute with proton RT (median dose 73.9 GyRBE) [31]. Here, planning constraints were cord surface D2% 64 GyRBE (60 GyRBE if >3 vertebral bodies) and central cord D2% 60 Gy RBE. At 66-month median follow-up, cumulative incidence of late myelopathy/neuropathy was 16%, all but one of which were Grade 1–2.

Marucci et al. reviewed 85 patients with C spine or cervical-occipital junction chordomas or chondrosarcomas treated between 1982 and 2000 [32]. Median dose was 76.3 GyRBE (range 68.9–83), and planning constraints were Dmax cord surface/center 67–70/55–58 GyRBE. At median 41-month follow-up, the rate of Grade 3 myelopathy was 4.7%; the only variable significantly associated with this outcome was number of prior surgeries.

Chowdhry et al. reviewed 68 patients with T/L spine tumors (43% chordoma) treated between 2002 and 2013 [33]. Median dose was 72 GyRBE (range 59.4–78.2); 24% of patients received pre-operative RT in addition to postoperative RT, and 15% received a dural plaque brachytherapy boost. In total, eight patients experienced Gr ≥ 3 spinal cord toxicity, of which four were attributed to surgery, three to tumor progression, and only one to RT.

Taken together with the safety data from the aforementioned prospective and retrospective studies, these data suggest that, in the context of appropriate institutional experience, doses significantly in excess of conventional cord tolerance can be delivered safely.

Finally, chordoma patients are at significant risk of treatment-related insufficiency fractures. Osler et al. described 62 sacral chordoma patients who received RT plus surgery (71%) or RT alone (29%) between 1992 and 2013 [34]. At a median follow-up of 22 months, fracture rate was 47%, including 76% in high sacrectomy + RT group, 0% in the low sacrectomy + RT group, and 22% in the RT alone group. These data suggest that, while RT undoubtedly contributes to fracture risk, surgery is also a major determinant of this outcome.

## Carbon Ion Therapy

CIRT has been performed in Germany and Japan for over 25 years. As of 2020, 12 CIRT facilities have been established worldwide, but CIRT remains unavailable in the United States. In chordomas of the spine and sacrum, CIRT has been used as definite-intent therapy for patients not undergoing surgery, as well as in the postoperative setting for surgical patients; there is no significant experience with preoperative CIRT. The two largest series describing outcomes in this setting come from German and Japan and are described below (Table 15.5).

At the Heidelberg Ion Beam Therapy Center (HIT), 68 sacrococcygeal chordomas (23% recurrent) were treated with CIRT between 2009 and 2013 [35]. 41% of patients were treated with CIRT alone and 59% with surgery followed by CIRT; of surgical patients, 65% had R2 and 35% R0/1 resections. Median total dose was 66 GyRBE (range: 60–74), delivered as CIRT only (3–4 Gy per fraction, $n = 46$) or as 50 Gy of photon IMRT (at 2 Gy/fx) with a CIRT boost at 3 Gy/fx ($n = 22$). At a median follow-up of 60 months, the 5-year OS, PFS, and LC were 74%, 53%, and 53%, respectively. Recurrent disease was associated with markedly worse LC compared to primary disease (HR 4.25, 95% CI 1.99–9.09, $p < 0.001$). The incidence of late toxicity ≥ Grade 3 was 21%. This included insufficiency fractures in 16% and radiation neuropathy in 5%. The comparatively modest outcomes in this study must be taken in the context of the high rate of R2 resection, which is known from other studies to be a strong negative prognostic factor.

A nationwide Japanese retrospective study (Fig. 15.2) reported the largest cohort of 218 sacral chordoma patients (3.2% with recurrent disease) who received definitive-intent CIRT alone between 2003 and 2014 [12], many of which had been previously reported in smaller series [36, 37]. All patients were treated with CIRT alone, without surgery; the most frequent dose fractionation was 67.2 Gy RBE in 16 fractions. At a median follow-up period of 56 months, 5-year OS, PFS, and LC were 84%, 48%, and 72%, respectively. Acute and late Grade ≥3 adverse events occurred in 4% and 6% of patients, respectively.

There are several ongoing CIRT studies. The ongoing single-institution Phase II ISAC trial at HIT (NCT01811394) randomizes patients with sacral chordoma who either have not undergone resection or have undergone R2 resection to proton therapy or CIRT [38]. In both arms, 64 GyRBE is delivered in 16 fractions. The study was opened in 2013 and is currently accruing. Another ongoing clinical trial, Surgery Versus Definitive Radiation Therapy in Primary Localized Disease (SACRO), was organized by the Italian Sarcoma Group. In this study, which includes both a randomized arm and a non-randomized registry arm, sacral chordoma patients undergo either (a) surgery with RT if R1 margins or without RT for R0 margins or (b) RT alone without surgery. RT in this trial can include carbon ions, protons, and photons. This study is currently accruing patients.

**Table 15.5** Carbon ion studies

| Study | Design | Center and years Enrolled | Number of Pts | Location | Histology (% chordoma) | % Surgery | Margins | Median RT dose (range) | Median f/u | Disease outcomes | Key subsets | Grade≥3 toxicity |
|---|---|---|---|---|---|---|---|---|---|---|---|---|
| Bostel et al. [35] | Ret-rospective | Heidelberg 2009–2013 | 68 | 100% sacrum | 100% | 59% | 35% R0/1, 65% R2 | 66 GyRBE (60–74)<br>Carbon: 3–4 Gy/fx<br>IMRT: 2 Gy/fx to 50 Gy with carbon boost ($n = 22$) | 60.3mo | LC5: 53%<br>PFS: 53%<br>OS5: 74% | Primary vs recurrent: LF HR 4.25; $p < 0.001$ | 21% |
| Demizu et al. [12] | Ret-rospective | Japan 2003–2014 | 218 | 100% sacrum | 100% | 0% | N/A | 67.2 GyRBE/16 Fx | 56mo | LC5: 72%<br>PFS5: 48%<br>OS5: 84% | | Acute: 4%<br>Late: 6% |

*Key: f/u* follow-up, *fx* fraction, *GyRBE* gray relative biological effectiveness, *HR* hazard ratio, *LC#* local control at # years, *mo* month, *N.R.* not recorded, *OS#* overall survival at # years, *PFS#* progression-free survival at # years, *pt* patient, *RT* radiotherapy, *yr* year

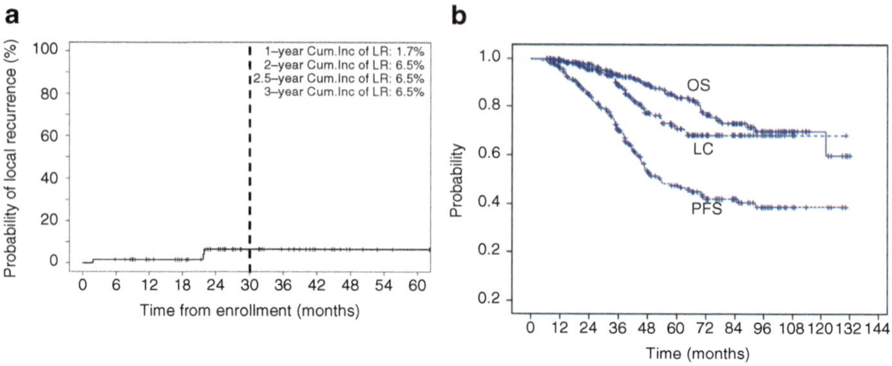


**Fig. 15.2** Outcomes following proton therapy or carbon ion therapy for chordoma. (**a**) Local failure of spine/sacral chordomas treated with proton therapy was 6.5% at 2.5 years (median follow-up 30 months) [11]. (**b**) Local control of sacral chordomas treated with carbon therapy was 72% at 5 years (median follow-up 56 months) [12]

## Conclusion

The foregoing data suggest several principles for the optimal coordination of radiation and surgery in spine and sacral chordomas.

1. Local control is a critical determinant of chordoma disease course. Local failures are highly morbid, difficult to salvage, and associated with higher rates of metastatic disease. Surgery alone, even if R0 and en bloc, results in unacceptably high rates of local recurrence. While no randomized study has compared surgery alone to surgery plus RT or to RT alone, the promising results detailed above suggest that RT should be considered in the management of all spine and sacral chordomas. Decisions regarding RT should be made by a radiation oncologist experienced in treating these tumors, in conjunction with the surgeon, prior to surgery. Patients should also be engaged in the many, often complex, decisions that need to be made to optimize their treatment outcome and satisfaction.
2. Advanced forms of RT delivery are required to permit an adequate RT dose to radioresistant tumor in close proximity to radiosensitive structures such as the spinal cord. Proton therapy, carbon ion therapy, and SBRT all have evidence supporting their use in spine and sacral chordomas.
3. Outcomes for locally recurrent disease are unsatisfactory regardless of treatment strategy. Therefore, every effort must be made to achieve local control at the initial presentation. The notion sometimes encountered that patients should have surgery first, with radiation reserved until the time of a local recurrence, is profoundly flawed and has no place in the curative-intent management of chordoma.
4. Intralesional/R2 procedures are associated with inferior outcomes despite RT. In contrast, unresected patients treated with definitive-intent RT alone can have favorable outcomes. Therefore, surgery should only be undertaken if an en bloc resection with at least R1, but preferably R0, margins is anticipated. One conse-

quence of this principle is that it is not optimal to refer a patient for radiation after the fact only if surgery does not achieve the desired results; on the contrary, it is critical for the surgeon and the radiation oncologist to design a comprehensive treatment approach together prior to any intervention. For patients in whom an oncologically sound surgery is not possible or unacceptably morbid (e.g., C spine or high sacral tumors), definitive-intent RT alone represents a promising option.

5. While no randomized data evaluates timing of RT relative to surgery, the extremely promising results obtained in several studies of preoperative RT, coupled with its theoretical and practical advantages (smaller treatment volumes, prevention of tumor seeding, mitigation of hardware artifacts, etc.) suggest that this strategy should be routinely considered in clinical practice as well as form the basis of future investigations.
6. Regardless of the specific RT modality employed, dose escalation is a critical determinant of local control. This also implies spinal cord doses higher than those commonly accepted in other scenarios. While significant data support the safety of this approach, it does require specialized expertise on the part of the treating radiation oncologist, as well as knowledge of the unique clinical behavior and patterns of spread of this disease. For this reason, as well as the importance of adequate oncologic management at initial diagnosis and the expert multi-disciplinary care required to ensure that all chordoma patients should be referred to a center with significant experience in this disease at the time of presentation.

## References


1. Radaelli S, Fossati P, Stacchiotti S, et al. The sacral chordoma margin. Eur J Surg Oncol. 2020;46:1415–22.
2. Schwab JH, Healey JH, Rose P, Casas-Ganem J, Boland PJ. The surgical management of Sacral Chordomas. Spine (Phila Pa 1976). 2009;34:2700–4.
3. Varga PP, Szövérfi Z, Fisher CG, et al. Surgical treatment of sacral chordoma: prognostic variables for local recurrence and overall survival. Eur Spine J. 2015;24:1092–101.
4. Kerekes D, Goodwin CR, Ahmed AK, Verlaan J-J, Bettegowda C, Abu-Bonsrah N, Sciubba DM. Local and distant recurrence in resected sacral chordomas: a systematic review and pooled cohort analysis. Glob Spine J. 2019;9:191–201.
5. McPherson CM, Suki D, McCutcheon IE, Gokaslan ZL, Rhines LD, Mendel E. Metastatic disease from spinal chordoma: a 10-year experience. J Neurosurg Spine. 2006;5:277–80.
6. Konieczkowski DJ, DeLaney TF, Yamada Y (Josh) J. Radiation strategies for spine chordoma: proton beam, carbon ions, and stereotactic body radiation therapy. Neurosurg Clin N Am. 2020;31:263–88.
7. Dial BL, Kerr DL, Lazarides AL, et al. The role of radiotherapy for chordoma patients managed with surgery: analysis of the National Cancer Database. Spine (Phila Pa 1976). 2020;45:E742–51.
8. Houdek MT, Rose PS, Hevesi M, et al. Low dose radiotherapy is associated with local complications but not disease control in sacral chordoma. J Surg Oncol. 2019;119:856–63.
9. DeLaney TF, Liebsch NJ, Pedlow FX, et al. Phase II study of high-dose photon/proton radiotherapy in the management of spine sarcomas. Int J Radiat Oncol. 2009;74:732–9.

10. DeLaney TF, Liebsch NJ, Pedlow FX, et al. Long-term results of phase II study of high dose photon/proton radiotherapy in the management of spine chordomas, chondrosarcomas, and other sarcomas. J Surg Oncol. 2014;110:115–22.
11. Konieczkowski DJ, Chen Y-LE, Bernstein KD, et al. Prospective phase II study of scanned beam proton therapy for spine sarcomas. Int J Radiat Oncol. 2018;102:e325–6.
12. Demizu Y, Imai R, Kiyohara H, et al. Carbon ion radiotherapy for sacral chordoma: a retrospective nationwide multicentre study in Japan. Radiother Oncol. 2021;154:1–5.
13. Kabolizadeh P, Chen Y-L, Liebsch N, Hornicek FJ, Schwab JH, Choy E, Rosenthal DI, Niemierko A, DeLaney TF. Updated outcome and analysis of tumor response in mobile spine and sacral chordoma treated with definitive high-dose photon/proton radiation therapy. Int J Radiat Oncol. 2017;97:254–62.
14. Jin CJ, Berry-Candelario J, Reiner AS, et al. Long-term outcomes of high-dose single-fraction radiosurgery for chordomas of the spine and sacrum. J Neurosurg Spine. 2020;32:79–88.
15. Krishnan J, Rao S, Hegde S, Shetty J. Evaluation of healthy tissue dose at different regions between volumetric-modulated arc therapy and intensity-modulated radiation therapy plans in the treatment of various cancers. J Med Phys. 2019;44:213–21.
16. Kandula S, Zhu X, Garden AS, et al. Spot-scanning beam proton therapy vs intensity-modulated radiation therapy for ipsilateral head and neck malignancies: a treatment planning comparison. Med Dosim. 2013;38:390–4.
17. Gottschalk B. Passive beam scattering. In: DeLaney TF, Kooy HM, editors. Prot. Charg. Part. Radiother. 1st ed. Philadelphia: Lippincott Williams & Wilkins; 2007. p. 33–40.
18. Pedroni E. Pencil beam scanning. In: DeLaney TF, Kooy HM, editors. Prot. Charg. Part. Radiother. 1st ed. Philadelphia: Lippincott Williams & Wilkins; 2007. p. 40–9.
19. Pompos A, Durante M, Choy H. Heavy ions in cancer therapy. JAMA Oncol. 2016;2:1539–40.
20. Gerweck L, Paganetti H. Radiobiology of charged particles. In: DeLaney TF, Kooy HM, editors. Prot. Charg. Part. Radiother. 1st ed. Philadelphia: Lippincott Williams & Wilkins; 2007. p. 8–18.
21. Murray FR, Snider JW, Schneider RA, Walser M, Bolsi A, Pica A, Lomax AJ, Weber DC. Prognostic factors for spinal chordomas and chondrosarcomas treated with postoperative pencil-beam scanning proton therapy: a large, single-institution experience. J Neurosurg Spine. 2020;32:921–30.
22. Müller BS, Ryang Y-M, Oechsner M, Düsberg M, Meyer B, Combs SE, Wilkens JJ. The dosimetric impact of stabilizing spinal implants in radiotherapy treatment planning with protons and photons: standard titanium alloy vs. radiolucent carbon-fiber-reinforced PEEK systems. J Appl Clin Med Phys. 2020;21:6–14.
23. Akiyama T, Ogura K, Gokita T, et al. Analysis of the infiltrative features of chordoma: the relationship between micro-skip metastasis and postoperative outcomes. Ann Surg Oncol. 2018;25:912–9.
24. Wagner TD, Kobayashi W, Dean S, et al. Combination short-course preoperative irradiation, surgical resection, and reduced-field high-dose postoperative irradiation in the treatment of tumors involving the bone. Int J Radiat Oncol. 2009;73:259–66.
25. Indelicato DJ, Rotondo RL, Begosh-Mayne D, Scarborough MT, Gibbs CP, Morris CG, Mendenhall WM. A prospective outcomes study of proton therapy for chordomas and chondrosarcomas of the spine. Int J Radiat Oncol. 2016;95:297–303.
26. Baumann BC, Lustig RA, Mazzoni S, et al. A prospective clinical trial of proton therapy for chordoma and chondrosarcoma: feasibility assessment. J Surg Oncol. 2019;120:jso.25502.
27. Youn SH, Cho KH, Kim J-Y, et al. Clinical outcome of proton therapy for patients with chordomas. Radiat Oncol J. 2018;36:182–91.
28. Beddok A, Saint-Martin C, Mammar H, et al. High-dose proton therapy and tomotherapy for the treatment of sacral chordoma: a retrospective monocentric study. Acta Oncol (Madr). 2020:1–7.
29. Rotondo RL, Folkert W, Liebsch NJ, et al. High-dose proton-based radiation therapy in the management of spine chordomas: outcomes and clinicopathological prognostic factors. J Neurosurg Spine. 2015;23:788–97.

30. Aibe N, Demizu Y, Sulaiman NS, et al. Outcomes of patients with primary sacral chordoma treated with definitive proton beam therapy. Int J Radiat Oncol. 2018;100:972–9.
31. Stieb S, Snider JW, Placidi L, Kliebsch U, Lomax AJ, Schneider RA, Weber DC. Long-term clinical safety of high-dose proton radiation therapy delivered with pencil beam scanning technique for extracranial chordomas and chondrosarcomas in adult patients: clinical evidence of spinal cord tolerance. Int J Radiat Oncol. 2018;100:218–25.
32. Marucci L, Niemierko A, Liebsch NJ, Aboubaker F, Liu MCC, Munzenrider JE. Spinal cord tolerance to high-dose fractionated 3D conformal proton-photon irradiation as evaluated by equivalent uniform dose and dose volume histogram analysis. Int J Radiat Oncol. 2004;59:551–5.
33. Chowdhry VK, Liu L, Goldberg S, Adams JA, Bernstein KDA, Liebsch NJ, Niemierko A, Chen Y-L, DeLaney TF. Thoracolumbar spinal cord tolerance to high dose conformal proton–photon radiation therapy. Radiother Oncol. 2016;119:35–9.
34. Osler P, Bredella MA, Hess KA, Janssen SJ, Park CJ, Chen YL, DeLaney TF, Hornicek FJ, Schwab JH. Sacral insufficiency fractures are common after high-dose radiation for sacral chordomas treated with or without surgery. Clin Orthop Relat Res. 2016;474:766–72.
35. Bostel T, Mattke M, Nicolay NH, Welzel T, Wollschläger D, Akbaba S, Mayer A, Sprave T, Debus J, Uhl M. High-dose carbon-ion based radiotherapy of primary and recurrent sacrococcygeal chordomas: long-term clinical results of a single particle therapy center. Radiat Oncol. 2020;15:206.
36. Imai R, Kamada T, Araki N, et al. Carbon ion radiation therapy for unresectable sacral chordoma: an analysis of 188 cases. Int J Radiat Oncol. 2016;95:322–7.
37. Demizu Y, Jin D, Sulaiman NS, et al. Particle therapy using protons or carbon ions for unresectable or incompletely resected bone and soft tissue sarcomas of the pelvis. Int J Radiat Oncol. 2017;98:367–74.
38. Uhl M, Edler L, Jensen AD, Habl G, Oelmann J, Röder F, Jäckel O, Debus J, Herfarth K. Randomized phase II trial of hypofractionated proton versus carbon ion radiation therapy in patients with sacrococcygeal chordoma-the ISAC trial protocol. Radiat Oncol. 2014;9:100.

# Systemic Therapy, Trials, and Future Directions for Chordoma of the Spine

# 16

Daniel J. Zabransky, Zach Pennington, and Christian Meyer

## Abbreviations

| | |
|---|---|
| CDK4/6 | Cyclin-dependent kinases 4 and 6 |
| CDKN2A | Cyclin-dependent kinase inhibitor 2A |
| DSS | Disease-specific survival |
| EGFR | Epidermal growth factor receptor |
| EZH2 | Enhancer of zeste 2 |
| FDA | Food and Drug Administration |
| HER2 | Human epidermal growth factor receptor 2 |
| JAK | Janus kinase |
| KIT | Tyrosine-protein kinase KIT |
| LAG-3 | Lymphocyte-activation gene 3 |
| mTOR | Mammalian target of rapamycin |
| ORR | Overall response rate |
| OS | Overall survival |
| PD1 | Programmed cell death protein 1 |
| PDGFB | Platelet-derived growth factor β |
| PDGFR | Platelet-derived growth factor receptor |
| PDGFRA | Platelet-derived growth factor receptor α |
| PDGFRB | Platelet-derived growth factor receptor β |
| PD-L1 | Program cell death ligand 1 |
| PFS | Progression-free survival |

D. J. Zabransky · C. Meyer (✉)
Department of Medical Oncology, The Johns Hopkins Sidney Kimmel Comprehensive Cancer Center, Baltimore, MD, USA
e-mail: cmeyer13@jhmi.edu

Z. Pennington
Department of Neurosurgery, Johns Hopkins University School of Medicine, Baltimore, MD, USA



D. M. Sciubba, J. H. Schwab (eds.), *Chordoma of the Spine*,
https://doi.org/10.1007/978-3-030-76201-8_16

| | |
|---|---|
| PI3K | Phosphoinositide-3-kinase (PI3K) |
| PR | Partial response |
| PRC2 | Polycomb repressive complex 2 |
| PTEN | Phosphatase and tensin homolog deleted on chromosome 10 |
| RB | Retinoblastoma |
| RTK(s) | Receptor tyrosine kinase(s) |
| SD | Stable disease |
| SMARCB1 | SWI/SNF related, matrix associated, actin dependent regulator of chromatin, subfamily b, member 1 |
| STAT | Signal transducer activator of transcription |
| SWI/SNF | Switch/sucrose non-fermentable |
| TBXT | T-box transcription factor T |
| TCR | T cell receptor |
| TKI(s) | Tyrosine kinase inhibitor(s) |
| VEGFR | Vascular endothelial growth factor receptor |
| VP-16 | Etoposide |

## Introduction

Surgical resection and adjuvant radiation can lead to long-term disease control in many patients with chordoma [1]. However, gross total resection is not always technically feasible, and subtotal resection is associated with disease recurrence, possible tumor seeding, and development of metastatic disease [2, 3]. Five-year conditional disease-specific survival (DSS) for patients with localized chordoma is 83%; however, 5-year conditional DSS is only 71% for those with metastatic disease [4]. The use of cytotoxic chemotherapy has been proposed and tested as an option for the treatment of metastatic chordoma; however, there has been little evidence to date supporting its clinical efficacy [5]. Furthermore, the rarity of chordoma precludes the study of systemic therapies using large-scale, prospective trials. Nonetheless, data from genomic, epigenomic, and transcriptomic analyses, along with the study of the chordoma tumor-immune microenvironment, have identified a number of promising new treatment targets.

## Cytotoxic Chemotherapy

Chordoma is considered unresponsive to cytotoxic chemotherapy, and there is no prospective data to support its clinical use. To date the only available clinical trial data is derived from a small phase II, prospective study by Chugh et al. studying this use of cytotoxic chemotherapy in patients with advanced chordoma. In this trial, the authors found that a regimen of the topoisomerase I inhibitor, rubitecan, in 15 patients with advanced chordoma was associated with moderate toxicity and little clinical benefit; only one patient had an objective response to treatment [6].

Multi-agent regimens have been described in a handful of case reports with varying degrees of reported success. In their report, Fleming et al. described complete remission in two patients with dedifferentiated sacral chordoma treated with neoadjuvant radiation, sacrectomy, and adjuvant systemic therapy. One patient was treated with ifosfamide, and the other was treated with a six-drug regimen including cisplatin, etoposide, vincristine, dacarbazine, cyclophosphamide, and doxorubicin [7]. Similarly, in a retrospective review of six pediatric patients with clival chordomas, Dhall et al. found the use of adjuvant ifosfamide and etoposide (VP-16) resulted in disease stability in two patients with a median follow-up of 9 years from diagnosis [8]. Ceruso et al. similarly documented both clinical and radiographic responses in a patient with advanced sacral chordoma that was treated with oral cyclophosphamide and prednisone given on a metronomic schedule (continuous administration of low doses of the active drugs) [9].

Despite these isolated case reports, there are no high-quality data to suggest that cytotoxic chemotherapy is an effective treatment for either conventional and chondroid chordoma. Thus, development of targeted and immune-based therapies has been a major focus of chordoma research.

## Molecular-Targeted Therapies: Receptor Tyrosine Kinases and Cell Signaling Pathways

Given the lack of demonstrated efficacy for conventional cytotoxic chemotherapy, there has been a drive to identify the key molecular changes associated with chordoma oncogenesis. Identification of the mutated or overexpressed genes and dysregulated molecular pathways has provided opportunities for the use of targeted therapies in the treatment of chordoma [10, 11]. Key changes that have been associated with chordoma tumorigenesis include increased expression and activation of receptor tyrosine kinases (RTKs) and alterations in both the downstream effectors of these RTKs and the negative regulators of RTK signaling [12, 13]. While no single, dominant molecular pathway has been implicated in the development of chordoma, analysis of patient chordoma samples has noted increased expression of the following RTKs: epidermal growth factor receptor (EGFR), tyrosine-protein kinase KIT (KIT), platelet-derived growth factor receptors A and B (PDGFRA and PDGFRB), and vascular endothelial growth factor receptor 2 (VEGFR2) [12, 14, 15].

Perhaps consistent with the relatively indolent growth pattern of chordomas, histopathology studies have found chordomas to have a relatively low burden of somatic mutations. Analysis of 37 chordoma tumor exomes or genomes revealed a median of 21 coding substitutions and 4 insertion-deletion mutations (indels) per case [16]. In spite of the relatively low mutation burden, alterations in a small number of pathways have been consistently identified. These include changes in the phosphoinositide-3-kinase (PI3K)/Akt/mammalian target of rapamycin (mTOR) pathway. Noted changes include activating mutations in the PIK3CA gene and truncations or deletions in its negative regulator – phosphatase and tensin homolog on chromosome 10 (PTEN). Alterations in genes encoding regulators of the cell cycle have also been identified, including mutations in cyclin D/cyclin-dependent kinases

4 and 6 (CDK4/6), retinoblastoma (RB), and the Janus kinase (JAK)/signal transducer activator of transcription (STAT) pathways. All have been postulated to be involved in tumorigenesis [16–19].

Numerous preclinical studies support the use of targeted small molecule inhibitors in chordomas harboring alterations in these pathways among others. Clinical implementation of these therapies has been attempted with the use of several tyrosine kinase inhibitors (TKIs). TKIs that have been previously described in the preclinical or clinical setting include the PDGFR inhibitor imatinib; the KIT inhibitor dasatinib; the EGFR/ human epidermal growth factor receptor 2 (HER2) inhibitors erlotinib, lapatinib, and gefitinib; and the VEGFR inhibitors sorafenib, pazopanib, and sunitinib. Other inhibitors that have been described include the anti-EGFR antibody cetuximab and the PI3K/Akt/mTOR pathway inhibitors temsirolimus, sirolimus, and everolimus (Fig. 16.1) [10]. These pathways present targets for molecular therapies that have been evaluated in preclinical and, in some cases, clinical studies [10, 20]. A summary of phase II trials of TKIs for the treatment of chordoma is presented in Table 16.1.

## PDGFR

Imatinib, a multi-kinase inhibitor with activity against BCR-ABL, KIT, and PDGFR, was the first molecular-targeted therapy to show clinical benefit in the treatment of chordoma. A phase II study of patients with advanced chordoma expressing platelet-derived growth factor β (PDGFB)/PDGF receptor β (PDGFRB) treated 56 patients with 800 mg/day of imatinib. While only one partial response (PR) was seen by at 6-month follow-up (ORR, 2%), 35 patients (70%) had stable disease (SD) for an overall clinical benefit rate of 64%. The median progression-free survival (PFS) and overall survival (OS) were 9.2 and 34.9 months, respectively [21]. Multiple other studies, including two other clinical trials, have investigated the use of imatinib, either as monotherapy or in combination with chemotherapy, in patients with chordoma [10, 22, 23].

Dasatinib, another PDGFR inhibitor that also has activity against Src, was studied in a phase II trial involving patients with locally advanced or metastatic sarcomas. Across the 32 included patients, median PFS was 6 months and OS was 43% and 18% at 2 and 5 years, respectively [24].

## mTOR

Multiple clinical case reports have found mTOR inhibitors to have clinically significant activity against chordoma [25–27]. The combination of the mTOR inhibitor everolimus and imatinib was recently examined in a phase II clinical trial by Stacchiotti and colleagues. The examined cohort comprised 43 patients with advanced or metastatic chordoma that had progressed following initial surgical, radiation, or medical treatment. Of note, 13 patients had previously been treated with imatinib. While the antitumor effect was modest, with an ORR of 22.5%, 6 of

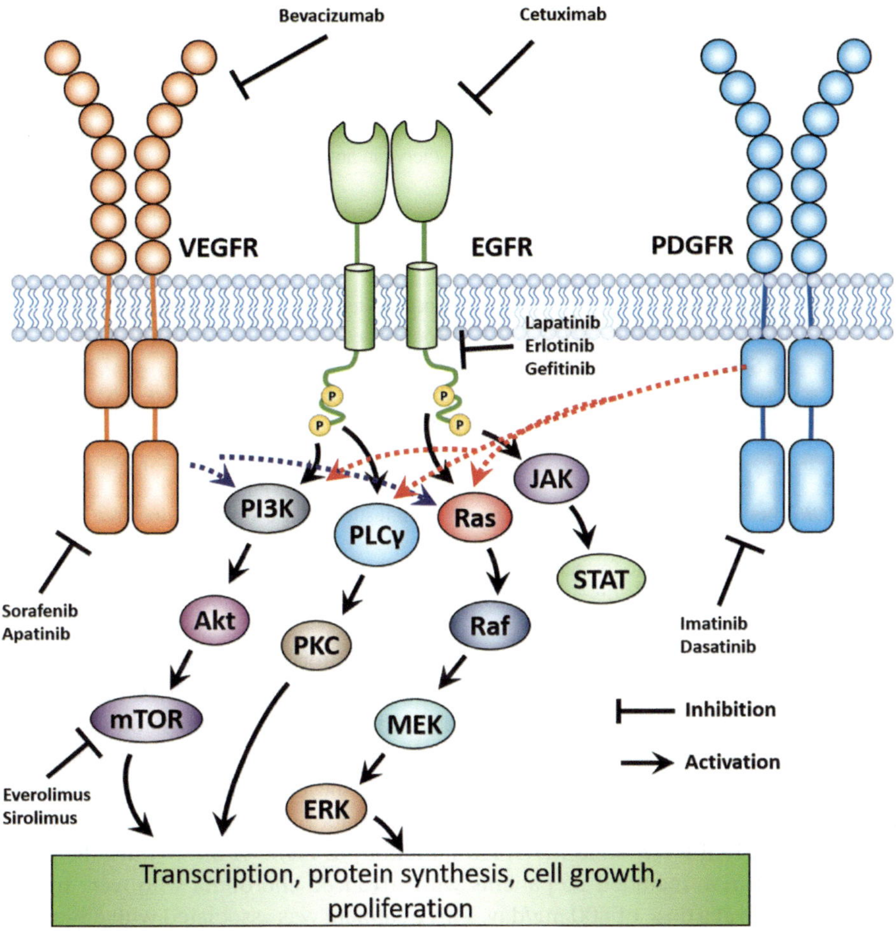


**Fig. 16.1** Selected molecular-targeted therapies against RTK signaling pathways for the treatment of chordoma

30 chemotherapy-naïve patients (20%) and 3 of 13 patients (23%) previously treated with imatinib demonstrated a partial response, as defined by Choi criteria [28]. Molecular characterization of this subgroup found that these patients had tumors with high levels of mTOR phosphorylation (present in ≥60% of tumor cells). Similar phosphorylation levels were not observed in the tumors from patients who did not benefit from treatment with everolimus and imatinib [29].

## VEGFR

VEGF protein expression is detected in chordoma samples [15, 30, 31]. Accordingly, multiple anti-VEGF therapies have been investigated for their clinical utility in patients with advanced or unresectable chordoma. Agents that have been previously

**Table 16.1** Phase II clinical trials of TKIs for the treatment of chordoma. Median PFS and OS in months using RECIST 1.1 criteria are reported unless otherwise noted

| Pathway targeted | Drug [trial reference] | Number of patients | PFS (months or otherwise noted) | OS (months or otherwise noted) | BORR (%) |
|---|---|---|---|---|---|
| PDGFR | Imatinib [21] | 56 | 9.2 | 34.9 | 2 |
| | Dasatinib [24] | 32 | 6.3[a] | Not reported[b] | 19[a] |
| mTOR | Everolimus + imatinib [29] | 43 | 14 | 47.1 | 22.5 |
| VEGFR | Sorafenib [38] | 9 | Not reported | Not reported | 44[c] |
| | Sorafenib [39] | 27 | Not reached | Not reached | 3.7 |
| | Sorafenib [40] | 26 | 72.9% at 9 months | 86.5% at 12 months | Not reported |
| | Apatinib [41] | 2 | 18 | 88% at 12 months | 3.7 |
| EGFR | Lapatinib [53] | 18 | 8 | 25 | 33.3 |

*Key: BORR* best overall tumor response rate, *OS* overall survival, *PFS* progression-free survival
[a]Evaluated by Choi criteria
[b]Reported values not specific for patients with chordoma included in the study
[c]Includes patients with stable disease

examined include the small molecule VEGF inhibitors sorafenib [32], pazopanib [23, 33, 34], and sunitinib [23], as well as the humanized anti-VEGF-A antibody, bevacizumab [35], and thalidomide, which modulates VEGF expression [36, 37].

Of these, the small molecule inhibitors have been most popular, and to date there have been four phase II clinical trials examining the clinical utility of anti-VEGF TKIs in patients with chordoma [38–41]. Two trials [38, 39] evaluated the use of sorafenib, a VEGFR1/2/3 and PDGFRB inhibitor [42]. One of these trials, the phase II Angionext trial, included 26 patients with advanced chordoma who were treated with sorafenib at a dose of 800 mg/day. This treatment was associated with a 9-month PFS of 72.9% [39]. Sunitinib was similarly examined in a trial of advanced non-GIST soft tissue sarcomas, including nine patients with chordoma. Patients were treated with 37.5 mg of daily sunitinib and examinations at 16 and 24 weeks demonstrated stable disease in 44% and 22% of chordoma patients, respectively [40], as defined by RECIST criteria [43]. Finally, a single-arm, phase II nonrandomized trial of apatinib, a VEGFR-2 inhibitor, was performed at a single institution [41, 44]. The results suggested it may have mild efficacy on disease control. Although only one patient had a partial response by RECIST criteria, median PFS was 18 months, 1-year OS was 88%, and 63% of patients had local disease control at 6 months.

## EGFR

The genes encoding EGFR and its ligands are highly expressed in patient-derived chordoma samples. Additionally, comparison of gene expression in fetal nucleus pulposus tissue and chordoma samples demonstrates significantly higher EGFR protein expression in tumor sample [17, 45]. Inhibition of EGFR and other human epidermal growth receptor family members has therefore been an attractive strategy for the treatment of chordoma. Case reports have detailed the use of small molecule inhibitors of EGFR, including erlotinib and gefitinib, as well as the anti-EGFR chimeric monoclonal antibody, cetuximab. These case reports have suggested anti-EGFR treatments to have clinical benefit both in terms of tumor response and improvement in neurologic symptoms secondary to chordoma mass effect [35, 46–52].

Another small molecule EGFR inhibitor, lapatinib, has also been evaluated in a phase II clinical trial. In this trial, lapatinib, a dual EGFR and HER2 inhibitor, was administered to 18 patients with locally advanced or metastatic, EGFR-expressing chordoma at a dose of 1500 mg/day (mean dose intensity of 1282 mg/day). Six of the 18 patients (33%) experienced partial disease response (ORR 33.3%), and seven others had stable disease by RECIST criteria with a minimum follow-up of 6 months. Median PFS in the cohort was 8 months, and the overall clinical benefit rate was reported at 22% [53]. Based upon these promising initial results, Stacchiotti et al. have begun a phase II, single-arm trial of the second-generation EGFR TKI, afatinib. The trial is currently enrolling patients with locally advanced or metastatic EGFR-expressing chordoma (NCT03083678).

## CDK4/6

Progression through the cell cycle is tightly controlled by a large network of proteins, and dysregulation of this cycle has been implicated in the tumorigenesis of multiple malignancies, including chordoma [54]. One key molecule is p16, encoded by the gene cyclin-dependent kinase inhibitor 2A (*CDKN2A*). p16 negatively regulates CDK4/6, which is responsible for stimulating cells to progress through the G1/S transition of the cell cycle [55]. CDK4/6 are often overactivated in chordoma samples due to loss of p16, resulting in increased cellular proliferation [56, 57]. Inhibition or downregulation of CDK4/6 may therefore represent a potential therapeutic target. Both strategies have proven effective in vitro, with CDK4/6 inhibition in p16-deleted cells resulting in decreased cellular proliferation and repression of other oncogenic properties [57, 58]. The CDK4/6 inhibitor used in these studies – palbociclib – is currently approved for the treatment of breast cancer [59] and is undergoing evaluation of its efficacy in a phase II study of patients with advanced or metastatic chordoma (NCT03110744).

## Epigenetic Therapies

In the past decade, epigenetic regulation of chromatin structure and gene expression has been increasingly recognized as an important driver in tumorigenesis [60]. Control of chromatin packing dynamics is therefore another potential target for novel chordoma therapies. Missense and nonsense mutations in SMARCB1, a member of the ATP-dependent SWI/SNF chromatin-remodeling complex, have been documented in chordoma samples [18]. Low expression of the SMARCB1 protein is additionally associated with poor prognosis in skull base chordomas [61]. SMARCB1 and the SWI/SNF complex play key roles in the epigenetic regulation of cell cycle progression and multiple signaling pathways [62]. Inactivation of SMARCB1, through either loss of protein expression or mutational inactivation, leads to increased activity of enhancer of zeste 2 (EZH2), a histone-lysine N-methyltransferase that forms the catalytic subunit of the polycomb repressive complex 2 (PRC2) [63, 64]. Increased PRC2 activity amplifies chromatin methylation, notably in regions encoding genes crucial to cell survival, proliferation, and invasion [65].

Curiosity about the efficacy of EZH2 inhibitors served as the basis of a phase I trial of tazemetostat, a selective EZH2 inhibitor [66]. In this trial of 46 patients with relapsed or refractory INI1-negative tumors, two children were being treated for chordoma. Though the chordoma cohort was too small to reach definitive conclusions, one of the chordoma patients was forced to withdraw from the study after experiencing worsening pain from her sacral mass. However, her tumor was found to be stable by RECIST 1.1 criteria at the time of discontinuation, and she experienced complete response of her pulmonary metastases. After withdrawing, she received radiation to the sacral mass, and radiographic follow-up at 4 months demonstrated persistent remission of her distant pulmonary metastases, suggesting that tazemetostat may induce an antitumor immune response [67]. This remains speculative though, and a phase II clinical trial is currently underway, which exams tazemetostat for the treatment of adult patients with SMARCB1-negative tumors, including poorly differentiated chordoma (NCT02601950).

## Immunotherapy

The immune system and its impact on the development and treatment of cancer has been studied since the nineteenth century [68]. Work over the previous three decades has led to a more complete understanding of the role the immune system plays in the detection and elimination of neoplastic cells. This process of immune surveillance is regulated by multiple factors, including T cell immune checkpoints, molecular interactions that negatively regulate T cell function. For example, the programmed cell death-ligand 1 (PD-L1) found on cancer cell membranes binds to the programmed cell death protein 1 (PD-1) on CD8+ effector T cells resulting in CD8+ T cell anergy [69]. Disruption of this anergy-inducing interaction has therefore been a focus of novel immunotherapies and has stimulated the development of drugs that alter immunosurveillance by inhibiting these immune checkpoints. These checkpoint inhibitors are rapidly becoming a key aspect of chemotherapy as they have been successfully used to treat patients with cancers in which chemotherapy had been ineffective. Their use in the treatment of chordoma is therefore also the subject of great interest and study [5, 70].

The FDA has approved use of multiple antibodies that target components of two key immune checkpoint pathways: the binding of cytotoxic T-lymphocyte-associated protein 4 (CTLA-4) to CD80/CD86 and the binding of PD-1 and PD-L1. These inhibitors include the anti-CTLA-4 antibody ipilimumab, the anti-PD-1 antibodies nivolumab and pembrolizumab, and the anti-PD-L1 antibodies atezolizumab, avelumab, and durvalumab [70]. Preclinical data has shown that chordoma cell lines express both PD-1 and PD-L1 at the gene and protein levels [71]. The chordoma tumor immune microenvironment may serve to increase the growth and invasive potential of chordoma cells. For instance, expression of the PD-L1 gene and protein is upregulated by exposure to pro-inflammatory cytokines such as IFN-γ [71]. Exposure to TNF-α also increases PD-L1 gene expression and upregulates expression of genes associated with the epithelial-mesenchymal transition, PI3K/AKT signaling, pro-angiogenesis, and anti-apoptotic pathways (Fig. 16.2) [72]. This suggests that chordomas may activate T cell checkpoints and decrease the activity of T cells in response to an otherwise immune stimulating environment.

Analysis of nine human chordoma tissue samples showed that 94.9% of the samples expressed PD-L1 as measured in a tissue microarray, and samples from patients with metastatic chordoma had higher expression of PD-L1 than those from patients with non-metastatic disease [73]. Infiltrating T lymphocytes (TILs) have also been examined. One study showing that 22% of TILs found in chordoma samples expressed PD-1, and a second observed detectable CTLA-4 on the majority of TILs in chordoma patient samples [74, 75]. Furthermore, treatment with avelumab, an anti-PD-L1 antibody, increased the immune-mediated killing of human-derived chordoma cell lines in vitro [76]. Taken together, these studies serve as rationale for targeting the immune system in the treatment of chordoma.

Recent case reports have shown that treatment with anti-PD-1 antibodies, such as pembrolizumab or nivolumab, led to reduction in tumor sizes and subjective clinical improvement. Notably, these improvements were observed even in patients with chordoma that was refractory to multiple earlier lines of therapy [77]. Both phase I and II clinical trials evaluating the use of anti-PD-1 antibodies alone, in conjunction with radiation or in combination with an inhibitor of another immune checkpoint, lymphocyte-activation gene 3 (LAG-3), are recruiting patients with chordoma (NCT03173950, NCT02989636, and NCT03623854).

Despite this, recent data has suggested that only a subset of patients with chordoma may be amenable to immunotherapy with checkpoint inhibitors. In order to be eliminated by the host immune system, tumor cells must not only downregulate anergy-inducing checkpoint molecules, but they must also actively express peptides novel peptides demonstrating them to be "non-self." This presentation is done through the interaction of human leukocyte antigen (HLA) class 1-peptide complexes on tumor cells and surface receptors on CD8+ effector T cells. Recently, Patel et al. [78] examined samples for surgically treated chordoma patients and found that 40% or more of chordoma samples may not express HLA class 1/peptide complexes. However, in vitro work has found proton- and photon-based radiation to increase HLA expression [79]. Consequently, paired radiotherapy and checkpoint

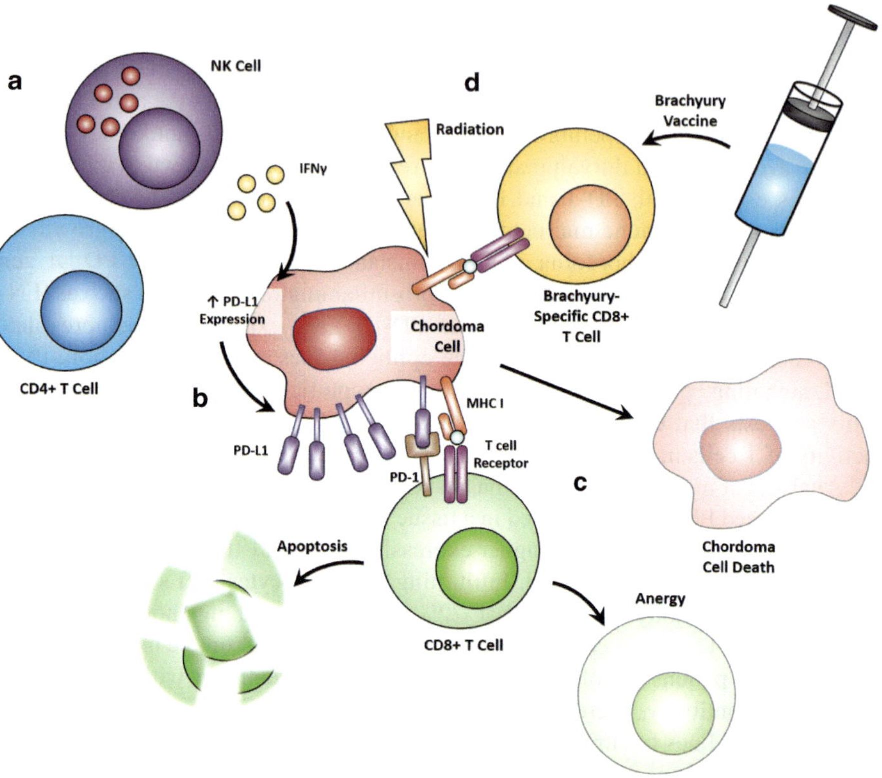


**Fig. 16.2** The chordoma tumor immune microenvironment. (**a**) In response to pro-inflammatory signals and cytokines such as INF-γ, chordoma cells increase expression of PD-L1. (**b**) Higher levels of PDL-1 expression lead to activation of T cell immune checkpoints through binding to PD-1 receptors on the T cell surface. (**c**) Activation of T cell immune checkpoints induces T cell anergy to tumor-specific antigens and apoptosis of effector T cells. (**d**) Brachyury vaccine strategies use epitopes from brachyury-derived tumor antigens to induce production and activation of brachyury antigen-specific CD8+ T cells. These T cells have an enhanced ability to recognize and possibly destroy chordoma cells. Clinical trials of brachyury vaccines have also incorporated the use of radiation with the goal of enhancing the anti-tumor immune response

inhibitor administration may improve tumor cell killing. This is currently undergoing investigation in a phase I trial (NCT02989636).

## Brachyury

Brachyury is a transcription factor encoded by the T-box transcription factor T gene (*TBXT*) located on the long arm of chromosome 6 [80]. Brachyury has a conserved role in development [81], and its expression has been established as a diagnostic marker in chordoma [82, 83]. Brachyury is highly expressed in patient chordoma samples, with the rare exception of a subset of dedifferentiated chordomas [84].

Chromosome 6 duplication and *TBXT* copy number gain have both been observed in chordoma cell lines and patient samples. The increased somatic copy number gain of *TBXT* has in turn been correlated with increased brachyury expression [85–88].

Preclinical studies have shown that brachyury is involved in numerous critical cellular pathways. These include pathways regulating cell growth, apoptosis, the epithelial-to-mesenchymal transition, and cellular differentiation [89–92]. In vivo experimental models have been used to demonstrate that disruption of brachyury expression or activity can prevent the formation of chordoma tumors or decrease the size of existing tumors [90, 92].

Based upon this preclinical evidence, brachyury has also become as an attractive target for systemic therapies. One such therapy is the chordoma Brachyury vaccine, originally described by Hamilton et al. in a murine model of metastatic colorectal adenocarcinoma [93]. The group found that treating mice transplanted with MC38 cells using a *Saccharomyces cerevisiae*-based brachyury vaccine produced robust brachyury-specific CD4+ and CD8+ T cell responses with minimal toxicity. Importantly, treated mice also showed a significant reduction in their lung metastasis burden. Based upon this, a phase I clinical trial of a yeast-based cancer Brachyury vaccine was launched in patients with chordoma or other advanced solid tumors (Fig. 16.2) [94]. The vaccine was well tolerated and induced the development or enhancement of brachyury-specific CD4+ and/or CD8+ T cells in 55% of patients. Of the ten patients with chordoma, none had evidence of disease progression at 5-month evaluation. Among these patients, the median PFS was 8.3 months, though only two patients had disease response (one with partial response and one with mixed response). Of note, both patients demonstrating disease response had received radiation treatment prior to their vaccination. This radiotherapy may have upregulated HLA class 1/brachyury complex expression, enhancing the "non-self" signal provided by the chordoma cells. Based upon this, two phase II trials have been initiated looking at concomitant treatment with radiotherapy and a Brachyury vaccine. One trial is examining patients with locally advanced, unresectable chordoma using concomitant radiotherapy and vaccination with the yeast-based Brachyury vaccine (NCT02383498) [95]. The second (NCT03595228) is using a poxvirus-based Brachyury vaccine (BN-Brachyury vaccine) with radiation in patients with chordoma. In this second study, the vaccine consists of two recombinant poxvirus vectors delivered in tandem as a prime-boost strategy. These viruses are modified to express brachyury as well as viral molecules known to increase immune cell activation [96].

## Conclusions

Treatment of chordoma after exhaustion of local therapy options remains challenging. Chordoma has no established standard of care therapy with conventional cytotoxic chemotherapy proving ineffective. Large randomized trials of systemic therapy are difficult to conduct owing to the rarity of chordoma, the heterogeneous nature of the disease, and the varying rates of progression observed across patients. Nevertheless, an enhanced understanding of the molecular drivers and tumor immune microenvironment in chordoma has opened the door for new, targeted treatment paradigms which may prove useful in long-term control or remission for those with advanced disease. Early results have been promising, but continued study is necessary, and the ultimate solution may rely on establishment of patient-specific regimens dictated by each tumor's unique genetic fingerprint.

## References

1. Catton C, O'Sullivan B, Bell R, Laperriere N, Cummings B, Fornasier V, Wunder J. Chordoma: long-term follow-up after radical photon irradiation. Radiother Oncol. 1996;41:67–72.
2. Hulen CA, Temple HT, Fox WP, Sama AA, Green BA, Eismont FJ. Oncologic and functional outcome following sacrectomy for sacral chordoma. J Bone Jt Surg. 2006;88:1532–9.
3. Chambers PW, Schwinn CP. Chordoma: a clinicopathologic study of metastasis. Am J Clin Pathol. 1979;72:765–76.
4. Huang J-F, Chen D, Zheng X-Q, Lin J-L, Wang X-Y, Wu A-M. Conditional survival and changing risk profile in patients with chordoma: a population-based longitudinal cohort study. J Orthop Surg Res. 2019;14:181.
5. Colia V, Stacchiotti S. Medical treatment of advanced chordomas. Eur J Cancer. 2017;83:220–8.
6. Chugh R, Dunn R, Zalupski MM, Biermann JS, Sondak VK, Mace JR, Leu KM, Chandler WF, Baker LH. Phase II study of 9-nitro-Camptothecin in patients with advanced chordoma or soft tissue sarcoma. J Clin Oncol. 2005;23:3597–604.
7. Fleming GF, Heimann PS, Stephens JK, Simon MA, Ferguson MK, Benjamin RS, Samuels BL. Dedifferentiated chordoma: response to aggressive chemotherapy in two cases. Cancer. 1993;72:714–8.
8. Dhall G, Traverso M, Finlay JL, Shane L, Gonzalez-Gomez I, Jubran R. The role of chemotherapy in pediatric clival chordomas. J Neuro-Oncol. 2011;103:657–62.
9. Spalato Ceruso M, Napolitano A, Silletta M, Vincenzi B. Unexpected benefit from an 'old' metronomic chemotherapy regimen in advanced chordoma. BMJ Case Rep. 2019;12:e228728.
10. Meng T, Jin J, Jiang C, Huang R, Yin H, Song D, Cheng L. Molecular targeted therapy in the treatment of chordoma: a systematic review. Front Oncol. 2019;9:30.
11. Ozair MZ, Shah PP, Mathios D, Lim M, Moss NS. New prospects for molecular targets for chordomas. Neurosurg Clin N Am. 2020;31:289–300.
12. Dewaele B, Maggiani F, Floris G, Ampe M, Vanspauwen V, Wozniak A, Debiec-Rychter M, Sciot R. Frequent activation of EGFR in advanced chordomas. Clin Sarcoma Res. 2011;1:4.
13. D'Agati G, Cabello EM, Frontzek K, Rushing EJ, Klemm R, Robinson MD, White RM, Mosimann C, Burger A. Active receptor tyrosine kinases, but not Brachyury, are sufficient to trigger chordoma in zebrafish. Dis Model Mech. 2019;12:dmm039545.
14. Tamborini E, Miselli F, Negri T, et al. Molecular and biochemical analyses of platelet-derived growth factor receptor (PDGFR) B, PDGFRA, and KIT receptors in chordomas. Clin Cancer Res. 2006;12:6920–8.
15. Akhavan-Sigari R, Gaab MR, Rohde V, Brandis A, Tezval H, Abili M, von Eckardstein K, Ostertag H. Expression of vascular endothelial growth factor receptor 2 (VEGFR-2), inducible nitric oxide synthase (iNOS), and Ki-M1P in skull base chordoma: a series of 145 tumors. Neurosurg Rev. 2014;37:79–88.
16. Tarpey PS, Behjati S, Young MD, et al. The driver landscape of sporadic chordoma. Nat Commun. 2017;8:890.

17. Tamborini E, Virdis E, Negri T, et al. Analysis of receptor tyrosine kinases (RTKs) and downstream pathways in chordomas. Neuro-Oncology. 2010;12:776–89.
18. Choy E, MacConaill LE, Cote GM, Le LP, Shen JK, Nielsen GP, Iafrate AJ, Garraway LA, Hornicek FJ, Duan Z. Genotyping cancer-associated genes in chordoma identifies mutations in oncogenes and areas of chromosomal loss involving CDKN2A, PTEN, and SMARCB1. PLoS One. 2014;9:e101283.
19. Wang L, Zehir A, Nafa K, et al. Genomic aberrations frequently alter chromatin regulatory genes in chordoma. Genes Chromosom Cancer. 2016;55:591–600.
20. Foundation C. Therapeutic targets in chordoma. 2020. https://www.chordomafoundation.org/targets. Accessed 1 Sept 2020.
21. Stacchiotti S, Longhi A, Ferraresi V, et al. Phase II study of Imatinib in advanced chordoma. J Clin Oncol. 2012;30:914–20.
22. Adenis A, Ray-Coquard I, Italiano A, et al. A dose-escalating phase I of imatinib mesylate with fixed dose of metronomic cyclophosphamide in targeted olid tumours. Br J Cancer. 2013;109:2574–8.
23. Lipplaa A, Dijkstra S, Gelderblom H. Efficacy of pazopanib and sunitinib in advanced axial chordoma: a single reference centre case series. Clin Sarcoma Res. 2016;6:19.
24. Schuetze SM, Bolejack V, Choy E, et al. Phase 2 study of dasatinib in patients with alveolar soft part sarcoma, chondrosarcoma, chordoma, epithelioid sarcoma, or solitary fibrous tumor. Cancer. 2017;123:90–7.
25. Stacchiotti S, Marrari A, Tamborini E, et al. Response to imatinib plus sirolimus in advanced chordoma. Ann Oncol. 2009;20:1886–94.
26. Ricci-Vitiani L, Runci D, D'Alessandris QG, et al. Chemotherapy of skull base chordoma tailored on responsiveness of patient-derived tumor cells to rapamycin. Neoplasia. 2013;15:773–82.
27. Lebellec L, Chauffert B, Blay J-Y, et al. Advanced chordoma treated by first-line molecular targeted therapies: outcomes and prognostic factors. A retrospective study of the French Sarcoma Group (GSF/GETO) and the Association des Neuro-Oncologues d'Expression Française (ANOCEF). Eur J Cancer. 2017;79:119–28.
28. Choi H, Charnsangavej C, Faria SC, Macapinlac HA, Burgess MA, Patel SR, Chen LL, Podoloff DA, Benjamin RS. Correlation of computed tomography and positron emission tomography in patients with metastatic gastrointestinal stromal tumor treated at a single institution with Imatinib Mesylate: proposal of new computed tomography response criteria. J Clin Oncol. 2007;25:1753–9.
29. Stacchiotti S, Morosi C, Lo Vullo S, et al. Imatinib and everolimus in patients with progressing advanced chordoma: a phase 2 clinical study. Cancer. 2018;124:4056–63.
30. Li X, Ji Z, Ma Y, Qiu X, Fan Q, Ma B. Expression of hypoxia-inducible factor-1α, vascular endothelial growth factor and matrix metalloproteinase-2 in sacral chordomas. Oncol Lett. 2012;3:1268–74.
31. Tauziède-Espariat A, Bresson D, Polivka M, et al. Prognostic and therapeutic markers in chordomas: a study of 287 tumors. J Neuropathol Exp Neurol. 2016;75:111–20.
32. Eroukhmanoff J, Castinetti F, Penel N, Salas S. Auto-immune thyroid dysfunction induced by tyrosine kinase inhibitors in a patient with recurrent chordoma. BMC Cancer. 2016;16:679.
33. Ribeiro MFSA, de Sousa MC, Hanna SA, Maldaun MVC, Kurimori CO, de Lima LGCA, Mattedi RL, Munhoz RR. Tumor reduction with Pazopanib in a patient with recurrent lumbar chordoma. Case Rep Oncol Med. 2018;2018:1–7.
34. Stein J, Milhem M, Vaena D. Clinical outcomes and toxicities of pazopanib administered orally in crushed form: case reports and review of the literature. J Oncol Pharm Pract. 2020;26:232–5.
35. Asklund T, Sandström M, Shahidi S, Riklund K, Henriksson R. Durable stabilization of three chordoma cases by bevacizumab and erlotinib. Acta Oncol (Madr). 2014;53:980–4.
36. Sherbet GV. Therapeutic potential of thalidomide and its analogues in the treatment of cancer. Anticancer Res. 2015;35:5767–72.

37. Chay WY, Teo M, Sittampalam K, Toh HC. Effective use of thalidomide in the treatment of recurrent metastatic chordoma. J Clin Oncol. 2011;29:e477–80.
38. Bompas E, Le Cesne A, Tresch-Bruneel E, et al. Sorafenib in patients with locally advanced and metastatic chordomas: a phase II trial of the French sarcoma group (GSF/GETO). Ann Oncol. 2015;26:2168–73.
39. Lebellec L, Bertucci F, Tresch-Bruneel E, et al. Circulating vascular endothelial growth factor (VEGF) as predictive factor of progression-free survival in patients with advanced chordoma receiving sorafenib: an analysis from a phase II trial of the french sarcoma group (GSF/GETO). Oncotarget. 2016;7:73984–94.
40. George S, Merriam P, Maki RG, et al. Multicenter phase II trial of sunitinib in the treatment of nongastrointestinal stromal tumor sarcomas. J Clin Oncol. 2009;27:3154–60.
41. Liu C, Jia Q, Wei H, et al. Apatinib in patients with advanced chordoma: a single-arm, single-centre, phase 2 study. Lancet Oncol. 2020;21:1244–52.
42. Wilhelm SM, Adnane L, Newell P, Villanueva A, Llovet JM, Lynch M. Preclinical overview of sorafenib, a multikinase inhibitor that targets both Raf and VEGF and PDGF receptor tyrosine kinase signaling. Mol Cancer Ther. 2008;7:3129–40.
43. Therasse P, Arbuck SG, Eisenhauer EA, et al. New guidelines to evaluate the response to treatment in solid tumors. J Natl Cancer Inst. 2000;92:205–16.
44. Liao Z, Li F, Zhang C, et al. Phase II trial of VEGFR2 inhibitor apatinib for metastatic sarcoma: focus on efficacy and safety. Exp Mol Med. 2019;51:1–11.
45. Chen H, Zhang K, Lu J, Wu G, Yang H, Chen K. Comprehensive analysis of mRNA-lncRNA co-expression profile revealing crucial role of imprinted gene cluster DLK1-MEG3 in chordoma. Oncotarget. 2017;8:112623–35.
46. Trapani D, Conforti F, De Pas T. EGFR inhibition in a pretreated sacral chordoma: a role for Erlotinib? Case report and a brief review of literature. Transl Med @ UniSa. 2017;16:30–3.
47. Houessinon A, Boone M, Constans J-M, Toussaint P, Chauffert B. Sustained response of a Clivus chordoma to Erlotinib after Imatinib failure. Case Rep Oncol. 2015;8:25–9.
48. Singhal N, Kotasek D, Parnis FX. Response to erlotinib in a patient with treatment refractory chordoma. Anti-Cancer Drugs. 2009;20:953–5.
49. Launay SG, Chetaille B, Medina F, Perrot D, Nazarian S, Guiramand J, Moureau-Zabotto L, Bertucci F. Efficacy of epidermal growth factor receptor targeting in advanced chordoma: case report and literature review. BMC Cancer. 2011;11:423.
50. Linden O, Ehinger M, Kinhult S, Relander T, Lundgren L, Engellau J, Kjellén E. Cetuximab and EGFR inhibitors in patients with neurological symptoms due to chordoma. J Clin Oncol. 2012;30:10024.
51. Hof H, Welzel T, Debus J. Effectiveness of Cetuximab/Gefitinib in the therapy of a sacral chordoma. Oncol Res Treat. 2006;29:572–4.
52. Lindèn O, Stenberg L, Kjellén E. Regression of cervical spinal cord compression in a patient with chordoma following treatment with cetuximab and gefitinib. Acta Oncol (Madr). 2009;48:158–9.
53. Stacchiotti S, Tamborini E, Lo Vullo S, et al. Phase II study on lapatinib in advanced EGFR-positive chordoma. Ann Oncol. 2013;24:1931–6.
54. Gordon E, Ravicz J, Liu S, Chawla S, Hall F. Cell cycle checkpoint control: the cyclin G1/Mdm2/p53 axis emerges as a strategic target for broad-spectrum cancer gene therapy - a review of molecular mechanisms for oncologists. Mol Clin Oncol. 2018;9:115–34.
55. Hamilton E, Infante JR. Targeting CDK4/6 in patients with cancer. Cancer Treat Rev. 2016;45:129–38.
56. Yakkioui Y, Temel Y, Creytens D, Jahanshahi A, Fleischeuer R, Santegoeds RGC, Van Overbeeke JJ. A comparison of cell-cycle markers in skull base and sacral chordomas. World Neurosurg. 2014;82:e311–8.
57. von Witzleben A, Goerttler LT, Marienfeld R, et al. Preclinical characterization of novel chordoma cell systems and their targeting by pharmocological inhibitors of the CDK4/6 cell-cycle pathway. Cancer Res. 2015;75:3823–31.

58. Liu T, Shen JK, Choy E, Zhang Y, Mankin HJ, Hornicek FJ, Duan Z. CDK4 expression in chordoma: a potential therapeutic target. J Orthop Res. 2018;36:1581–9.
59. Serra F, Lapidari P, Quaquarini E, Tagliaferri B, Sottotetti F, Palumbo R. Palbociclib in metastatic breast cancer: current evidence and real-life data. Drugs Context. 2019;8:1–16.
60. Ahuja N, Sharma AR, Baylin SB. Epigenetic therapeutics: a new weapon in the war against cancer. Annu Rev Med. 2016;67:73–89.
61. Li M, Zhai Y, Bai J, Wang S, Gao H, Li C, Gui S, Du J, Zhang Y. SNF5 as a prognostic factor in skull base chordoma. J Neuro-Oncol. 2018;137:139–46.
62. Kohashi K, Oda Y. Oncogenic roles of SMARCB1/INI1 and its deficient tumors. Cancer Sci. 2017;108:547–52.
63. Kim KH, Roberts CWM. Mechanisms by which SMARCB1 loss drives rhabdoid tumor growth. Cancer Genet. 2014;207:365–72.
64. Geller JI, Roth JJ, Biegel JA. Biology and treatment of Rhabdoid tumor. Crit Rev Oncog. 2015;20:199–216.
65. Gan L, Yang Y, Li Q, Feng Y, Liu T, Guo W. Epigenetic regulation of cancer progression by EZH2: from biological insights to therapeutic potential. Biomark Res. 2018;6:10.
66. Chi S, Fouladi M, Shukla N, et al. Abstract A175: phase 1 study of the EZH2 inhibitor, tazemetostat, in children with relapsed or refractory INI1-negative tumors including rhabdoid tumors, epithelioid sarcoma, chordoma, and synovial sarcoma. Mol Cancer Ther. 2018;17:A175.
67. Gounder MM, Zhu G, Roshal L, Lis E, Daigle SR, Blakemore SJ, Michaud NR, Hameed M, Hollmann TJ. Immunologic correlates of the abscopal effect in a SMARCB1/INI1-negative poorly differentiated Chordoma after EZH2 inhibition and radiotherapy. Clin Cancer Res. 2019;25:2064–71.
68. Esfahani K, Roudaia L, Buhlaiga N, Del Rincon SV, Papneja N, Miller WH Jr. A review of cancer immunotherapy: from the past, to the present, to the future. Curr Oncol. 2019;27:S87–97.
69. Qin W, Hu L, Zhang X, Jiang S, Li J, Zhang Z, Wang X. The diverse function of PD-1/PD-L pathway beyond cancer. Front Immunol. 2019; https://doi.org/10.3389/fimmu.2019.02298.
70. Waldman AD, Fritz JM, Lenardo MJ. A guide to cancer immunotherapy: from T cell basic science to clinical practice. Nat Rev Immunol. 2020;20:651–68.
71. Mathios D, Ruzevick J, Jackson CM, et al. PD-1, PD-L1, PD-L2 expression in the chordoma microenvironment. J Neuro-Oncol. 2015;121:251–9.
72. Gulluoglu S, Tuysuz EC, Sahin M, Yaltirik CK, Kuskucu A, Ozkan F, Dalan AB, Sahin F, Ture U, Bayrak OF. The role of TNF-α in chordoma progression and inflammatory pathways. Cell Oncol. 2019;42:663–77.
73. Feng Y, Shen J, Gao Y, Liao Y, Cote G, Choy E, Chebib I, Mankin H, Hornicek F, Duan Z. Expression of programmed cell death ligand 1 (PD-L1) and prevalence of tumor-infiltrating lymphocytes (TILs) in chordoma. Oncotarget. 2015;6:11139–49.
74. Liang WS, Millis SZ, Gatalica Z, Reddy SK, Little A, Van Tine BA. Identification of actionable targets in chordomas using a multiplatform molecular analysis, and response with targeted therapy. J Clin Oncol. 2015;33:e22215.
75. He G, Liu X, Pan X, Ma Y, Liu X. Cytotoxic T lymphocyte antigen-4 (CTLA-4) expression in chordoma and tumor-infiltrating lymphocytes (TILs) predicts prognosis of spinal chordoma. Clin Transl Oncol. 2020;22:2324–32.
76. Fujii R, Friedman ER, Richards J, Tsang KY, Heery CR, Schlom J, Hodge JW. Enhanced killing of chordoma cells by antibody-dependent cell-mediated cytotoxicity employing the novel anti-PD-L1 antibody avelumab. Oncotarget. 2016;7:33498–511.
77. Migliorini D, Mach N, Aguiar D, Vernet R, Landis BN, Becker M, McKee T, Dutoit V, Dietrich P-Y. First report of clinical responses to immunotherapy in 3 relapsing cases of chordoma after failure of standard therapies. Onco Targets Ther. 2017;6:e1338235.
78. Patel SS, Nota SP, Sabbatino F, Nielsen GP, Deshpande V, Wang X, Ferrone S, Schwab JH. Defective HLA class I expression and patterns of lymphocyte infiltration in chordoma tumors. Clin Orthop Relat Res. 2020; https://doi.org/10.1097/CORR.0000000000001587.

79. Gameiro SR, Malamas AS, Bernstein MB, et al. Tumor cells surviving exposure to proton or photon radiation share a common immunogenic modulation signature, rendering them more sensitive to T cell–mediated killing. Int J Radiat Oncol. 2016;95:120–30.
80. Edwards YH, Putt W, Lekoape KM, Stott D, Fox M, Hopkinson DA, Sowden J. The human homolog T of the mouse T(Brachyury) gene; gene structure, cDNA sequence, and assignment to chromosome 6q27. Genome Res. 1996;6:226–33.
81. Le Gouar M, Guillou A, Vervoort M. Expression of a SoxB and a Wnt2/13 gene during the development of the mollusc Patella vulgata. Dev Genes Evol. 2004;214:250–6.
82. Karpathiou G, Dumollard JM, Dridi M, Dal Col P, Barral F-G, Boutonnat J, Peoc'h M. Chordomas: a review with emphasis on their pathophysiology, pathology, molecular biology, and genetics. Pathol - Res Pract. 2020;216:153089.
83. Schwab JH, Boland PJ, Agaram NP, et al. Chordoma and chondrosarcoma gene profile: implications for immunotherapy. Cancer Immunol Immunother. 2009;58:339–49.
84. Vujovic S, Henderson S, Presneau N, Odell E, Jacques T, Tirabosco R, Boshoff C, Flanagan A. Brachyury, a crucial regulator of notochordal development, is a novel biomarker for chordomas. J Pathol. 2006;209:157–65.
85. Presneau N, Shalaby A, Ye H, et al. Role of the transcription factor T (brachyury) in the pathogenesis of sporadic chordoma: a genetic and functional-based study. J Pathol. 2011;223:327–35.
86. Hallor KH, Staaf J, Jönsson G, et al. Frequent deletion of the CDKN2A locus in chordoma: analysis of chromosomal imbalances using array comparative genomic hybridisation. Br J Cancer. 2008;98:434–42.
87. Rinner B, Froehlich EV, Buerger K, et al. Establishment and detailed functional and molecular genetic characterisation of a novel sacral chordoma cell line, MUG-Chor1. Int J Oncol. 2011;40:443–51.
88. Otani R, Mukasa A, Shin M, Omata M, Takayanagi S, Tanaka S, Ueki K, Saito N. Brachyury gene copy number gain and activation of the PI3K/Akt pathway: association with upregulation of oncogenic Brachyury expression in skull base chordoma. J Neurosurg. 2018;128:1428–37.
89. Nelson AC, Pillay N, Henderson S, et al. An integrated functional genomics approach identifies the regulatory network directed by brachyury ( T ) in chordoma. J Pathol. 2012;228:274–85.
90. Shah SR, David JM, Tippens ND, et al. Brachyury-YAP regulatory Axis drives Stemness and growth in cancer. Cell Rep. 2017;21:495–507.
91. Jäger D, Lechel A, Tharehalli U, Seeling C, Möller P, Barth TFE, Mellert K. U-CH17P, -M and -S, a new cell culture system for tumor diversity and progression in chordoma. Int J Cancer. 2018;142:1369–78.
92. Sharifnia T, Wawer MJ, Chen T, et al. Small-molecule targeting of brachyury transcription factor addiction in chordoma. Nat Med. 2019;25:292–300.
93. Hamilton DH, Litzinger MT, Jales A, Huang B, Fernando RI, Hodge JW, Ardiani A, Apelian D, Schlom J, Palena C. Immunological targeting of tumor cells undergoing an epithelial-mesenchymal transition via a recombinant brachyury-yeast vaccine. Oncotarget. 2013;4:1777–90.
94. Heery CR, Singh BH, Rauckhorst M, et al. Phase I trial of a yeast-based therapeutic cancer vaccine (GI-6301) targeting the transcription factor Brachyury. Cancer Immunol Res. 2015;3:1248–56.
95. Menon H, Ramapriyan R, Cushman TR, et al. Role of radiation therapy in modulation of the tumor stroma and microenvironment. Front Immunol. 2019;10:193.
96. García-Arriaza J, Esteban M. Enhancing poxvirus vectors vaccine immunogenicity. Hum Vaccin Immunother. 2014;10:2235–44.

# Index




D. M. Sciubba, J. H. Schwab (eds.), *Chordoma of the Spine*, https://doi.org/10.1007/978-3-030-76201-8

GPSR Compliance

*The European Union's (EU) General Product Safety Regulation (GPSR) is a set of rules that requires consumer products to be safe and our obligations to ensure this.*

*If you have any concerns about our products, you can contact us on ProductSafety@springernature.com*

In case Publisher is established outside the EU, the EU authorized representative is:

Springer Nature Customer Service Center GmbH
Europaplatz 3
69115 Heidelberg, Germany

**Batch number: 10726135**

Printed by Printforce, the Netherlands